R FACTOR

R FACTOR

Drug Resistance Plasmid

Edited by
Susumu Mitsuhashi

UNIVERSITY PARK PRESS
Baltimore·London·Tokyo

UNIVERSITY PARK PRESS
Baltimore · London · Tokyo

Library of Congress Cataloging in Publication Data
Main entry under title:

R factor, drug resistance plasmid.

  Includes indexes.
    1. R factors. I. Mitsuhashi, Susumu, 1917–
[DNLM: 1. Drug resistance, Microbial. 2. Extrachromo-
somal inheritance. QW52 R103]
QR177.R18   616.01′4   77-13934
ISBN 0-8391-1182-7

Originally published by
UNIVERSITY OF TOKYO PRESS

FOREWORD

Salvador E. Luria
Massachusetts Institute of
Technology Center for Cancer Research

One of the most intriguing discoveries in bacteriology since the introduction of antibiotic substances for treating bacterial infections has been the occurrence and spread of the resistance (R) factors. Apart from their implications for the epidemiology of certain infections, these factors have broadened our perspective on the role that genetic exchanges play in the natural history of bacterial species. It is not an exaggeration to state that a novel era of bacterial ecology has been opened by the study of the R factors.

This field has acquired added significance from the discovery of restriction enzymes produced by the factors as they replicate as episomes in the bacterial cells. Restriction enzymes are being used in a variety of experimental procedures to produce recombinant DNA molecules, an exciting if controversial area of genetic engineering. More important from the biological standpoint is the light that the restriction and modification phenomena may throw on the mechanisms that control and limit interactions between the genomes of different species and possibly on the evolution of the procaryotic genome itself.

The authors of this volume have been among the most productive leaders in the field of R factor research. They are to be congratulated for having produced a valuable and informative book. Microbiologists and molecular biologists will be particularly grateful to Professor Mitsuhashi, who was the guiding force in making this book a reality.

FOREWORD

Bernard D. DAVIS
Harvard Medical School

The discovery and analysis of resistance-transfer factors have been perhaps the most significant development in microbiology in the past decade, important equally for theoretical studies in molecular and microbial genetics and chemotherapeutic action, and for epidemiology and the practice of medicine. It is fitting that this achievement should now be summarized by one of the main contributors, Dr. Susumu Mitsuhashi; and as his former teacher, I am pleased to think that his experience in my laboratory may have provided some of the background for this work.

Dr. Mitsuhashi was a member of our group in 1953 and 1954, along with two other investigators whose subsequent distinguished careers are well known: Charles Gilvarg, now at Princeton University, and Werner Maas, now at New York University Medical School. We were in a small, self-contained laboratory unit, supported as a branch of the Tuberculosis Control Division of the U.S. Public Health Service, and housed in a district health center of New York City, as guests of the Department of Public Health of Cornell University Medical College. This unit was originally intended to work on problems of tuberculosis. However, shortly after setting it up in 1947, I discovered an efficient method of using penicillin to isolate auxotrophic mutants of bacteria; and my chief, Dr. Carroll Palmer, generously permitted us to shift to full-time work on these mutants, since they seemed to have certain advantages over the *Neurospora* mutants with which Beadle and Tatum had established biochemical genetics as a flourishing field. In retrospect I would say, somewhat nostalgically, that our work probably gained from our relatively isolated location, free of distraction.

We worked mostly on biosynthetic pathways. We were particularly intrigued by the pathway of aromatic biosynthesis, which was opened up when certain mutants that required a group of aromatic metabolites were found to respond also to shikimic acid (a product of the shikimi tree in Japan). Dr. Mitsuhashi characterized the two enzymes that converted quinic acid, *via* 5-dehydroquinic acid, to 5-dehydroshikimic acid. We also did a certain amount of genetic work with our new mutants, including the use of a U-tube with a fritted glass disk to separate the two parental cultures in a bacterial mating, thus demonstrating the need for cell contact in Lederberg's system for gene transfer in *E. coli* K12. I have been interested to see that Dr. Mitsuhashi later used the same device to establish the essential role of conjugation in resistance transfer. My original description of this device as a "bacterial contraceptive" was rejected by an editor as inappropriately frivolous, but by now perhaps tastes have so changed that at last my little joke can see print!

Japanese microbiologists can justly be proud of their highly original achievements with the resistance-transfer factors. Indeed, its very originality is responsible for the striking lag of workers elsewhere in taking up this valuable lead. For there was a long struggle to eliminate Lamarckism from bacterial genetics, and the key Luria-Delbruck experiment had convinced most of us that drug-resistant strains could arise only by spontaneous mutation, followed by selection by the drug. Hence, when Dr. Mitsuhashi wrote me describing an emergence of drug resistance much too rapid for mutation and selection, I was skeptical, and my response must have been very discouraging. But this is now water under the bridge—and the bridge itself, as described in the previous monograph and this book, is truly a handsome edifice. Indeed, its stature and beauty remind us that a certain degree of isolation may help us to escape from the orthodox preconceptions that tend to limit the range of our imagination.

PREFACE

In spite of improved sanitary conditions and the concomitant use of antibiotics for clinical treatment, the incidence of infections caused by *Shigellae* had not decreased to any great extent by the mid-1960s. Thus, much attention was focused upon bacillary dysentery, and research committees were organized in Japan to study it from both the epidemiological and the clinical viewpoints. The rapid appearance of resistant *Shigella* strains and the isolation of multiply resistant strains attracted our attention first from the clinical and second from the genetic viewpoint.

The first report of the transmissibility of multiple resistance by mixed cultivation created a stir among microbiologists and geneticists in Japan, although the mechanism was not fully understood at that time. In addition, it was found by chance that multiple resistance was spontaneously lost from *Shigella* strains. Using a U-tube with a fritted glass disk devised by Dr. B. D. Davis to separate the two parental cultures, we found that drug-resistance determinants exist extrachromosomally and are transmissible by conjugation, similar to the F factors, and we offered the term R (resistance) factors to describe these determinants. In 1971, I published a monograph, "Transferable Drug Resistance Factor R" in order to introduce the many papers and reports published during the 1960s in Japan, so that they might become stepping-stones for future progress in R-factor research.

The great importance of R plasmid in chemotherapy and in microbial genetics has caused rapid progress in plasmid research and publication of many new papers. In publishing this second monograph, it is my purpose to introduce the many fundamental and creative new findings in R plasmid research conducted since the publication of my first monograph.

The R factor and its genetics offer many clues to solving the problems of gene evolution and the origin of plasmid. Questions about plasmid, including lysogeny and the latency of viral infections such as oncogenic viruses, are now fundamental problems in modern biology, and progress in research in these fields is of great importance in the medical world.

The authors are deeply indebted to Drs. H. Umezawa, B. D. Davis, and S. E. Luria for their thoughtful encouragement, which has made this monograph possible. Some of the authors' investigations were supported by research grants from the Japanese Ministry of Education, the Japan Society for the Promotion of Science, the U.S. National Science Foundation, the Japan Science Promotion Fund, and the World Health Organization.

Susumu Mitsuhashi
Department of Microbiology
School of Medicine, Gunma University
Reference Laboratory of
Drug-resistant Bacteria
Episome Institute

CONTENTS

xiv

DRUG RESISTANCE IN BACTERIA

1 EPIDEMIOLOGY OF BACTERIAL DRUG RESISTANCE

Susumu MITSUHASHI

Department of Microbiology, School of Medicine, Gunma University, Maebashi, Japan

1. History of Bacterial Drug Resistance

In 1907 Ehrlich (*12*) described the trypanocidal activity of *p*-rosaniline, and in the same year his research group (*14*) reported that *Trypanosome brucei* became resistant by repeated exposure to the drug. Knowledge of drug resistance in microorganisms is therefore as old as the history of chemotherapy itself. It has since been shown that microorganisms can develop resistance following repeated exposure to chemical substances. Initially, however, the importance of this phenomenon, called "adaptation," was not readily apparent to clinicians. Drug resistance of bacteria was also reported by Morgenroth and Kaufmann (*54*) soon after the discovery of the antipneumococcal effect of ethyldihydrocupreine hydrochloride (optochin), indicating that pneumococci could also develop resistance to drugs. Following the introduction of a number of chemotherapeutic agents and antibiotics, many observations on bacterial drug resistance were reported as shown by reports of resistance to sulfanilamide (SA) by Maclean *et al.* (*38*), to penicillin (PC) by

Abraham *et al.* *(2)*, and to streptomycin (SM) by Murray *et al.* *(55)*. Studies have shown, moreover, that the rate of appearance of bacterial drug resistance is tremendously high when compared with the rate of mutation in higher organisms. This high rate could be accounted for by the following factors: (a) short generation time, (b) presence of enormous numbers of microorganisms, (c) mechanisms of high rate of gene transfer, such as transduction and plasmid infection, (d) infectivity of microorganisms themselves, and (e) the widespread use of large amounts of antibacterial agents increasing the frequency of contact with microorganisms, thus creating a strong selection tendency among the drug-resistant members of the population. Furthermore, since microorganisms, unlike the germ cells in higher organisms, are fully and directly exposed to the full effect of antibacterial agents, the result is an exaggeratedly high rate of appearance of resistant strains.

Many drug-resistant strains of bacteria reported in earlier papers were obtained mostly *in vitro* under experimental conditions. Using experimental animals, bacteria may be rendered drug-resistant by single, repeated, or continuous exposure to antibacterial agents *in vitro* or *in vivo* even though the mutation rate differs for each strain. Although many studies, especially on the biochemical mechanism of drug action, were made with interesting results, bacterial drug resistance still did not arouse clinical medical interest. However, with the increasing incidence of infections caused by resistant strains of bacteria, drug resistance has now become a problem of prime clinical importance with the clinical and pharmaceutical sciences giving it the attention it deserves. Moreover, studies on the genetic and biochemical mechanisms of bacterial drug resistance have shown that there are many differences between resistant strains obtained in the laboratory and those isolated from clinical sources. For example, inactivation of penicillin by staphylococcal strains which develop resistance in *in vitro* experiments is not caused by β-lactamase, whereas many wild strains which have high β-lactamase activity, the main factor responsible for resistance to PC, are isolated from clinical sources *(15, 64, 65)*. By repeated exposure of staphylococci to chloramphenicol (CM), the strains become resistant to the agent but the resistance mechanism cannot be accounted for by inactivation of the drug. In clinical cases, many staphylococcal strains which are resistant to CM inactivate it by acetylation using intrinsic acetyl CoA *(35, 68)*. Similarly, the clinical isolates of Enterobacteriaceae

which are resistant to chloramphenicol also inactivate the drug by acetylation (52, 61, 62). Resistance to tetracycline (TC), CM, SM, and
SA, or combinations thereof in many clinical isolates of *Shigella* and
Escherichia coli is caused mostly by the presence of various R factors
and nonconjugative(r) plasmids in the bacterial cell. The differences
between the drug resistance of strains of human and animal origin and
the *in vitro* developed resistance of laboratory strains may be caused by
the following factors: (a) several different biochemical mechanisms exist
for resistance to a single drug. A resistant strain which is adapted for
evolution must survive the noxious environment and carry bacteriological properties adapted for both parasitism and infectivity. Thus, the
strain will be selected from an extremely large and heterogeneous population of microorganisms which has been exposed to the drug *in vivo*.
In contrast, the strains of microorganisms used in *in vitro* laboratory
experiments are quite limited, hence the resistant strains do not always
present themselves as frequently as those from natural sources. (b)
Natural resistance also occurs in mixed bacterial flora where microorganisms of different species and strains coexist multiply and simultaneously. Under such conditions gene transfer takes place frequently,
through conjugation, transduction with bacteriophages, and transformation through bacterial DNA. For example, the nontransferable drug
resistance determinant acquires transferability by the formation of recombinants between resistance determinant and conjugative plasmids
(sex factors), such as F, R, and T factors (7, 18, 19, 26, 31, 32) (see
Chapter 12). The resistance determinant is integrated into the host
chromosome and transmitted by chromosomal transfer in the presence
of sex factors, such as F, Col, R, and T (27, 43, 66). Nontransmissible
genetic elements which exist extrachromosomally also acquire transmissibility in cooperation with sex factors, such as Col and T (26, 53,
63). Drug resistance in staphylococci is transduced with bacteriophages
which are derived from lysogenic donor strains of resistance (50), and
many resistant determinants are jointly transduced (20, 28, 42, 51, 57).
These facts strongly suggest that in a mixed culture of staphylococci
the transfer of drug resistance is through transduction. Hence the author
has predicted that among the staphylococci, lysogenization and transduction of resistance with prophages are mainly responsible for the
acquisition of resistance, for the wide distribution of multiple-resistant
strains, and for changes in the phage typing patterns (41, 50). Novick

has proved that sensitive strains of staphylococci acquire drug resistance in experimental animals by injection with the phage lysates obtained from drug-resistant strains (*58*). Studies of drug resistance in strains isolated from clinical sources have revealed the presence of R factors, the wide distribution of T factors (*53*), the formation of recombinants between resistance determinants and conjugative plasmids, and the distribution of drug resistance through transduction.

In fact, there may be two types of drug resistance in bacteria, constitutive and inducible resistance (*15, 20, 22, 24, 33, 34, 64, 72, 79*). Drug resistance in the former type is stable and inheritable, while in the latter it is unstable and high resistance is demonstrated only when the strain is pretreated with subinhibitory concentrations of a drug. The resistance of the induced cells is lost when they are grown in the absence of inducers. In other words, the antibacterial agent is the active inducer and the properties of inducible resistance are inheritable. Both types of resistance are based on mutation and can be accounted for by present concepts in genetics. Hinshelwood (*21*) has suggested that the gradual production of increased resistance is not based simply on spontaneous mutation, but involves an inheritable physiologic alteration of the cellular enzyme pattern in which the drug plays a directing, as well as a selecting, role. With respect to the morphologic characteristics studied by earlier biologists, the concept, *i.e.*, Lamarckism, has long been eliminated, and the mechanism of development of bacterial drug resistance is generally considered to be accounted for by mutation. A resistant variant appears spontaneously during the course of bacterial multiplication, without regard to the presence or absence of drug. The drug acts merely as a selective agent which inhibits the cells that have failed to develop the mutation but allows the growth of a mutant that has developed the appropriate mutation. This genetic concept can be applied easily to instances of one-step mutation, such as dramatic change in drug resistance in which cultures of staphylococci, *Shigella, E. coli*, and *Hemophilus influenzae*, sensitive to SM, produced colonies resistant to 1,000 μg/ml of the drug after overnight incubation on plates containing the drug. The gradual and limited elevation of drug resistance of *Staphylococcus aureus* to PC has also been interpreted along genetic lines, *i.e.*, mutation, indicating that the process of gradual elevation of drug resistance also involves a whole series of mutations, *i.e.*, multi-steps of mutation (*10*).

Definitive evidence on this problem of bacterial resistance, *i.e.*, physiological adaptation or mutation, was furnished by fluctuation analysis and later by the replica-plating method. Fluctuation analysis is a statistical method for studying resistance to bacteriophage which was reported by Luria (*37*), and subsequently by Demerec (*11*) to study drug resistance. The results of both fluctuation analysis and the replica-plating method indicated that drug-resistant mutants appear spontaneously before exposure to the drug and the drug only acts as a selective agent which allows the growth of a drug-resistant mutant. It is a known fact that the development of resistance to one drug is independent of resistance to another if the mechanisms of both resistances are different. Therefore, theoretically the chance of simultaneously developing the resistance to both drugs in a single cell is very small. However, it is possible to successively develop resistance to one drug in organisms already resistant to another and so on. Based on such mutation phenomena it can be predicted that multiple-resistant strains may appear, multiply and spread in a noxious environment such as occurs in the widespread use of large amounts of various antibacterial agents. In practice, recent surveys have disclosed that many strains isolated from clinical sources are multiple-resistant and such multiple resistance is predominant in the clinical isolates of such species as the staphylococci, *E. coli*, *Klebsiella-Aerobacter*, *Proteus*, and *Shigella*. The fact that such bacterial strains can persist within the body following treatment and clinical cure with antibacterial agents also will serve to promote the development of multiple resistance if these strains are now exposed to contact with other drugs. The conspicuous fact that these bacterial strains continue to survive in the body and spread steadfastly among infectious lesions can be accounted for by the following factors: (a) virulence, (b) host does not acquire immunity after infection, (c) high infectivity and ability to successfully parasitize, (d) increased resistance to disinfectants, and (e) acquisition of multiple resistance to antibacterial agents.

Based on evolutionary theory, it can be predicted that such bacterial strains multiply and spread even under unfavorable conditions brought about by the widespread use of prophylactic treatment, improvement in sanitary conditions, and development of newer antibacterial agents. Another important factor responsible for the wide spread of multiple resistance is gene transfer from cell to cell among the strains that are encountered most frequently in pathological lesions. For example, pneumococci demonstrated from clinical sources are mostly drug-sensitive or singly resistant to tetracycline, although they can develop resistance to various antibacterial agents when inoculated into a medium containing the drug. Consequently, through evolution they are no longer prominent in infectious lesions, while strains which can easily acquire multiple resistance survive and persist in pathological lesions, even in the presence of antibiotic and chemotherapeutic agents. Among most genera of Enterobacteriaceae (*6, 23, 43*), the R factors are the most important elements responsible for resistance to TC, CM, SM, SA, ampicillin (APC), and kanamycin (KM). It is also clinically important that R factors are transmissible by cell-to-cell contact among the strains which are encountered most frequently in pathologic lesions and can replicate autonomously *in vivo* in such strains. These facts strongly suggest that the presence of plasmids and bacteriophages play an important role in bacterial evolution, in addition to mutation based on bacterial chromosomes. To paraphrase an old philosophical point, "genetics proposes and nature disposes." In the interplay of environment with DNA in the bacteria, the organisms appear to have fallen back on reserve mechanisms of plasmid replication, plasmid transfer, and phage methods in order to survive against increased environmental pressure from antibiotics. Only time will reveal the final outcome.

2. Drug Resistance of Gram-negative Bacteria Isolated in Japan

In spite of improved sanitary conditions and prophylactic inoculation, the incidence of infections caused by *Shigella* strains did not decrease remarkably in Japan until 1970, with the situation remaining much the same as it is in developing countries of the tropics. Importance, therefore, was placed upon bacillary dysentery, and many research committees were organized to study this problem which included drug resistance.

    Shigella strains isolated since 1962 were collected by research teams working on projects entitled: "Drug Resistance of *Shigella* Strains" (chief, M. Abe, Tokyo Municipal Hospital, Ebara), with the cooperation of 15 participating laboratories (*1*) and "Studies on the Drug Resistance of *Shigella* Strains" (chief, T. Ezaki, Tokyo Municipal

Hospital, Toyotama), with the cooperation of 17 participating laboratories from 1965 through 1968 (*13*).

The strains of gram-negative bacteria isolated since 1965 were collected and stocked in our laboratory. They were isolated from infected lesions taken from inpatients in hospitals throughout Japan participating in the following research projects: "Studies on the Infection of Gram-negative Bacteria" (chief, S. Ishiyama, School of Medicine, Nihon University, Tokyo), with the cooperation of 16 participating laboratories from 1965 through 1968 (*23*) and "Studies on the Drug Resistance of Bacteria Which Cause Intestinal Tract Infections" (chief, H. Hiraishi, Tokyo Municipal Hospital, Komagome), with the cooperation of 30 participating laboratories from 1969 to the present.

a) Drug resistance of the Shigella strain

Soon after the discovery of SA, it was found that derivatives of SA were effective against bacillary dysentery as well as the infectious diseases caused by gram-positive bacteria. As a result, large amounts of SA have been used in Japan since 1940. But its effectiveness lasts only about 10 years and SA-resistant *Shigella* strains appeared rapidly and reached a maximum of 80–90% of *Shigella* isolates resistant to SA (Fig. 1).

Fortunately the production of antibiotics such as SM, TC, and CM, which were quite effective against bacillary dysentery, started at

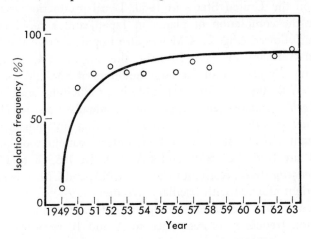

Fig. 1. Isolation frequency of SA-resistant *Shigella*.

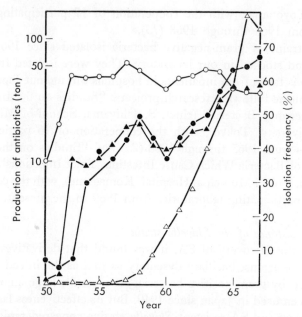

Fig. 2. Production of antibiotics and appearance of antibiotic-resistant *Shigella*. ○ SM; ● CM; ▲ TC; △ *Shigella*.

that time. SM production in Japan commenced in 1950 and by 1953
production had increased rapidly to meet demand. TC was first imported from the United States in 1950. Local production started in
1953 after the completion of plants in Japan, and a rapid increase
production followed (Fig. 2). CM was also imported from the United
States and Germany in 1950. In 1954, the output of CM in Japan
increased rapidly in spite of the large amounts of SM and TC being
produced. With the increase of antibiotic production, antibiotic-resistant *Shigella* strains began to appear and gradually increased (Fig. 2).

Isolation of multiple-resistant strains. The first isolation of a multiple-resistant *Shigella* strain from a dysenteric patient took place in
1952, and involved TC, SM, and SA (*67*). In 1955 a quadruple-
resistant *Shigella* strain, resistant to TC, SM, SA, and CM, was isolated
from a patient afflicted with bacillary dysentery (*29*).

Viewed from a theoretical standpoint, when 10^{-a} and 10^{-b} show
the mutation frequency of resistance to A and B, respectively, and
the development of resistance to the one is independent of that of

resistance to the other, $10^{-(a+b)}$ shows the mutation rate of simultaneous resistance to both drugs. This indicates an infinitesimal chance of simultaneously developing both mutations in a single cell. This is the theoretical justification of combined chemotherapy. Therefore, the report of a quadruply resistant *Shigella* strain attracted much attention from clinical and genetic viewpoints.

The next report of the isolation of a multiple-resistant strain from a case of dysentery caused by *Shigella flexneri* 2b was made in 1956 (*30*). However, no other cases of bacillary dysentery caused by multiple-resistant strains were reported in 1956 from about 100,000 reported cases of bacillary dysentery. Isolation of multiple-resistant strains of enteric bacteria in Japan from 1952 to 1959 is shown in Table I. At that time the spread of multiple-resistant *Shigella* strains in Japan was not accounted for by an epidemic spread of a strain resistant to the four drugs because of the difference in serotypes of such strains.

In 1957 our laboratory reported the first isolation of multiply resistant *Shigella* and *E. coli* strains in our district from specimens obtained during an epidemic at a tuberculosis sanatorium. From 100 tuberculosis patients suffering from bacillary dysentery, *S. flexneri* 3a strains resistant to four drugs, TC, CM, SM and SA, were isolated from 87 patients. The source of the strain causing the epidemic was traced to the six-member family of a bean-curd dealer. *S. flexneri* 3a strains were isolated from specimens taken from four members (A, B, C, and D) of the family (Fig. 3). *S. flexneri* 3a strains isolated from C and D were drug-sensitive. *S. flexneri* 3a and *E. coli* strains, resistant to TC, CM, SM, and SA, were isolated from A who had suffered from varicella one month prior to the epidemic and who had been treated with a total amount of 1,250 mg of CM. *S. flexneri* 3a, sensitive to the four drugs, and *E. coli*, resistant to the four drugs, were isolated from B after treatment with CM for one day. After 4 more days of treatment with CM, followed by one day with TC, *S. flexneri* 3a and *E. coli* strains resistant to the four drugs, were isolated from A (*40, 43, 48*). In 1958 we also isolated *E. coli* and *Escherichia freundii* strains resistant to TC, CM, SM, SA from specimens obtained during an epidemic caused by *S. flexneri* 2a 9 days after the administration of CM. An *E. coli* strain resistant to the four drugs was isolated from another patient after being completely cured of dysentery by treatment with CM (*40, 43, 49*).

TABLE I. Isolation of Multiple-resistant Strains of Gram-negative Rod Bacteria

Time	Place	Strain
1952 Aug.	Kyoto	*S. flexneri* 1b
1955 July	Tokyo	*S. flexneri* 4a
1956 Aug.	Tokyo	*S. flexneri* 2b
1957 June	Tokyo	*S. flexneri* 1b
		S. flexneri 2b
1957	Tokyo	*S. flexneri* 1b
		S. flexneri 2a
		S. flexneri 2b
		S. flexneri 3a
		S. flexneri v.Y
1957 Sep.	Nagoya	*S. flexneri* 3a
1957 Oct.	Tokyo	*S. flexneri* 2a
1957 Dec.	Gunma	*S. flexneri* 3a
		S. flexneri 3a ⎱ *a*
		E. coli ⎰
1959 Nov.	Gunma	*S. flexneri* 2a ⎱ *a*
		E. coli ⎰
1959 Nov.	Gunma	*E. freundii* ⎱ *a*
		E. coli ⎰

a Two strains carrying the same resistance pattern were isolated from a patient.

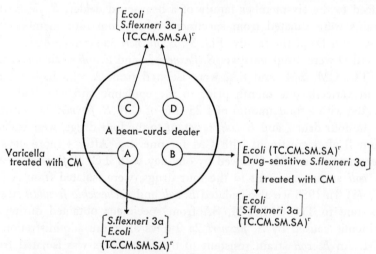

Fig. 3. An epidemic of bacillary dysentery and first isolation of
E. coli strains resistant to (TC. CM. SM. SA). r, resistant.

Cases	Resistance pattern	Reference
1	TC. SM. SA	Suzuki *et al.* (*67*)
1	TC. CM. SM. SA	Kitamoto *et al.* (*29*)
51 (mass)	TC. CM. SM. (SA)	Kobari (*30*)
3	TC. CM. SM. (SA)	See Refs. *40, 43*
2	TC. CM. SM. (SA)	
1	TC. CM. SM. (SA)	
3	TC. CM. SM. (SA)	
2	TC. CM. SM. (SA)	
2	TC. CM. SM. (SA)	
1	TC. CM. SM. (SA)	
66 (mass)	TC. CM. SM. SA	Ochiai *et al.* (*59*)
24 (mass)	TC. CM. SM. (SA)	
87 (mass)	TC. CM. SM. SA	Mitsuhashi *et al.* (*40, 43, 48, 49*)
2	TC. CM. SM. SA	
1	CM. SM. SA	
1	TC. CM. SM. SA	

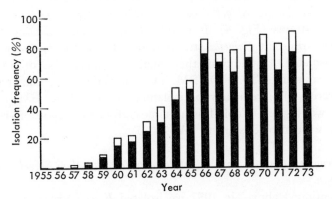

Fig. 4. Yearly changes of appearance of antibiotic-resistant *Shigella* strains in Japan, ☐ antibiotic-resistant strains (TC. CM. SM); ■ multiple-resistant strains among antibiotic-resistant strains.

TABLE II. Isolation of Antibiotic-resistant *Shigella* Strains in Japan

Year	1952	53	54	55	56	57
Number of strains examined	3,500	4,900	4,876	5,327	4,399	4,873
Number of antibiotic-resistant strains	3	7	11	5	14	98
Patterns of antibiotic resistance (%)						
TC. CM. SM	0	0	0	(1)	(1)	37
TC. SM	(1)	0	0	0	0	2
CM. SM	0	0	0	0	0	2
TC. CM	0	0	0	0	(1)	0
TC	(1)	(2)	0	0	(4)	46
SM	(1)	(5)	(11)	(4)	(8)	13
CM	0	0	0	0	0	0

Number in parenthesis indicates the real number of isolates. Percentage was not

The observations indicated that multiple resistance was not a problem restricted to *Shigella* strains, but involved all enteric bacteria, and on the basis of the observations interest in the origin of this multiple resistance was stimulated.

Most of the resistant *Shigella* isolated prior to 1956 were resistant only to SM or to TC, and the first isolation of multiple-resistant *Shigella* was reported in 1965. However, the frequency of multiple-resistant *Shigella* strains isolated being increased and, in 1967, 97% of the antibiotic-resistant *Shigella* isolates were multiply resistant among resistant strains (Fig. 4). It is interesting to note that, among the antibiotic-resistant *Shigella* strains, those resistant to CM alone were never isolated. In addition, the isolation of single TC or SM or of double-resistant (CM. TC), (SM. TC), or (CM. SM) strains has been very rare. The frequency of isolation of (TC. CM. SM)-resistant strains was highest (Table II) and almost all of these multiple-resistant strains were also resistant to SA (70–75).

b) *Drug resistance of gram-negative bacteria, other than Shigella, isolated in Japan*
As mentioned above, in 1957 we isolated *E. coli* strains resistant to four drugs, TC, CM, SM, and SA, during an epidemic caused by *S. flexneri* 3a resistant to the same drugs. Subsequently in 1958, we found

58	59	60	61	62	64	66	68	70	72
6,563	547	497	659	6,853	3,588	4,292	1,237	562	824
240	48	97	143	2,140	1,888	3,392	963	496	745
80	82	75	79	77	85	95.5	82.3	83.7	84
1	2	4	1	2	1	0.5	1.7	1	0.3
3	0	5	6	6	4	1.0	15	12.3	8.5
0	2	1	0	1	1	0.1	0	0.6	1.3
8	8	6	12	10	7	0.7	0.5	0.2	0.7
8	6	9	2	4	2	2.2	0.5	2	2.4
0	0	0	0	0	0	0	0	0.2	2.4

computed when the number of strains was fewer than 20.

E. coli, E. freundii, and *S. flexneri* 2a resistant to TC, CM, SM, SA
in a patient. From another patient afflicted with a *S. flexneri* 2a resistant to CM, SM, SA, *E. coli,* resistant to the same agents, was
isolated (Table I). These observations stimulated our interest in the
genetics and the origin of this multiple drug resistance *(40, 43, 49).*

A survey by this laboratory showed that of 1,145 healthy human
subjects 1.4% carried multiple-resistant *E. coli* strains *(49).* Another
survey in 1960 disclosed that of a group of healthy human subjects
studied 1.3% carried multiple-resistant *E. coli* strains *(80).* In contrast,

TABLE III.   Demonstration of Drug-resistant *E. coli* Strains from Human Subjects

Human subjects		Total number examined	Isolation of resistant *E. coli* (%)
Healthy human subjects		1,145	1.4
Healthy human subjects		1,000	1.3
Inpatients	treated with CM[a]	89	61.0
	with tuberculosis and treated with SM	132	20.5
	with bacillary dysentery	163	9.8
Outpatients		201	0.5

[a] Unpublished observation (Mitsuhashi and Takahashi, 1963).   Drug resistance involved TC, CM, and SM.

61.0% of the tuberculosis inpatients treated with CM and 20.5% of the tuberculosis inpatients treated with SM carried multiple-resistant strains of *E. coli*. The results are shown in Table III. Of 93 drug-resistant *E. coli* strains isolated from tuberculosis patients, 81.5% were multiple-resistant, *i.e.*, resistant to TC, CM, SM, SA; TC, SM, SA; or CM, SM, SA (Table IV).

It has been well recognized that there is an increasing incidence of infections with bacteria that normally live within the host, and that drug resistance of *E. coli* and other gram-negative rods belonging to the Enterobacteriaceae is becoming a clinically serious problem.

A survey of drug resistance of isolated enteric bacteria other than *Shigella* is now being conducted at hospitals throughout Japan (*23*). The isolation frequency of gram-negative rod bacteria from clinical sources is shown in Fig. 5; included are *Escherichia*, 45.5%; *Pseudomonas*, 26.4%; *Proteus*, 13.2%; *Klebsiella*, 10.9%; *Aerobacter* culture, 3.4%; and others, 0.6%. *Escherichia* cultures included *E. coli*, 45.5%

TABLE IV. Resistance Patterns of *E. coli* Strains

Resistance patterns		Number of strains	Isolation frequency among resistant strains (%)
Quadruple	TC. CM. SM. SA	117	36.7
Triple	TC. SM. SA	25	
	CM. SM. SA	11	11.9
	TC. CM. SM	2	
Double	SM. SA	61	
	TC. SM	9	
	TC. SA	8	25.7
	CM. SA	2	
	CM. SM	1	
	TC. CM	1	
Single	SA	62	
	TC	14	25.7
	SM	5	
	CM	1	

Three hundred and nineteen drug-resistant strains were demonstrated from 461 *E. coli* strains isolated from 1971 to 1973. A CM-resistant *E. coli* strain was also resistant to APC.

TABLE V. Resistance Patterns of Gram-negative Rod Bacteria to TC, CM, SM, and SA

Resistance pattern	Isolation frequency (%)			
	E. coli	Klebsiella	Proteus	Salmonella
Quadruple	25.3	26.2	14.7	2.2
Triple	8.2	9.2	16.8	12.6
Double	17.8	9.7	17.1	10.0
Single	17.8	19.5	24.3	54.3
Sensitive	30.8	35.4	27.2	20.8
Number of strains examined	461	535	397	1,980

Quadruple resistance, TC. CM. SM. SA; triple resistance, CM. SM. SA, TC. SM. SA, TC. CM. SA, TC. CM. SM; double resistance, TC. CM, SM. SA, CM. SM, TC. SM, CM. SA, TC. SA; single resistance, TC, CM, SM, SA. Summary of results from 3,373 strains isolated from 1965 to 1973.

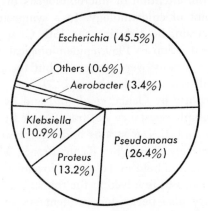

Fig. 5. Isolation frequency of gram-negative rod bacteria from clinical sources. Results based on surveys conducted by a research project "Studies on the Infection of Gram-negative Bacteria" (chief, S. Ishiyama, School of Medicine, Nihon Univ., Tokyo). Summary of results from 1,786 strains isolated from 1965 to 1967.

and *E. freundii*, 2.2%. Others included *Serratia*, 0.3%; *Salmonella*, 0.1%; *Arizona*, 0.1%; and *Hafnia*, 0.1%.

Of 1,306 strains isolated from 1965 to 1967, drug-resistant strains, with special reference to four drugs, TC, CM, SM, and SA, included

E. coli, 71.2%; *E. freundii,* 60.0%; *Klebsiella,* 63.0%; *Aerobacter,* 62.3%; and *Proteus* culture, 35.1%. Among them, quadruply (TC. CM. SM. SA)-resistant strains were isolated most frequently and included *E. coli,* 38.8%; *E. freundii,* 45.0%; *Klebsiella,* 41.0%; *Aerobacter,* 31.6%; and *Proteus* culture, 16.2%. It should be noted that the isolation frequency of drug-sensitive strains was rather high when compared with that of *Shigella* strains. This may be accounted for by the fact that infections with enteric bacteria other than *Shigella* are often caused by strains from sources which have never had contact with antibiotics while shigellosis is caused often by strains from carriers treated with antibiotics.

3. Discovery of R Factors

Appearance of multiple-resistant *Shigella* strains and their rapid increase in number attracted the attention of microbiologists in Japan, especially from the standpoint of epidemiology. In a symposium on drug resistance of *Shigella* strain, held during the 15th General Assembly of Japan Medical Association in 1959, epidemiological aspects of multiple-resistant *Shigella* strains were presented but the genetic approach to this problem still remained unsolved (*3, 30*).

In 1959 independent reports by Ochiai *et al.* (*60*) and by Akiba *et al.* (*4, 5*) indicated that multiple resistance was transferable by mixed cultivation between *Shigella* and *E. coli* strains and *vice versa.* This problem was discussed extensively during the Kanto Branch Meeting of Japan Bacteriological Association held in Tokyo in November, 1959, but questions about the mechanisms involved in the transmission were not answered. Our laboratory also began independent studies on a genetic approach to the problem of multiple resistance of *Shigella* and *E. coli* strains. Culture filtrates of many quadruple-resistant *Shigella* strains or of strains that had been subjected to ultraviolet irradiation were not able to transfer their multiple resistance to drug-sensitive *E. coli* strains. Deoxyribonucleic acid extracts from such strains were not able to mediate the transfer of multiple resistance when drug-sensitive *E. coli* strains were inoculated in culture media containing such extracts. We confirmed the findings of Ochiai *et al.* and Akiba *et al.* that multiple resistance was transferred after mixed cultivation of both drug-resistant and -sensitive strains. Then we recalled the fact that the bacterial chromosome is transferred from one cell to another by direct cell-to-cell contact (*36*) and that the presence of the episome was established in 1958 by Jacob and Wallman (*25*). I recalled also the U-shaped tube fitted with ultrafine fritted glass devised by B. D. Davis, who used it to prove the transmission of the F factor by cell-to-cell contact, called the conjugal process (*9*). Using this method, we discovered that the transfer of multiple resistance was not mediated by the filtrable agents, *i.e.*, bacteriophages, deoxyribonucleic acids, *etc.* (*44*). Drug resistance was transmitted by mixed cultivation from drug-resistant *E. coli* K12 F⁻ or Hfr to sensitive *Shigella* regardless of the polarity of the F agent. Between substrains of *E. coli* K12, drug resistance was found to be transmitted similarly by mixed cultivation without regard to the polarity of the F agent (*44*). These facts indicated to us that transferable drug resistance is transmitted independently of the chromosomal transmission of the donor strain and that this agent is different from the F factor. Furthermore, we found by chance that the transferable drug resistance agent was spontaneously lost from resistant strains of *Shigella* or *E. coli* during storage in a cooked meat medium (*45*). Similarly, the transferable drug resistance property was artificially lost from resistant strains of *Shigella* or *E. coli* upon treatment with acriflavin (*46, 47*). This fact was confirmed later by Watanabe and Fukasawa (*78*) who also found that the transmission of drug resistance was interrupted when the mixed culture was subjected to blender treatment (*77*). These findings indicated to us that the transfer of drug resistance was mediated by cell-to-cell contact, namely by conjugation, and that the transferable drug resistance agent exists independently of the host chromosome. It was found that a mixed incubation of a small number of bacterial cells carrying transmissible drug resistance results in the rapid acquisition of multiple drug resistance by a majority of the recipient cells. This observation favors the view that transmissible drug resistance is a property which replicates at a faster rate than the bacterial chromosome. I proposed the term "R (resistance) factor" for the property of transmissible drug resistance (*39*). At that time, Watanabe and Nakaya used the abbreviations of *rtf* (resistance transfer factor) (*76*) and *rta* (resistance transfer agent) (*56*), respectively. At a conference on infective heredity held in 1962 at the National Institute of Genetics in Mishima, Japan, Japanese geneticists discussed the transmissible drug resistance property

TABLE VI. Discovery of R Factor

Subject	Presentation	Reference
Drug resistance is transferable by mixed cultivation	1959 Nov.	Ochiai *et al.* (*60*)
	1959 Nov.	Akiba *et al.* (*4, 5*)
Transfer of drug resistance is not mediated by filtrable agents	1960 Jan.	Mitsuhashi *et al.* (*44*)
Drug resistance is transmitted regardless of the polarity of F agent	1960 Jan.	Mitsuhashi *et al.* (*44*)
Transferable drug resistance property is eliminated spontaneously during storage	1960 March	Mitsuhashi *et al.* (*45*)
Transferable drug resistance agent is eliminated by treatment with acriflavin	1960 June	Mitsuhashi *et al.* (*46*)
Transmission of drug resistance is interrupted by blender treatment		Watanabe *et al.* (*77*)
The term "R factor" suggested to indicate the transferable drug resistance property	1960	Mitsuhashi (*39*)
The range of transmission includes all species of the *Enterobacteriaceae*, *Vibrio comma*, and *P. pestis*	1960	Harada *et al.* (*17*)
	1961, 1963	Baron *et al.* (*8*)
		Ginoza *et al.* (*16*)
Bordetella bronchiseptica	1974	Terakado and Mitsuhashi (*69*)

and agreed to use the term "R factor". The history of the discovery of R factor is shown in Table VI.

It was found that R factors are transferable among all species of the family Enterobacteriaceae (*17*), the *Vibrio* group (*8*), and *Pasteurella pestis* (*16*). These properties of the R factor, *i.e.*, autonomous replication and a wide range of transmission among enteric bacteria, are of great importance in public health and animal husbandry.

REFERENCES

1 Abe, M. 1964. *Nihon Iji Shimpo*, No. 2115, 21–27 (in Japanese).
2 Abraham, E. P., Chain, E., Fletcher, C. M., Florey, H. W., Gardener, A. D., Heatley, N. G., and Jennings, M. A. 1941. *Lancet*, **ii**, 177.
3 Akiba, T. 1959. *Proc. 15th Gen. Assem. Japan. Med. Assoc.*, **5**, 299–305 (in Japanese).

4 Akiba, T., Koyama, T., Isshiki, Y., Kimura, S., and Fukushima, T. 1960. *Nihon Iji Shimpo*, No. 1886, 45–50 (in Japanese).

5 Akiba, T., Koyama, K., Isshiki, Y., Kumura, S., and Fukushima, T. 1960. *Japan. J. Microbiol.*, **4**, 219–227.

6 Anderson, E. S. and Datta, N. 1965. *Lancet*, **i**, 407–409.

7 Anderson, E. S. and Lewis, M. J. 1965. *Nature*, **208**, 843–849.

8 Baron, L. S. and Falkow, S. 1961. *Rec. Genet. Soc. Am.*, **30**, 59.

9 Davis, B. D. 1950. *J. Bacteriol.*, **60**, 507–508.

10 Demerec, M. 1945. *Proc. Natl. Acad. Sci. U.S.*, **31**, 16–24.

11 Demerec, M. 1948. *J. Bacteriol.*, **56**, 63–74.

12 Ehrlich, P. 1907. *Ber. Klin. Wochschr.*, **44**, 233–236.

13 Ezaki, T. 1967. *Japan. J. Infect. Dis.*, **41**, 99–107 (in Japanese).

14 Franke, E. and Roehl, W. 1907. Quoted by Ehrlich, P. 1907.

15 Geronimus, L. H. and Cohen, S. 1957. *J. Bacteriol.*, **73**, 28–34.

16 Ginoza, H. S. and Matney, T. S. 1963. *J. Bacteriol.*, **85**, 1177–1178.

17 Harada, K., Suzuki, M., Kameda, M., and Mitsuhashi, S. 1960. *Japan. J. Exp. Med.*, **30**, 289–299.

18 Harada, K., Kameda, M., Suzuki, M., and Mitsuhashi, S. 1964. *J. Bacteriol.*, **88**, 1257–1265.

19 Harada, K., Kameda, M., Suzuki, M., and Mitsuhashi, S. 1967. *Japan. J. Microbiol.*, **11**, 143–151.

20 Hashimoto, H., Oshima, H., and Mitsuhashi, S. 1968. *Japan. J. Microbiol.*, **12**, 321–327.

21 Hinshelwood, C. N. 1946. *In* Chemical Kinetics of the Bacterial Cell, pp. 1–204, Clarendon Press, Oxford.

22 Inoue, M., Hashimoto, H., and Mitsuhashi, S. 1969. *J. Antibiot.*, **23**, 68–74.

23 Ishiyama, S. 1967. *Chemotherapy*, **15**, 581–587 (in Japanese).

24 Izaki, K., Kiuchi, K., and Arima, K. 1966. *J. Bacteriol.*, **91**, 628–633.

25 Jacob, F. and Wallman, E. L. 1958. *Compt. Rend. Acad. Sci.*, **247**, 154–156.

26 Kameda, M., Harada, K., Suzuki, M., and Mitsuhashi, S. 1969. *Japan. J. Microbiol.*, **13**, 255–262.

27 Kameda, M., Harada, K., Suzuki, M., and Mitsuhashi, S. 1970. *Japan. J. Microbiol.*, **14**, 423–426.

28 Kasuga, T., Hashimoto, H., and Mitsuhashi, S. 1968. *J. Bacteriol.*, **95**, 1764–1766.

29 Kitamoto, O., Takigami, T., Kasai, N., Fukaya, I., and Kawashima, A. 1956. *Japan. J. Infect. Dis.*, **3**, 403–405 (in Japanese).

30 Kobari, K. 1959. *Proc. 15th Gen. Assem. Japan. Med. Assoc.*, **5**, 317–323 (in Japanese).

31 Kondo, E. and Mitsuhashi, S. 1964. *J. Bacteriol.*, **88**, 1266–1276.

32 Kondo, E. and Mitsuhashi, S. 1966. *J. Bacteriol.*, **91**, 1787–1794.

33 Kono, M., Hashimoto, H., and Mitsuhashi, S. 1965. *Japan. J. Bacteriol.*, **20**, 122–123 (in Japanese).

34 Kono, M., Hashimoto, H., and Mitsuhashi, S. 1966. *Japan. J. Microbiol.*, **10**, 59–66.

35 Kono, M., Ogawa, K., and Mitsuhashi, S. 1968. *J. Bacteriol.*, **95**, 886–892.

36 Lederberg, J. and Tatum, E. L. 1946. *Cold Spring Harbor Symp. Quant. Biol.*, **11**, 113–114.

37 Luria, S. E. 1947. *Bacteriol. Rev.*, **11**, 1–40.

38 Maclean, I. H., Rogers, K. B., and Fleming, A. 1939. *Lancet*, **i**, 562–568.

39 Mitsuhashi, S. 1960. *Science (Tokyo)*, **30**, 628–633 (in Japanese).

40 Mitsuhashi, S. 1963. *Protein, Nucleic Acid, Enzyme*, **8**, 216–228 (in Japanese).

41 Mitsuhashi, S. 1967. *Japan. J. Microbiol.*, **11**, 49–68.

42 Mitsuhashi, S. 1968. *Asian Med. J.*, **11**, 59–68.

43 Mitsuhashi, S. 1969. *J. Infect. Dis.*, **119**, 89–100.

44 Mitsuhashi, S., Harada, K., and Hashimoto, H. 1960. *Japan. J. Exp. Med.*, **30**, 179–184.

45 Mitsuhashi, S., Hashimoto, H., Harada, K., Suzuki, M., Kameda, M., and Matsuyama, T. 1960. *Japan. J. Bacteriol.*, **15**, 844–848 (in Japanese).

46 Mitsuhashi, S., Harada, K., and Kameda, M. 1960. *Tokyo Iji Shinshi*, **77**, 462 (in Japanese).

47 Mitsuhashi, S., Harada, K., and Kameda, M. 1961. *Nature*, **189**, 947.

48 Mitsuhashi, S., Harada, K., Hashimoto, H., and Egawa, R. 1961. *Japan. J. Exp. Med.*, **31**, 47–52.

49 Mitsuhashi, S., Harada, K., Hashimoto, H., and Egawa, R. 1961. *Japan. J. Exp. Med.*, **31**, 53–60.

50 Mitsuhashi, S., Oshima, H., Kawaharada, U., and Hashimoto, H. 1965. *J. Bacteriol.*, **89**, 967–976.

51 Mitsuhashi, S., Hashimoto, H., Kono, M., and Morimura, M. 1965. *J. Bacteriol.*, **89**, 988–992.

52 Mitsuhashi, S., Kono, M., and Harada, K. 1967. *5th Int. Congr. Chemother.*, Vienna, Austria, C2/9, 499–509.

53 Mitsuhashi, S., Kameda, M., Harada, K., and Suzuki, M. 1969. *J. Bacteriol.*, **97**, 1520–1521.

54 Morgenroth, J. and Kaufmann, M. 1912. *Z. Immunitaetsforsch.*, **15**, 610–618.

55 Murray, R., Kilham, L., Wilcox, C., and Finland, M. 1964. *Proc. Soc. Exp. Biol. Med.*, **63**, 470–474.

56 Nakaya, R., Nakamura, A., and Murata, Y. 1960. *Biochem. Biophys. Res. Commun.*, **3**, 654–659.
57 Novick, R. P. and Morse, S. I. 1967. *J. Exp. Med.*, **125**, 45–59.
58 Novick, R. P. 1967. *Fed. Proc.*, **27**, 29–38.
59 Ochiai, K., Totani, T., and Toshiki, Y. 1959. *Nihon Iji Shimpo*, No. 1837, 25–37 (in Japanese).
60 Ochiai, K., Yamanaka, K., Kimura, K., and Sawada, O. 1959. *Nihon Iji Shimpo*, No. 1861, 34–46 (in Japanese).
61 Okamoto, S. and Suzuki, Y. 1965. *Nature*, **208**, 1301–1303.
62 Okamoto, S., Suzuki, Y., Mise, K., and Nakaya, R. 1967. *J. Bacteriol.*, **94**, 1616–1622.
63 Ozeki, H., Stocker, A. D., and Smith, S. M. 1962. *J. Gen. Microbiol.*, **28**, 671–687.
64 Pollock, M. R. 1950. *Br. J. Exp. Pathol.*, **31**, 739–753.
65 de Reuck, A. V. S. and Cameron, M. P. (eds.). 1962. Resistance to Penicillins, Little Brown, Boston.
66 Sugino, Y. and Hirota, Y. 1962. *J. Bacteriol.*, **84**, 902–910.
67 Suzuki, S., Nakazawa, S., and Ushioda, T. 1956. *Chemotherapy*, **4**, 336–338 (in Japanese).
68 Suzuki, Y., Okamoto, S., and Kono, M. 1966. *J. Bacteriol.*, **92**, 798–799.
69 Terakado, N. and Mitsuhashi, S. 1974. *Antimicrob. Agents Chemother.*, **6**, 836–840.
70 Tanaka, T., Hashimoto, H., Nagai, Y., and Mitsuhashi, S. 1967. *Japan. J. Microbiol.*, **11**, 155–162.
71 Tanaka, T., Nagai, Y., Hashimoto, H., and Mitsuhashi, S. 1969. *Japan. J. Microbiol.*, **13**, 187–191.
72 Tanaka, T., Tsunoda, M., and Mitsuhashi, S. 1973. *Japan. J. Microbiol.*, **17**, 291–295.
73 Tanaka, T., Kobayashi, A., Ikemura, K., Hashimoto, H., and Mitsuhashi, S. 1974. *Japan. J. Microbiol.*, **18**, 343–347.
74 Tanaka, T., Ikemura, K., Tsunoda, M., Sasagawa, I., and Mitsuhashi, S. 1976. *Antimicrob. Agents Chemother.*, **9**, 61–64.
75 Tanaka, T., Tsunoda, M., and Mitsuhashi, S. 1975. *In* Microbial Drug Resistance, ed. by S. Mitsuhashi and H. Hashimoto, pp. 187–199, University of Tokyo Press, Tokyo / University Park Press, Baltimore and London.
76 Watanabe, T. and Fukasawa, T. 1960. *Biochem. Biophys. Res. Commun.*, **3**, 660–665.
77 Watanabe, T. and Fukasawa, T. 1960. *Medicine and Biology*, **56**, 98–100 (in Japanese).

78 Watanabe, T. and Fukasawa, T. 1961. *J. Bacteriol.*, **81**, 679–683.
79 Weaver, J. R. and Pattee, P. A. 1964. *J. Bacteriol.*, **88**, 574–580.
80 Zenyoji, H., Nakagami, C., Benoki, M., Mitsuhashi, S., Harada, K., and Kakinuma, Y. 1961. *Japan. J. Bacteriol.*, **16**, 1015–1016 (in Japanese).

2 EPIDEMIOLOGY OF R FACTORS

Susumu Mitsuhashi
Department of Microbiology, School of Medicine, Gunma University, Maebashi, Japan

Improved sanitary conditions and preventive medicine in developed countries have protected human beings from the threat of infectious diseases caused by pathogenic bacteria seen in text book. Furthermore, the rapid progress of chemotherapeutic agents and worldwide use of the drugs have caused many changes in the kind of bacteria which play a leading role in infectious diseases. The properties of these microorganisms are characteristic in infectivity, skilful parasitism and multiple drug resistance. It should be noted further that human beings, livestocks and fishes cannot acquire high immunity against infections with these microorganisms, probably due to the antigenic properties of bacterial toxins and cell components.

Selection of drug-resistant bacteria through practical use of chemotherapeutic agents is increasing the chance of infection with such microorganisms at hospitals and farms, called hospital- and farm-infection. The selective force of drugs, in addition to infectivity and parasitic ability, has caused the emergence of bacteria prevalent and fixed at hospitals and farms, *i.e.*, hospital- and farm-strain.

The presence of conjugative(R) and nonconjugative(r) resistance plasmids gives us an additional trouble in practical medicine, livestock hygiene, and culture fish industry due to the horizontal spread of drug resistance from bacteria to bacteria in addition to the infectious spread of bacteria themselves. Thus, drug resistance plasmids accompanied by hospital- and farm-strains have become a new biological hazard at hospitals and farms.

1. Demonstration of R Factors in Japan

Drug resistance of *Shigella* strains has been extensively studied in Japan by the Research Committee on Drug Resistance of *Shigella* Strains (chief, T. Ezaki) with 17 participating laboratories (7) and by the Research Committee on Intestinal Infections Caused by Bacteria (chief, H. Hiraishi) with 30 participating laboratories. All *Shigella* strains isolated by the committees were sent to the Department of Microbiology, School of Medicine, Gunma University and their drug resistance and distribution of R factors were investigated.

In relation to resistance to tetracycline (TC), chloramphenicol (CM), streptomycin (SM), and sulfanilamide (SA), the isolation frequency of the strains with quadruple resistance was highest, followed by those with single, triple, and double resistance (Table 1 and Fig. 1A). The isolation frequencies of *Escherichia coli* strains with resistance to the four drugs were quite similar to that of *Shigella* strains (Fig. 1B) (*33–35, 37*).

Among *Shigella* strains resistant to TC, CM, SM, and SA, and combinations thereof, 75.0% carried R factors. The demonstration frequency of R factors in the triple-resistant strains was the highest (86.7%), followed by the strains with quadruple, double, and single resistance (Table I). Among the single-resistant strains, the strains with SA-resistance were isolated most frequently and those with resistance to other drugs, *i.e.*, TC, CM, and SM were isolated rather infrequently (Fig. 1). Among the triple-resistant strains, the strains with (CM. SM. SA) resistance were isolated most frequently, followed by those with (TC. SM. SA) resistance. But there were very few the strains with triple resistance to other combinations of the four drugs. The strains with (SM. SA) resistance were isolated most frequently among double-resistant strains, followed by those with (TC. SA) resistance. There were very few strains isolated with other combinations

TABLE I. Drug Resistance Patterns of *Shigella* Strains and Isolation Frequency of R Factors

Resistance pattern[a]		Number of strains (%)		Demonstration frequency of R factors in resistant bacteria (%)	
Quadruple	TC. CM. SM. SA	8,660	(77.1)		(75.5)
Triple	CM. SM. SA	405 (3.3)		(90.6)	
	TC. SM. SA	110 (0.9)	535 (4.7)	(70.4)	(86.7)
	TC. CM. SA	20 (0.2)		(77.8)	
Double	SM. SA	235 (1.9)		(18.0)	
	TC. SA	68 (0.5)		(88.9)	
	TC. CM	6 (0.05)	121 (1.1)	5/6[b]	(35.1)
	CM. SA	8 (0.06)		6/8	
	TC. SM	3 (0.02)		2/3	
	CM. SM	1 (0.01)		1/1	
Single	SA	1,850 (14.9)		(5.6)	
	TC	41 (0.3)	1,917 (17.0)	(34.6)	(9.6)
	CM	25 (0.2)		(36.0)	
	SM	1 (0.01)		0/1[b]	
Sensitive		1,220			

Results of survey of 12,453 *Shigella* strains isolated from 1965 to 1973 (*32–34, 37*).

[a] In relation to resistance to TC, CM, SM, and SA.

[b] Percentage was not computed when the number of strains was fewer than 10.

[c] (%), among resistant strains.

Numerator, number of R⁺ strains ; denominator, total number of strains.

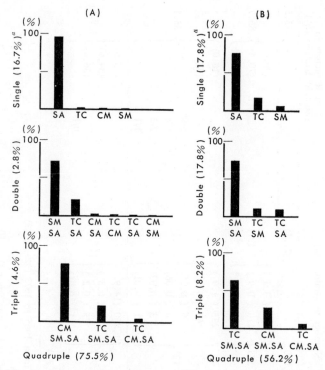

Fig. 1. Drug resistance patterns of *Shigella* and *E. coli* strains isolated in Japan. In relation to resistance to TC, CM, SM, and SA. Results of survey of 12,453 *Shigella* strains isolated from 1965 to 1973(A). Results of survey of 338 *E. coli* strains isolated from 1970 to 1973(B). [a] In relation to resistance to TC, CM, SM, and SA.

of double resistance. These results indicate that there is a selective step in the formation of multiple resistance, that is in the combinations (SM. SA) and (TC. SA), (CM. SM. SA) and (TC. SM. SA), and (TC. CM. SM. SA).

The demonstration of R factors in strains of *Shigella* isolated in Japan from 1945 to 1955 was very rare, but the isolation frequency of R factors increased rapidly thereafter with an increase in the number of multiple-resistant strains.

Drug resistance patterns of R factors in *Shigella* strains isolated in Japan are shown in Table I and Fig. 2. Of 12,453 strains isolated from 1965 to 1973, the R factors in 9,412 were demonstrated. Of those

TEBLE II. Distribution of R Factors among Drug-resistant Strains of Enteric Bacteria

Microorganism	Number of strains examined	Strains carrying R factors	
		Number	%
Shigella	1,700	1,275	75.0
E. coli	520	301	58.0
E. freundii	65	47	72.5
Salmonella	1,312	420	32.0
Klebsiella	170	120	70.5
Proteus	78	32	42.0
P. aeruginosa[a]	204	70	34.3

The strains resistant to TC, CM, SM, SA, and combinations thereof were selected at random from our stock cultures and the distribution of R factors was examined. [a] *P. aeruginosa* strains highly resistant to TC, CM, SM, and SA were selected from 1,200 stock cultures of *P. aeruginosa* (*11, 12*).

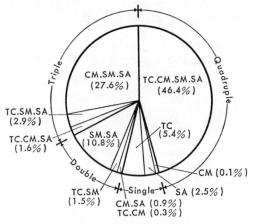

Fig. 2. Resistance patterns of R factors from *Shigella* strains isolated in Japan. 9,412 R factors were demonstrated in 12,453 *Shigella* strains isolated from 1965 to 1973. Drug resistance was examined with special reference to four drugs, TC, CM, SM, and SA.

R factors with resistance to the four drugs, 46.4% were quadruple-resistant, 32.1% triple-resistant, 13.5% double-resistant, and 8.0% single-resistant (*33, 34, 37*).

The isolation frequency of *Shigella* strains resistant to drugs other

TABLE III. Isolation Frequency of KM- or APC-resistant Strains and Demon-

Organism	Isolation frequency (%) of strains resistant to			
	KM	APC	CPC	GM
Shigella	0.4	2.9		
E. coli	1.5	4.7		
Salmonella	2.1	1.4		
K. pneumoniae	6.3	14.0		
P. aeruginosa	16.1		16.1	16.6

Summary of results from 12,242 strains of *Shigella*, 338 strains of *E. coli*, 2,920
[a] The number of R$^+$ strains/total number of KM- or APC-resistant strains.

than the four mentioned previously, *i.e.*, kanamycin (KM), and ampicillin (APC), was rather low (Table III). But the demonstration frequency of R factors with KM or APC resistance were rather high
among the strains with KM or APC resistance.

TABLE IV. Isolation Frequency of R Factors from *Shigella* Strains of Various
Serotypes

Serotype of strains		Number of strains tested	R$^+$ strains		
			Number	%	
S. sonnei		841	480		(57.1)
S. flexneri	1a	27	6	(22.2)	
	1b	21	6	(28.6)	
	2a	366	236	(64.5)	
	2b	51	22	(43.1)	
	3a	85	58	(68.2)	
	3b	13	6	(46.2)	(57.1)
	3c	4	2		
	4	26	9	(34.6)	
	6	2	2		
	X	17	9	(52.9)	
	Y	36	4	(11.1)	
S. dysenteriae		3	1		
S. boydii		1	1		

Strains tested are the same as those described in 1973 (*34*). Percentage was not
computed when the number of strains was fewer than 10.

stration of R Factors

Isolation frequency (%) of R factors carrying KM or APC resistance							
From total strains examined				From KM- or APC-resistant strains			
KM	APC	CPC	GM	KM	APC	CPC	GM
0.3	2.2			85.7[a]	77.5		
1.5	3.8			100	81.3		
1.3	0.6			65.5	48.7		
2.0	5.6			33.3	40.4		
10.3		11.7	5.8	63.6		72.7	35.2

strains of *Salmonella*, 335 strains of *K. pneumoniae* and 204 strains of *P. aeruginosa*. GM, gentamicin C, complex; CPC, carbenicillin.

The isolation frequency of R factors in *Shigella* strains of various serotype are shown in Table IV. The R factors in *Shigella flexneri* 3a, 2a and *Shigella sonnei* showed characteristic high frequency. It was found that some *Shigella* strains in a hetero-R state carried two types of R factor in a cell (*32*). R (SM. SA) factors were demonstrated most frequently in the strains in a hetero-R state (Table V).

TABLE V.   Isolation of *Shigella* Strains in Hetero-R State

Type of drug resistance	Number of R+ strains examined	Number of strains in hetero-R state and their resistance patterns (%)	
TC. CM. SM. SA	438	51 (11.6)	TC. CM. SM. SA / SM. SA
		5 (1.1)	TC. CM. SM. SA / TC
		3 (0.7)	TC. CM. SM. SA / CM. SM. SA
CM. SM. SA	241	4 (1.7)	CM. SM. SA / SM. SA
TC. SM. SA	38	3 (7.9)	TC. SM. SA / SM. SA
SM. SA	27	4 (14.8)	SM. SA / SA
TC. SA	32	2 (6.3)	SA[a] / TC

[a] The gene governing SA resistance was located on nontransferable plasmid(r) and r(SA) was conjugally transferred by the concomitant presence of R(TC) plasmid.

Drug resistance and distribution of R factors among enteric bacteria other than *Shigella* strains were extensively studied in Japan by the Research Committee of Gram-negative Bacteria (chief, S. Ishiyama) with 15 participating laboratories (*10*). All strains isolated by the committee were sent to the Department of Microbiology, School of Medicine Gunma University, and their biological and biochemical properties, drug resistance and distribution of R factors were examined. The distribution of R factors from enteric bacteria is shown in Table II. More than 60% of *Shigella, Escherichia coli, Escherichia freundii,* and *Klebsiella* strains resistant to TC, CM, SM, SA, and to combinations thereof carried R factors. The R factors had not been demonstrated in *Pseudomonas aeruginosa* strains for a long time using *E. coli* as a recipient, although very few papers reported the transfer of resistance in *P. aeruginosa* to other species of gram-negative bacilli (*24, 30, 42*). But it was found that the R factors could be easily demonstrated

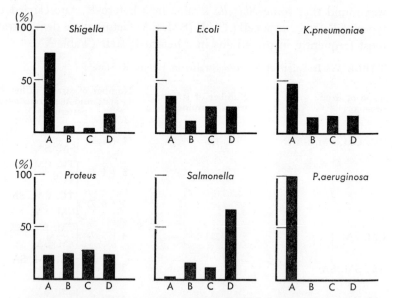

Fig. 3. Drug resistance patterns of enterobacteria isolated from clinical sources. Results based on surveys of 13,984 strains, including 11,433 *Shigella*, 319 *E. coli*, 292 *K. pneumoniae*, 171 *Proteus* group, 1,568 *Salmonella*, and 201 *P. aeruginosa*. Resistance patterns to resistance to TC, CM, SM, and SA. A, quadruple resistance; B, triple resistance; C, double resistance; D, single resistance.

in *P. aeruginosa* strains to *P. aeruginosa* recipients using intraspecies conjugation system *(11–14)*.

Drug resistance patterns of R factors from enteric bacteria isolated in Japan are shown in Fig. 3. More than 70% of the R factors were quadruple-resistant, 14.5% triple-resistant, 7.1% double-resistant, and 7.4% single-resistant.

Drug resistance patterns of enterobacteria in relation to resistance to TC, CM, SM, and SA are shown in Fig. 3. The strains with quadruple resistance were isolated most frequently from *Shigella, E. coli,* and *Klebsiella pneumoniae*. In *Salmonella* strains, the isolation frequency of single TC resistance was the highest. But the percentage

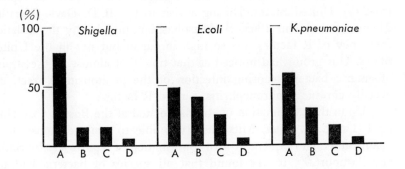

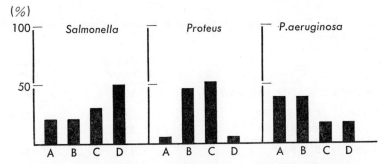

Fig. 4. Resistance patterns of R factors in relation to resistance to TC, CM, SM, and SA. Results based on surveys of 3,610 R factors, including 1,671 from *Shigella*, 338 from *E. coli*, 335 from *Klebsiella*, 965 from *Salmonella*, 231 from *Proteus*, and 70 R factors from *P. aeruginosa*. A, R factors carrying quadruple resistance; B, R factors carrying triple resistance; C, R factors carrying double resistance; D, R factors carrying single resistance.

of isolation of strains of *Salmonella* with four types of resistance pattern, *i.e.*, A, B, C, and D, were equal. These data reflect the resistance patterns of R factors demonstrated in each bacterial species; they being the *Coli-Shigella*, *Salmonella*, and *Proteus* types (Fig. 4). The resistance patterns of R factors in *K. pneumoniae* and *P. aeruginosa* are of the *Coli-Shigella* type.

2. Demonstration of R Factors in Other Countries

R factors were originally demonstrated in Japan, but were also found by workers in Europe in enteropathogenic strains of *E. coli* and *Salmonella* (2–5) of human and animal origin. There were no reports from the United States. During a visit to Dr. B. D. Davis (Harvard Medical School) in 1965, S. Mitsuhashi inquired why the isolation frequency of R factors was so high in Japan but not in the United States. Our group had noticed at that time that almost all the strains of enteric bacteria causing infection of the genitourinary tract, especially chronic nephronephritis, carried R factors.

Upon the examination of strains isolated at the Boston City Hospital (Dr. E. H. Kass) Mitsuhashi was able to easily demonstrate R factors at a high frequency(6). In confirmation of reports also by Smith and Armour(27), it was found that all species of bacteria had the

TABLE VI. Drug Resistance Patterns of R Factors Isolated in the United States and in Europe

Resistance pattern		Number of R factors	Isolation frequency (%)
Quadruple	TC. CM. SM. SA	93	69.9
Triple	CM. SM. SA	4	12.0
	TC. SM. SA	12	
Double	SM. SA	13	10.5
	TC. CM	1	
Single	TC	7	7.5
	SA	1	
	CM	2	

Drug resistance pattern of 133 R factors is shown with special reference to four drugs, TC, CM, SM, and SA (*4, 6, 8, 15–19, 25–27, 29*).

TABLE VII. Distribution of R Factors among Drug-resistant Strains of Enteric Bacteria

Strains	Number of strains examined	Strains isolated in	Strains carrying number	R factor %
Shigella	1,700	Japan (*21*, *33*)	1,275	75.0
	23	Greece (*15*, *16*)	22	95.8
E. coli	303	Japan (*21*)	201	66.3
	202	Japan (*35*)	60	29.7
	25	U.S.A. (*25*, *26*)	17	68.0
	42	U.S.A. (*27*)	32	76.1
	54	Greece (*15*, *16*)	40	74.0
	10	U.S.A. (*6*)	7	70.0
	85	Germany (*18*, *19*)	17	20.0
E. freundii	65		47	70.5
Klebsiella	76	Japan	56	73.7
	8	U.S.A. (*27*)	6	75.0
	20	Greece (*15*, *16*)	12	60.0
	21	U.S.A. (*6*)	7	33.0
Aerobacter	29	Japan	13	44.8
	1	U.S.A. (*6*)	1	
Enterobacter	162	Japan	66	40.7
	28	U.S.A. (*25*, *26*)	19	67.8
	5	Germany (*19*)	4	80.0
Proteus	169	Japan	50	29.6
	17	U.S.A. (*27*)	10	58.8
	8	U.S.A. (*6*)	2	25.0
	5	Germany (*19*)	2	20.0
Salmonella	1,568	Japan (*36*)	326	20.8
	22	Greece (*15*, *16*)	21	95.4
	298	France (*4*), Netherland (*20*)	53	17.7
	35	U.S.A. (*8*)	25	71.0
	7	U.S.A. (*6*)	3	43.0
Pseudomonas	204	Japan (*6*, *12*)	70	
	7	U.S.A. (*27*)	0	34.3
	1	U.S.A. (*6*)	0	

The strains tested in Japan were selected at random from the stock culture (*10*) in the Department of Microbiology, School of Medicine, Gunma University, which were resistant to TC, CM, SM, SA, and various combinations thereof. *Shigella* strains isolated in Japan were the same isolates shown in Table I. In Japan 1,316, other strains were isolated from 1965 to 1967.

capacity to transfer part or all of their resistance genes. These results are clear indications that R factors are widespread all over the world and play a major role in the resistance of all pathogenic gram-negative bacteria. Drug-resistance patterns of R factors isolated in the United States and in Europe are shown in Table VI. Of 133 R factors reported in these areas, 69.9% were quadruple-resistant, 12.0% triple-resistant, 10.5% double-resistant, and 7.5% single-resistant. The distribution of R factors among the strains of enteric bacteria of human origin is summarized in Table VII.

3. R Factors Carrying Resistance to KM or APC

The R factor carrying KM resistance was reported in 1963 by Lebek (*17*) in West Germany. When transferred this R factor was able to establish resistance to five drugs, including TC, CM, SM, SA, and KM. The R factor carrying APC resistance was isolated in 1965 by Datta (*5*). Thereafter, R factors carrying KM or APC resistance were isolated frequently in the United States and Europe, but only rarely in Japan. In 1966 our laboratory isolated R factors carrying KM or APC resistance (*9, 31*), but except for *K. pneumoniae* and *P. aeru-*

Organism	No. of strains examined	Isolation frequency (%)		Isolation frequency of R+ strains (%) 50 100
Shigella	12,453	KM	0.4	
		APC	3.0	
E.coli	461	KM	5.0	
		APC	11.9	
K.pneumoniae	535	KM	9.7	
		APC	21.9	
Proteus	397	KM	11.1	
		APC	36.8	
Salmonella	1,980	KM	2.6	
		APC	1.0	
P.aeruginosa	204	KM	16.1	
		CPC	16.1	
		GM	16.6	

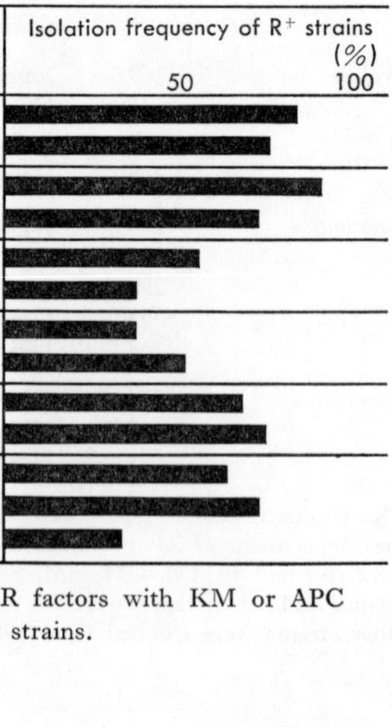

Fig. 5. Demonstration frequency of R factors with KM or APC resistance from KM- or APC-resistant strains.

TABLE VIII. Resistance Patterns of R factors Carrying KM or APC Resistance

R factor carrying	Resistance pattern	R factors isolated	
		Number	%
APC resistance	TC. CM. SM. SA. KM. APC	20	5.4
	TC. CM. SM. SA. APC	270	76.7
	Quadruple resistance	41	11.6
	Triple resistance	27	7.6
	Double resistance	7	
	APC resistance	5	
Total		370	
KM resistance	TC. CM. SM. SA. APC. KM	20	15.6
	TC. CM. SM. SA. KM	9	7.0
	Quadruple resistance	32	25.0
	Triple resistance	48	37.5
	Double resistance	18	14.0
	KM resistance	1	
Total		128	

The R factors were demonstrated in 15,704 strains of gram-negative enteric bacteria including *Shigella, E. coli, Salmonella, K. pneumoniae,* and *P. aeruginosa.* Resistance patterns to TC, CM, SM, SA, KM, and APC.

ginosa (Table III) the isolation frequencies of strains resistant to KM and APC were not so high in Japan. But the demonstration frequencies of R factors with KM or APC resistance were rather high in the strains resistant to the drugs (Fig. 5). As shown in Table VIII, the R factors possessing APC resistance were mostly multiple-resistant and 76.7% of them were quintuple-resistant, *i.e.,* (TC. CM. SM. SA. APC), followed by quadruple- and triple-resistant, in that order. The R factors with triple resistance, including KM, were isolated most frequently, and followed by quadruple, quintuple (TC. CM. SM. SA. KM), and double resistance, in that order.

4. *Distribution of R Factors in Strains Isolated from Domestic Animals*

Anderson *et al. (2, 3)* reported that strains of *Salmonella typhimurium* of phage type 29 are multiple-resistant, predominant in bovine infection in Britain, and cause many other infections which are almost certainly bovine in origin. They pointed out that its prevalence in cattle is due to a combination of two major factors; one, low standards of hygiene in intensive farming, in the cattle market, and in the transport of animals, and, two, the widespread use in animal husbandry of antibiotics and synthetic antibacterial drugs. They reported on the R factors in *S. typhimurium* in man and domestic animals in Britain (*2, 3, 5*), and found that 61% of 450 strains examined by them between December 1964 and February 1965 were resistant to one or more drugs. In a high proportion of these strains the resistance was of the infective type.

Other surveys in England disclosed that multiple-resistant strains of *E. coli* were isolated from the faeces of healthy pigs and calves on several farms in northwestern England. Many of these farms used feed for their animals which contained antibiotics and chemically synthesized drugs (*38*).

Other surveys in England (*28*) and in Japan (*22*) disclosed that a high incidence of drug resistance was found among *E. coli* strains isolated from healthy animals and from calves and sheep suffering from neonatal diarrhea or bacteremia, pigs suffering from neonatal or postweaning diarrhea or bowel edema and fowls suffering from coli-septi-

TABLE IX.   Isolation Frequency of Resistance to TC, CM, SM, SA, APC, and NM in Drug-resistant *E. coli* Strains Isolated from Domestic Animals

Resistant to	Strains from (%)				Reference
	Pig	Calf	Sheep	Fowl	
TC	61	75	66	58	*28* (Great Britain)
	84	nd[a]	nd	72	*22* (Japan)
CM	11	22	0	0	*28*
	4	nd	nd	2	*22*
SM	64	78	66	10	*28*
	90	nd	nd	61	*22*
SA	36	85	99	58	*28*
	65	nd	nd	75	*22*
APC	0	21	0	0	*28*
NM	11	0	33	0	*28*

[a] Not done.

TABLE X. Detection of R Factors from Drug-resistant *E. coli* Strains Isolated from Domestic Animals

R factors in strains from (%)				Reference
Pig	Calf	Sheep	Fowl	
75			80	Mitsuhashi[a]
75	91	66	66	Smith[b]
58			44	Walton[c]

[a] Incidence of R factors among resistant *E. coli* strains (*22*).
[b] Incidence of R factors among resistant strains of *E. coli* isolated from diseased domestic animals (*28*).
[c] Incidence of R factors from multiple-resistant strains of *E. coli* (*38*).

caemia. The isolation frequency of resistance to TC, CM, SM, SA, APC, and neomycin (NM) (or KM) in drug-resistant *E. coli* strains isolated from domestic animals are shown in Table IX. Isolation frequency of resistance to TC, SM, and SA was high but isolation frequency of resistance to CM was less than that in human beings. Isolation frequency of triple- or double-resistant strains was much higher than that of single-resistant strains (*22*). However, surveys in England disclosed that single-resistant strains were isolated more frequently

TABLE XI. Demonstration of R Factors in Cultured Fish

Fish	Demonstration frequency of R factors	Resistance patterns of R factors	
Hamachi (*Seriola quinqueradiata*)	54.3	TC. CM. SM. SA	(100)
Anago (*Oncorhynchus rhodurus macrostomus*)	52.9	CM. SM. SA	(100)
Mud turtle (*Trionyx sinensis japonicus*)	54.2	CM. TC. SA	(7.1)
		TC. SA	(85.7)
		SA	(4.7)
		TC	(2.4)
Eel (*Angilla japonica*)	26.0	TC. CM. SM. SA	(8.0)
		TC. SM. SA	(8.0)
		TC. SA	(80.0)
		TC	(4.0)
Trout (*Salmo gairdneri irideus*)	6.5	TC. SM. SA	(100)

than those in Japan (*28*), and as shown in Table X a high incidence of transferable drug resistance was found among drug-resistant strains of *E. coli* isolated from domestic animals (*22, 28, 38*).

Walton (*38*) reported that 99 of 134 multiple-resistant strains transferred their drug resistance to sensitive recipient strains. These R factors carried the resistance patterns of TC, CM, SM, SA, KM, and APC, and combinations thereof.

These surveys indicate a definite association between the drugs applied to the animals and the isolation from their faeces of strains of *E. coli* resistant to these drugs and capable of transferring this resistance.

The R factors were also demonstrated in cultured fishes owing to the widespread use of food containing antibiotics and chemically synthesized drugs for the purpose of growth promotion and animal husbandary (*1, 23, 40*). The high demonstration frequencies of R factors

TABLE XII.   Demonstration of R Factors in Fish Pathogens

Bacteria	Resistance patterns of R factors
A. liquefacience	CM. SM. SA
	TC. SA
A. salmocida	CM. SM. SA
Vibrio	TC. CM. SM. SA
	TC. SM. SA
	TC. SA
Citrobacter	TC. CM. SM. SA
	TC. SM. SA
	TC. SA
	CM. SA
Aerogenes	TC. SM. SA
Cloaca	TC. SM. SA
Enterobacter	TC. CM. SM. SA
	TC. CM. SA
	TC. SA
	TC
Klebsiella	TC. CM. SM. SA

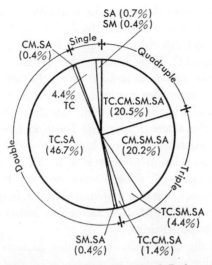

Fig. 6. Resistance patterns of R factors in bacteria isolated from cultured fish. Results based on surveys of 272 R factors isolated from 1970 to 1973. With reference to resistance to TC, CM, SM, and SA.

TABLE XIII. Carcass Samples Positive for Total Coliforms, Resistant Coliforms, and Percentage of Resistant Coliforms of Fecal Origin

Carcasses	Number of samples	Coliform positive	Resistant coliforms	Fecal coliform[a]
Pork				
Slaughterhouse 1				
Outside	100	84	76	72
Inside	100	77	62	72
Slaughterhouse 2				
Outside	100	97	74	69
Inside	100	73	56	73
Beef				
Slaughterhouse 1				
Outside	100	31	5	100
Inside	100	54	15	100
Slaughterhouse 2				
Outside	100	50	19	57
Inside	100	73	42	82

[a] These figures represent the percentage of resistant coliforms of fecal origin (*39*).

in anago and mud turtle can be explained by the intensive farming and culturing of them in ponds without sufficient fresh water supply. The use of running fresh water in trout culturing results in a low incidence of R factors in them (Table XI). High isolation frequencies of *Aeromonas liquefacience*, *Aeromonas salmocida* and *Vibrio* are characteristic in bacteria from cultured fish; resistance patterns of R factors from fish are shown in Table XII and Fig. 6. Comparing this data with those from human beings, it is characteristic that the isolation frequencies of R factors with double resistance are very high, followed by triple and quadruple resistance, in relation to resistance to TC, CM, SM, and SA. Among the R factors with double resistance, the R factors possessing (TC. SA) resistance were demonstrated most frequently, and the isolation frequency of R (SM. SA) factor was rather low, in contrast to the data from human beings.

Walton (*39*) examined the distribution of resistant bacteria in carcass samples and found a high percentage of resistant coliforms in pork carcasses (Table XIII).

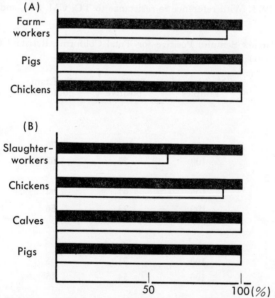

Fig. 7. Percentage of individuals with resistant enterobacteria. A, results achieved in Japan (S. Mitsuhashi and K. Suzuki, 1975, unpublished observation); B, results achieved in West Germany (*41*). ■ resistant bacteria; □ R⁺ bacteria.

We selected 95 pig farms at random and investigated the distribution of resistant enterobacteria in farm workers and pigs. As shown in Fig. 7, we were able to demonstrate drug-resistant enterobacteria in the faeces of all workers, and showed that their resistance was due to the presence of R factors. Similarly, we were able to demonstrate drug-resistant enterobacteria and R-bearing bacteria in all pigs examined. It should be noted that the drug resistance patterns of R factors demonstrated in farm workers and pigs from the same farm were almost the same. We were also able to demonstrate drug-resistant enterobacteria and R-bearing bacteria in all chickens on farms at various geographical locations. The surveys performed in West Germany also disclosed the high distribution of resistant enterobacteria and R plasmids in chickens, calves, and pigs (*39*, *41*).

Foods containing various kinds of antibiotics and chemically synthesized drugs have been used in many countries for the purpose of growth promotion and animal husbandry. This continuous use of drugs has brought about the appearance of drug resistance plasmids in farm animals and the selection of drug-resistant bacteria, resulting in the pollution of farms with resistant bacteria and in the infection of newly introduced animals with resistant bacteria.

REFERENCES

1 Aoki, T., Egusa, S., Ogata, Y., and Watanabe, T. 1971. *J. Gen. Microbiol.*, **65**, 343–349.

2 Anderson, E. S. and Datta, N. 1965. *Lancet*, **i**, 407–409.

3 Anderson, E. S. and Lewis, M. J. 1965. *Nature*, **208**, 843–849.

4 Chabbert, Y. A. and Baudens, J. G. 1965. *Antimicrob. Agents Chemother.*, 380–383.

5 Datta, N. 1962. *J. Hyg.*, **60**, 301–310.

6 Egawa, R., Hara, Y., Mitsuhashi, S., and Cohen, S. N. 1969. *Japan. J. Microbiol.*, **13**, 241–245.

7 Ezaki, T. 1965. *Japan. J. Infect. Dis.*, **41**, 99–107.

8 Gill, F. A. and Hook, E. W. 1966. *J. Am. Med. Assoc.*, **198**, 1267–1269.

9 Hashimoto, H., Ike, Y., Hosoda, T., and Mitsuhashi, S. 1970. *Japan. J. Microbiol.*, **14**, 227–231.

10 Ishiyama, S. 1967. *Chemotherapy*, **15**, 581–587 (in Japanese).

11 Iyobe, S., Hasuda, K., Fuse, A., and Mitsuhashi, S. 1974. *In* Progress

in Chemotherapy, Vol. 1, ed. by G. K. Daikos, Hellenic Society of Chemotherapy, Athens.

12 Iyobe, S., Hasuda, K., Sagai, H., and Mitsuhashi, S. 1975. *In* Microbial Drug Resistance, ed. by S. Mitsuhashi and H. Hashimoto, pp. 321–327, University of Tokyo Press, Tokyo / University Park Press, Baltimore and London.

13 Kawakami, Y., Mikoshiba, S., Nagasaki, S., Matsumoto, H., and Tazaki, T. 1972. *J. Antibiot.*, **25**, 607–609.

14 Knothe, H., Krčméry, V., Sietzen, W., and Borst, J. 1973. *Chemotherapy*, **18**, 229–234 (in Japanese).

15 Kontomichalou, P. 1967. *Pathol. Microbiol.*, **30**, 71–93.

16 Kontomichalou, P. 1967. *Pathol. Microbiol.*, **30**, 185–200.

17 Lebek, G. 1963. *Zentralbl. Bakteriol. Parasitenk.*, *Abt. 1*, **188**, 494–505.

18 Lebek, G. 1963. *Zentralbl. Bakteriol. Parasitenk.*, *Abt. 1*, **149**, 255–266.

19 Lebek, G. 1967. *Pathol. Microbiol.*, **30**, 1015–1036.

20 Manten, A., Guinee, P. A. M., and Kampelacher, E. H. 1966. *Zentralbl. Bakteriol. Parasitenk.*, *Abt. 1*, **200**, 13–20.

21 Mitsuhashi, S., Hashimoto, H., Egawa, R., Tanaka, T., and Nagai, Y. 1967. *J. Bacteriol.*, **93**, 1242–1245.

22 Mitsuhashi, S., Hashimoto, H., and Suzuki, K. 1967. *J. Bacteriol.*, **94**, 1166–1169.

23 Mitsuhashi, S. 1974. Symp. on Problems of Protein Sources in Japan, Tokyo, pp. 35–49.

24 Roe, E., Jones, R. J., and Lowbury, E. J. L. 1971. *Lancet*, **i**, 149–152, 1971.

25 Salzman, T. C., Scher, C. D., and Moss, R. 1967. *J. Pediatr.*, **71**, 21–26.

26 Salzman, T. C. and Klemm, L. 1966. *Antimicrob. Agents Chemother.*, 212–220.

27 Smith, D. H. and Armour, S. E. 1966. *Lancet*, **ii**, 15–18.

28 Smith, H. W. 1966. *J. Hyg. Camb.*, **64**, 465–474.

29 Smith, H. W. 1966. *Br. Med. J.*, **1**, 266–269.

30 Sykes, R. B. and Richmond, M. H. 1970. *Nature*, **226**, 952–954.

31 Tanaka, T., Nagai, Y., Sawa, T., Hashimoto, H., and Mitsuhashi, S. 1966. *Japan. J. Bacteriol.*, **21**, 591 (in Japanese).

32 Tanaka, T., Hashimoto, H., Nagai, Y., and Mitsuhashi, S. 1967. *Japan. J. Microbiol.*, **11**, 155–162.

33 Tanaka, T., Nagai, Y., Hashimoto, H., and Mitsuhashi, S. 1969. *Japan. J. Microbiol.*, **13**, 187–191.

34 Tanaka, T., Tsunoda, M., and Mitsuhashi, S. 1973. *Japan. J. Microbiol.*, **17**, 291–295.

35 Tanaka, T., Kobayashi, A., Ikemura, K., Hashimoto, H., and Mitsuhashi, S. 1974. *Japan. J. Microbiol.*, **18**, 343–347.
36 Tanaka, T., Ikemura, K., Tsunoda, M., Sasagawa, I., and Mitsuhashi,
   S. 1976. *Antimicrob. Agents Chemother.*, **9**, 61–64.
37 Tanaka, T., Tsunoda, M., and Mitsuhashi, S. 1975. *In* Microbial Drug
   Resistance, ed. by S. Mitsuhashi and H. Hashimoto, pp. 187–199, University of Tokyo Press, Tokyo / University Park Press, Baltimore and
   London.
38 Walton, J. R. 1966. *Lancet*, **ii**, 1300–1302.
39 Walton, J. R. 1971. *Ann. N.Y. Acad. Sci.*, **182**, 358–361.
40 Watanabe, T., Aoki, T., Ogata, Y., and Egusa, S. 1971. *Ann. N.Y.
   Acad. Sci.*, **182**, 383–410.
41 Wiedemann, B. and H. Knothe. 1971. *Ann. N.Y. Acad. Sci.*, **182**, 380–
   382.
42 Witchitz, J. L. and Chabbert, Y. A. 1972. *Ann. Inst. Pasteur*, **122**, 367–
   378.

GENETIC AND BIOMOLECULAR PROPERTIES OF R PLASMIDS

3 GENETICS OF R FACTORS

Shizuko IYOBE and Susumu MITSUHASHI
Department of Microbiology, School of Medicine, Gunma University, Maebashi, Japan

The extrachromosomal genetic elements, R (or r) plasmids, are capable of conferring on their host bacteria resistance to various chemotherapeutic agents and heavy metal ions (*51, 53, 67*). R plasmids carry multiple drug resistance genes and are transmissible by conjugation among various species of bacteria. We were able to isolate R plasmids from the bacteria of clinical isolates and transfer them to recipient bacteria such as *Escherichia coli* K12 for the convenience of genetic analysis. The genetic properties of R plasmids, *i.e.*, conjugal transferability, incompatibility, replication, *etc.*, in the same host bacteria have been precisely investigated. Nonconjugative drug resistance(r) plasmids were first demonstrated in *Staphylococcus aureus* (*52, 58, 59*) and thereafter were isolated from various species of bacteria including gram-positive and gram-negative bacteria (*55*). They encode mostly single resistance and, infrequently, double resistance, and their DNA size is usually smaller than that of R plasmids because of the lack of determinants governing conjugal transferability. The transformation or transduction technique is applied therefore for their genetic analysis.

Here we will deal with the cytoplasmic existence of R (or r) plasmids, the expression of drug resistance and their interaction with other plasmids or host bacteria from the view point of a host-parasite relationship.

1. Cytoplasmic Inheritance of Drug Resistance Genes

1) Evidence of the cytoplasmic existence of drug resistance genes

In addition to finding both rapid increase in multiple resistance and transmission of drug resistance by mixed cultivation, we noticed by chance that multiple resistance in *Shigella* strains was spontaneously lost during storage in cooked meat media (see Chapter 1). These findings encouraged us to study the genetic problems of multiple resistance in *Shigella* strains, and later in other gram-negative bacteria and *S. aureus* strains.

In order to know about the extrachromosomal existence of drug resistance genes, we first determined whether they are spontaneously or artificially eliminated from their host, and second the stability of their inheritance in the recombination-deficient (rec^-) host. Biomolecular studies using ultracentrifugation and electron microscopy enabled us to investigate the physical and molecular properties of R plasmid DNA.

It is known from experience that R (or r) plasmids are spontaneously lost by their host after long storage of bacteria, and some R (or r) plasmids isolated from *Proteus mirabilis* (*89*), *Salmonella typhimurium* (*93*), or *E. coli* (*47*) are unstable at elevated temperatures and are easily eliminated from their hosts. Artificial elimination of R (or r) plasmids is carried out by two mechanisms. The first is the selective killing of bacteria carrying R plasmids by the use of drugs, such as EDTA, sodium dodecylsulfate (SDS) or macarbomycin, to which these bacteria are susceptible (*2, 57, 79, 96*). These drugs are known to act on the bacterial cell surface, where some changes occur after infection of R plasmids to render the bacteria susceptible to the drugs. Consequently, these drugs allow the selective growth of bacteria without R plasmids which spontaneously appear in a population of bacteria carrying R plasmids, resulting in the elimination of R plasmids from the bacterial population. When *E. coli* strains are infected with R plasmids, the transfer organ pilus and its subunit pilin are produced on

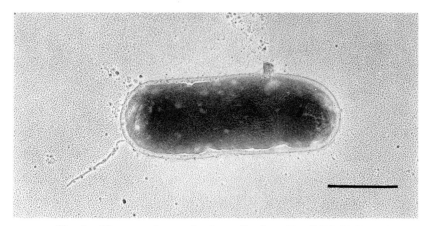

Fig. 1.   Electron micrograph of sex pilus from *E. coli* W3630 R$_{ms201}^{+}$.
Bar represents 1 μm. (Photographed by H. Hashimoto.)

the surface and in the outer membrane of bacterial cells (Fig. 1) (*7, 10*). Macarbomycin effectively kills bacteria which produce pili in a derepressed state, and the mutants which have lost their susceptibility to the drug are incapable of pili production (*42, 43*).

The second type of elimination is the direct curing of R (or r) plasmids by inhibition of their replication. DNA-intercalating agents, acriflavine and ethidium bromide, and an inhibitory agent for RNA synthesis, such as rifampicin, are effective curing-agents because of their inhibitory activity on DNA synthesis (*6, 28, 46, 54, 63*). Many antitumor agents with DNA-intercalating activity are also effective in the elimination of R (or r) plasmids (*23*). There is, however, another mechanism for the direct elimination of R plasmids. Pinney and Smith (*73*) reported that thymine starvation of bacteria could eliminate R plasmids, thus suggesting that it induces the synthesis of a nuclease which acts more specifically on the R plasmid DNA than on the host chromosome (*91*).

Although it is not widely applicable, the extrachromosomal existence of drug resistance genes can be proven by their stable existence in a *rec⁻* host. When a *recA* mutant of *E. coli* is used as a recipient for conjugation or transduction of genetic materials, the introduced DNA segments are incapable of recombination with the chromosome in the recipient strain. Therefore, the genes on the chromosome can be trans-

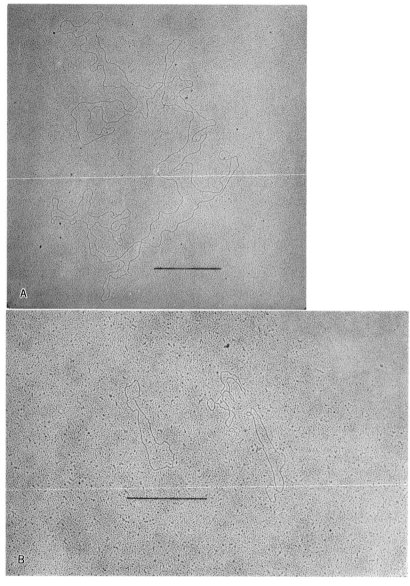

Fig. 2. Electron micrograph of the open circular molecules of plasmid DNA. Bar represents 1 μm. (A) R_{ms151} (TC. CM. SA. GM. KM. APC) from *E. coli* K12 *(30)*. (B) r(APC) derived from R_{ms201} *(27)*. GM: gentamicin. See the text for the abbreviations of other drugs.

ferred only to a *rec*+ strain but not to a *rec*‾ strain, because they cannot survive without integration into the host chromosome (*36*). However, genes on plasmids are transferable to a *rec*‾ strain by conjugation or transduction and can survive cytoplasmically in that cell (*34, 36, 84*). This method is very useful for the detection of r plasmids, when we have a transduction system using a *rec*‾ mutant. In fact, using this method we have proven that almost all drug resistance genes in *S. aureus* strains exist on r plasmids (*34*).

The direct method of proving the cytoplasmic existence of drug resistance genes is the physical isolation of plasmid DNA. The R (or r) plasmids can be isolated as a satellite DNA different from the chromosomal DNA by centrifugation, or can be demonstrated as covalently closed circular (CCC) or open circular (OC) DNA by means of electron microscopy (*14, 33*) (Fig. 2).

2) Molecular background in the cytoplasmic existence of R (or r) plasmids

The size of R (or r) plasmids is estimated by sedimentation velocity of the DNA in sucrose gradients or by electron microscopy, and cytoplasmic existence can be investigated from the viewpoint of molecular genetics.

The molecular weight of most R plasmids ranges from 30 to 50 Mdal. (Fig. 3). The smallest R plasmid with a molecular weight of 26 Mdal. is R_{6K} originating from *E. coli*, and it has a characteristically large copy number which reaches from 13 to 38 (*49*). The largest R plasmid with a molecular weight of 120 Mdal. is R*ts*1 (*22*) which was isolated from *P. mirabilis*, and is characteristically thermosensitive in its replication (*90*).

The copy number of R plasmids in a cell is generally stringently controlled to be 1 or 2 in *E. coli*, when estimated as CCC DNA. Since it is impossible to isolate all plasmid DNAs in CCC form, more than two plasmids can be expected to exist in a cell. We reported that the copy number of an R plasmid R_{100-1} was presumed to be about four to eight per chromosome by estimation of the chloramphenicol (CM) acetyltransferase activity expressed by the CM resistance (*cml*) gene on the R plasmid when compared with that expressed by the *cml* gene integrated into the host chromosome (*41*).

When the two kinds of mutant R plasmids, originating from the

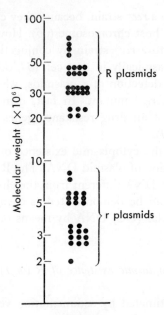

Fig. 3. Molecular weight of R(or r) plasmid DNA.

same R plasmid but possessing different resistance markers, coexist in the same cell, mutual exclusion occurs between them, and this phenomenon is called incompatibility (see Chapters 10, 11). When two incompatible R plasmids exist in a cell, the recombinant molecule between them can be obtained at a high frequency of 10% (*26*). However, some types of R plasmids are compatible with each other and can coexist stably in the same cell in a hetero-R state (*86*). According to a survey of drug resistance in *Shigella* strains in Japan, about 15% of R⁺ strains are in the hetero-R state (*86*), and both R (TC (tetracycline). CM. SM (streptomycin). SA (sulfanilamide)) and R (SM. SA) plasmids are isolated most frequently from such cells. The hetero-R state was also found in 50% of *E. coli* and *Salmonella* strains, in which multiple drug resistance was conferred by two types of R plasmids coexisting in a cell (*74*).

The molecular weight of r plasmids is as small as less than 10 Mdal. and the number of copies per chromosome is about 5 to 30 (see Chapter 8). The small size of r plasmids as compared to R plasmids is mainly due to the absence of the region encoding conjugal transferability. The large copy number of r plasmids reflects the difference in their replication system from that of R plasmids.

The drug resistance genes, such as *tet* (tetracycline) or *amp* (ampicillin, APC), can be separated together with the *rep* (replication) gene from R plasmids, resulting in the formation of r plasmids. The r(*tet*) plasmid pSC101 with a molecular weight of 5.8 Mdal. was separated from R_{6-5} plasmid with a molecular weight of 65 Mdal. after shearing of DNA (*16*). The r(*amp*) plasmid was also separated from an R plasmid as a translocatable unit to other R plasmids (*31*). The molecular weight of the r(*amp*) plasmid is within 1.7 to 3.9 Mdal.

Epidemiological surveys have disclosed the existence of r plasmids encoding resistance to SA, TC, SM, and (SM. SA) in gram-negative bacteria and of r plasmids governing resistance to SA, TC, PC (penicillin), Mac (macrolide antibiotics) or (Mac. PC) in gram-positive bacteria (*5, 13, 18, 35, 55, 58, 59, 82*). They can coexist with large copy numbers in the same bacterial cells and are capable of conferring multiple resistance on their host. A wide distribution of r plasmids should be noted to solve the origin of R plasmids (see Chapter 12).

It is interesting that many r (SM. SA) plasmids exist together naturally in bacterial cells carrying R (SM. SA) plasmids (*5*), and an r (APC) plasmid, RSF1030, was isolated from bacterial cells possessing R_{111} carrying an APC resistance gene in addition to other resistance genes (*32*). These results suggest that r plasmids can be derived from R plasmids by the loss of the genes encoding conjugal transferability, or that R plasmids can be formed by cointegration of r plasmids with the transfer (T) factor possessing the genes encoding both transferability and replication (*56*). It was in fact reported that an r (APC) plasmid had been separated from R_{ms201} (TC. CM. SM. SA. APC) and was able to replicate as a nonconjugative plasmid with a large number of copies in a cell (*27*). In addition, R_{100}-*kan* and T-*tet-kan* plasmids were isolated by combination of an r(KM) plasmid with either an R_{100} or T-*tet* plasmid, respectively (*47*).

3) Two modes of transferring drug resistance

The drug resistance determinants of R plasmids are conjugally and jointly transferred to a recipient even when selected for either one of their drug resistance markers, and R plasmids in the recipient are also transferable as a whole as well as in the first donor cells. Furthermore, the drug resistance genes and the genes encoding conjugal transferability on R plasmids are transduced with bacteriophages as a unit when phages are large enough to carry a whole genome of R plasmids, indicating that the region governing drug resistance is connected stably with the region concerning genome encoding plasmid autonomy, such as transferability and replication. On the other hand, it was found that a *S. typhymurium* strain resistant to (TC. SM. SA. APC) transferred (SM. SA), APC, and TC resistance separately (*3*). After successive transfers, the nonconjugative plasmids r (SM. SA), r (APC) and conjugative plasmids $\mathit{\Delta}$-TC and $\mathit{\Delta}$ were obtained. In this case, r (SM. SA) and r (APC) plasmids were considered to be mobilized by $\mathit{\Delta}$, and the $\mathit{\Delta}$-TC seemed to be a recombinant between r (TC) and $\mathit{\Delta}$. The $\mathit{\Delta}$ is a transferable plasmid without drug resistance genes and conferred transferability on r plasmids coexisting in the same bacterial cells. The T factor corresponding to $\mathit{\Delta}$ was demonstrated in our laboratory with a frequency of 40% among many strains of bacteria isolated from clinical sources (*56*). The r plasmids are mobilized by T factors or R plasmids coexisting in the same cells, or transferred by the formation of recombinants with various transferable plasmids.

2. Drug Resistance Genes on Plasmids

1) Genetic symbols for drug resistance genes

As described above, R (or r) plasmids carry genes governing resistance to various drugs, *i.e.*, TC, CM, SM, SA, Mac, KM (kanamycin) and other aminoglycoside antibiotics, APC and other β-lactam antibiotics, and heavy metal ions such as Ni^{2+}, Co^{2+}, Cd^{2+}, and Hg^{2+}. Up to the present genotypes for drug resistance have been expressed by the first three letters of a drug according to the system recommended by Demerec *et al.* (*20*), for example, *tet*, *str*, *sul*, *amp*, or *kan* were used for genotypes of resistance to TC, SM, SA, APC, or KM, respectively. For the genotype of CM resistance, *cml* was used instead of *chl*, because *chl* was already used for the genotype of chlorate resistance (*87*).

Recently, changes in genotype symbols in some cases of drug resistance became necessary because the enzymatic background of drug resistance has been clarified. In the case of KM resistance, it is expressed by various types of KM-inactivating enzymes, *i.e.*, aminoglycoside 3'-phosphotransferase-1, aminoglycoside 3'-phosphotransferase-2, or aminoglycoside 2''-nucleotidyltransferase (see Chapter 9). Therefore, it seems reasonable that the abbreviations for each enzymes capable of inactivating drugs are used as genotype designations instead of the names of drugs. The genotype expressed by one KM-inactivating enzyme, aminoglycoside 3'-phosphotransferase-1, confers on the host bacteria resistance to NM (neomycin), RM (ribostamycin), PM (paromomycin) and LV (lividomycin) in addition to KM, because all of these aminoglycosides are inactivated by this enzyme (55). Similarly, the plasmid carrying the gene encoding β-lactamase formation con-

TABLE I. Genetic Symbols for Drug Resistance Encoded by R (or r) Plasmids

Phenotype	Genotype	Effect[a]	
		Resistance	Enzyme formation
CM	cml (cat cam)	Chloramphenicol	CM-acetyltransferase
TC	tet	Tetracycline	
SA	sul	Sulfonamide	
SM	aph (3'') (str aphC)	Streptomycin	APH (3'')
SM	aad (3'') (str aadA)	Streptomycin	AAD (3'')
SP	aad (3'') (spc aadA)	Spectinomycin	AAD (3'')
GM	aac (6') (aacA)	Gentamicin	AAC (6')-II
GM	aac (2') (aacB)	Gentamicin	AAC (2')
GM	aac (3) (aacC)	Gentamicin	AAC (3)
GM	aad (2'') (aadB)	Gentamicin	AAD (2'')
KM	aph (3') (kan aphA)	Kanamycin	APH (3')-I
KM	aac (6') (kan aacA)	Kanamycin	AAC (6')-I
KM	aad (2'') (kan aadB)	Kanamycin	AAD (2'')
EM	mac (ery ero erm)	Macrolide antibiotics	Ribosomal Ribonucleic acid Methylase
FA	fus	Fusidic acid	
APC	amp (bla pen)	Ampicillin	β-Lactamase
CPC	bla	Carbenicillin	β-Lactamase
CER	bla	Cephalosporin	β-Lactamase
PC	pen (bla amp)	Penicillin	β-Lactamase
Co	cob	Cobaltous ion	
Hg	mer	Mercuric ion	Mercuric reductase
Ni	nic	Nickelous ion	

[a] Details, see Chapter 9.

fers on the host bacteria resistance to APC, CPC (carbenicillin) and other PC derivatives at the same time (see Chapter 9).

In consideration of these facts, a uniform nomenclature for genotypes and phenotypes conferred by plasmids was recently proposed by several plasmid researchers (*59a, 68;* see Chapter 3). Genetic symbols for drug resistance encoded by R (or r) plasmids are listed in Table I, and are used in this book.

2) Level of drug resistance

The difference in drug resistance level can be accounted for either by the difference in resistance genes or by the number of resistance genes. It is expected that genes encoding the formation of different drug-inactivating enzymes express different resistance levels in strains resistant to aminoglycoside or β-lactam antibiotics, and that the presence of different resistance genes responsible for both inactivation and impermeability of the drug confer a high level of resistance to the drug on their host bacteria (see Chapter 9).

A large copy number of resistance genes also confers a high level of resistance on the host bacteria. There exists a parallelism between the copy number of *cml* genes and their product, CM-acetyltransferase, in a cell, in which the *cml* genes derived from an R plasmid are integrated into various sites on the chromosome (*41*). In general, increase in the activity of drug-inactivating enzymes raised the resistance level to the drug.

The increase in the gene copy number occurs as a result of partial amplification of resistance genes on a plasmid (*27, 76*), or the increase in the copy number of whole plasmids after mutation (*62, 66*). The levels of both CM and SM resistance were elevated in a *P. mirabilis* strain carrying a plasmid R_{NR1} (TC. CM. SM. SA), resulting from an increase in the copy number of the region carrying both *cml* and *str* genes on R_{NR1} called transition (see Chapter 8). The increase in the copy number of *amp* genes caused an expression of high level APC resistance, resulting from replication of the *amp* gene on an r plasmid after segregation from the parent R plasmid R_{ms201} (TC. CM. SM. SA. APC) (*27*). In contrast, an increase in the copy number of whole R plasmids was reported after transfer to a different host or after mutation. The minimum inhibitory concentration (MIC) (μg/ml) level of APC resistance conferred by R_{6K} or R_{28K} increased when these plasmids were transferred to *E. coli* from *P. mirabilis* (*49*). In the replication mutants of R plasmids with a large copy number, the levels of both CM and SM resistance increased but, in contrast, the TC resistance level decreased (*62*). This can be explained by the fact that the expression of TC resistance is governed by at least two genes on the R plasmid, *i.e.*, the structural gene for TC resistance and the regulatory gene whose product repressor acts on the function of the structural gene, and that the level of TC resistance conferred by the mutant plasmid with a large copy number is decreased by the production of a large quantity of the repressor.

3) Genetic structure of R plasmids

R plasmids carry both the genes encoding resistances to various drugs and the genes concerning plasmid autonomy such as *rep*, *inc* (incompatibility), *tra* (transferability), and *eex* (entry exclusion). The genetic linkage of these genes was investigated by recombination analysis using point mutants of R plasmids (*25, 26*) or deletion analysis using the transduction technique (*30*). Many types of R plasmid mutants can be obtained by spontaneous mutation or by treatment with UV light or mutagenic agents. R mutants sensitive to TC or CM are selected from R plasmids carrying resistance to these drugs by a PC-screening method, because PC selectively kills bacterial cells capable of growing in the medium containing TC or CM. Using point mutants of an R plasmid R_{100-1}, Hashimoto and Mitsuhashi (*26*) determined the linkage order of TC and CM resistance genes. The deletion mutants of R plasmids can be obtained by transduction with phage P1 in *E. coli* because P1 transduces the same size of DNA as its own DNA and whole genome is not transduced by P1 when the plasmid DNA is larger than that of P1 phage DNA (60 Mdal.). Therefore, various types of R plasmid segments are obtained in transductants, and the joint transduction of genetic markers indicates the linkage order of genes on the R plasmid. When the drug resistance genes are not transduced with the genes governing autonomous replication, they cannot survive in the recipient cells except in cases of integration into the replicons, such as host chromosome, the resident plasmids in recipient cells or phage P1. A new attempt for the mapping of an R plasmid was carried out by Yoshikawa by transduction with phage P1 using the strain in which R_{100-1} was integrated into the chromosome (see Section 2, this

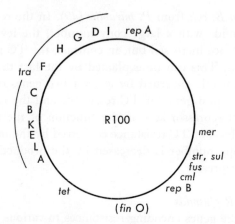

Fig. 4.   Genetic structure of an R_{100} factor. Genotypes for drug resistance, see Table I. *tra*, transferability; *rep*, replication.

chapter), and he was able to demonstrate two *rep* genes on the R plasmid (*94*). The fine structure of R_{100} was further determined by physical methods, such as the heteroduplex method (*81*) and partial denaturation method (*80*). The genetic map of R_{100} was determined by Dempsey and Willetts (*27*) (Fig. 4), and its similarity to that of the F plasmid (*1, 69*) was discussed.

3.   Relationship between R (or r) Plasmids and Other Genetic Elements

1)   Mobilization of the host chromosome by R plasmids

Chromosome mobilization mediated by R plasmids is called R-mating (*83*) which takes place by two processes. The first one is similar to the F factor-mediated chromosome transfer, in which the chromosome is transferred without polarity and at a low frequency. When the donor strain carries R_{100-1}, a derepressed mutant of R_{100} in transferability, the chromosome markers are transferred at a frequency of about 10^{-5} to 10^{-6}, and R_{100-1} itself is transferred at a frequency of 10^{0} to 10^{-1}. This chromosome transfer frequency is rather high compared to that mediated by other R plasmids. Most R plasmids, including R_{100}, are in a repressed state in transferability, and their transfer frequency is about 10^{-2} to 10^{-4}, and the bacterial chromosome is transferred by them at a frequency of about 10^{-7} to 10^{-8}. These facts indicate that chromosomal transfer frequency by R-mating is paralleled with that of R-transfer.

Another type of chromosome transfer is the polarized transfer as seen in the transfer by the F prime, namely the F plasmid carrying a chromosomal segment. In this case, the specific region of the chromosome is transferred at a high frequency. For example, the R_1 plasmid can transfer the chromosomal region near *trp* at a frequency of 10^{-4} to 10^{-5}, and its derepressed mutant R_1 *drd-19* transfers the *trp* gene at a frequency of 10^{-2} to 10^{-3} (*72*). It was suggested that the specific chromosomal affinity of R plasmid is concerned with the polarized transfer of the chromosome.

We prepared a strain in which the *cml* gene on R_{100} plasmid was integrated into the chromosome, near *lac*, and investigated R-mating by R_{100-1} (*38*). When this strain harbors R_{100-1}, a homologous region, including *cml* gene, is established on both the host chromosome and R plasmid, and the chromosomal region, including both *pur* and *gal* genes located near *lac*, is effectively transferred at a frequency of 10^{-2} to 10^{-3} (Fig. 5). In contrast, the *pur* and *gal* genes are transferred at the same frequency as other genes (about 10^{-5}) when either the chromosome does not carry the *cml* gene or the R plasmid deletes the *cml* gene. It seems that recombination is necessary for R-mating between the homologous regions of the chromosome and the R plasmid

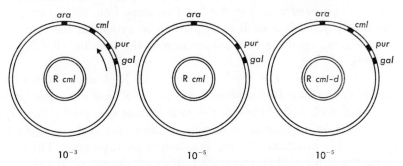

Fig. 5. The frequency of R-mating with various combinations of donor cells. The arrow indicates the direction of the chromosome transfer. The frequency of R-mating is expressed by the number of the recipient strains which accepted *pur* or *gal* gene per that of donor cells. *cml*, CM resistance gene; *cml-d*, deletion of CM resistance gene.

because the effective transfer of the *pur* and *gal* regions does not occur when the *recA* mutant is used as a donor strain, although the *cml* gene exists on both the chromosome and the R plasmid in this strain. The absence of the recombination in the *recA* host is proved using the strain with point mutations on the *cml* genes on both the chromosome and the R plasmid although these point mutants are capable of recombination in the *rec+* strain. In general, the recombination between chromosome and R plasmid seems to be necessary for the polarized transfer of the chromosome but not in transfer without polarity (*15, 60*).

2) *Integration of R plasmids into the host chromosome*

The phenomenon of R-mating suggests the presence of homologous regions between R plasmids and the host chromosome, and such regions will make possible the integration of R plasmids, partially or as a whole into the host chromosome.

The examples of the partial integration of R plasmids are seen in R_{11} or R_{100}, in which the *tet* or *cml* gene, respectively, is incorporated into the host chromosome (*24, 37*). The integrated *cml* genes could not return to the cytoplasmic state by themselves, indicating that the replication gene was lost from the *cml* gene by recombination with the chromosome. The chromosomal *cml* genes are, therefore, unstable and lost from their host strain after detachment from the chromosome; they are, however, capable of surviving in the cytoplasm by incorporation into a replicon such as the R or F plasmid. In such a strain, the *pro* genes near *cml* were lost at a low frequency from the chromosome and incorporated into an R (TC) plasmid in cytoplasm together with the *cml* gene, resulting in the formation of the R-prime, R (TC)-*cml pro* (*39*).

Another example of the integration of an R plasmid into the host chromosome using Rts1 and *galE* mutant of *E. coli* was reported by Terawaki *et al.* (*88*). Although the *galE* mutant is normally incapable of growing on a galactose-containing medium, it can do so when the *gal* operon is inactivated by the insertion of an R plasmid. The strain where the R plasmid is integrated into its *gal* operon on the chromosome, can, therefore, be easily isolated on the galactose-containing medium. In this mutant the plasmid Rts1 lost both temperature sensitivity in its replication and the inhibitory activity on the host growth at a high temperature.

The integration of R plasmids with their replication genes in a *ts* (temperature-sensitive) mutant cencerning the initiation of chromosome replication has been reported (*61, 64*). When this strain is infected by an R plasmid and grows at a nonpermissive temperature, temperature-resistant revertants are obtained. Most of these revertants have Hfr properties and can promote chromosome transfer at a high frequency. In these Hfr strains, R plasmids are integrated into the host chromosome and the replication of the chromosome is under the control of R plasmids at a nonpermissive temperature by the mechanism called "integrative suppression." Two *rep* genes on an R plasmid responsible for integrative suppression and for autonomous replication (*94*) were identified. An R-prime carrying a *lac* gene was isolated from the strain under integrative suppression after transduction by phage P1 (*65*).

3) Restriction and modification systems conferred by R plasmids
It was reported that some groups of R plasmids inhibit the growth of phages such as λ, P1, T_1, T_7, and W31; this phenomenon was called

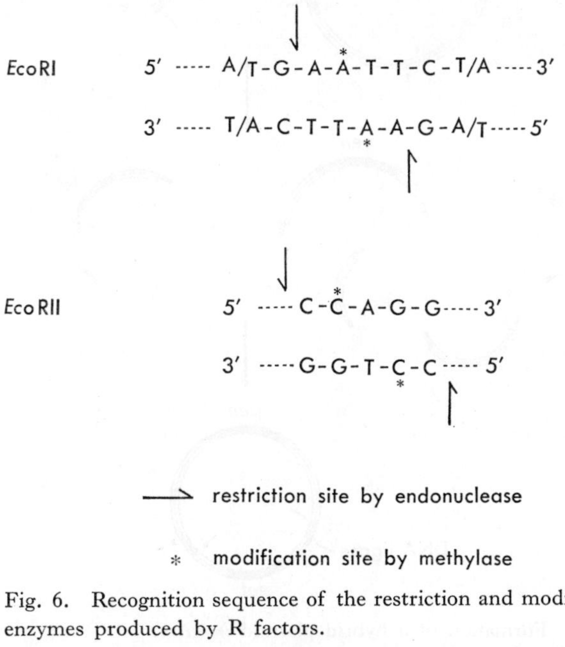

EcoRI
$$5' \; \text{-----} \; \text{A/T-G-A-} \overset{*}{\text{A}} \text{-T-T-C-T/A} \; \text{-----} \; 3'$$
$$3' \; \text{-----} \; \text{T/A-C-T-T-A-A-G-A/T} \; \text{-----} \; 5'$$

EcoRII
$$5' \; \text{-----} \; \text{C-} \overset{*}{\text{C}} \text{-A-G-G} \; \text{-----} \; 3'$$
$$3' \; \text{-----} \; \text{G-G-T-C-C} \; \text{-----} \; 5'$$

⟶ restriction site by endonuclease

＊ modification site by methylase

Fig. 6. Recognition sequence of the restriction and modification enzymes produced by R factors.

spp (suppression of phage plaque formation) (*95*). Since the adsorption of phages on bacterial cell was not affected by the presence of these R plasmids, one of the mechanisms in connection with *spp* may be due to the replication inhibition of the infected phage DNA at any step of transcription or translation and another is interpreted as restriction by endonuclease produced by R plasmids (*97*). The latter mechanism was first proved using a cell-free system with phage λ in which the degradation of DNA was observed in a cell extract from the bacterial cells carrying R plasmids (*85*). Furthermore, it was reported that the DNA could be modified by a residual R plasmid, escaping from the action of endonuclease. These facts indicate that R plasmids have restriction and modification systems as are seen in other genetic elements, such as bacterial chromosome or phages (*8*). Two enzymes

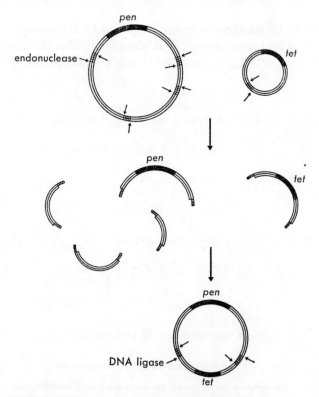

Fig. 7. Formation of a hybrid plasmid *in vitro*.

concerned with restriction and modification, endonuclease and methylase, are demonstrated in the strain carrying R plasmids. They are capable of discriminating the specific sequence of double-strand DNA consisting of a symmetrical pair of several bases. Two types of restriction-modification enzymes are found in each of the two R plasmids, and can be distinguished from each other according to their different recognizable base sequences in DNA. They are called *Eco*RI and *Eco*RII enzymes, and their attack sites in DNA are shown in Fig. 6. Both types of endonucleases cause nicks in each strand of DNA at opposite points as shown in the figure, resulting in the formation of DNA segments with several bases on both ends that can associate with each other by hydrogen bonding. The free 3'-hydroxyl and 5'-phosphate ends can be covalently joined by the action of the enzyme DNA ligase. In fact, a new plasmid consisting of both an *E. coli* plasmid pSC101 (*tet*) and PC-resistance gene derived from an r plasmid in *S. aureus* is produced *in vitro*, and its stable maintenance in *E. coli* was proved after infection by DNA transformation (Fig. 7) (*11*). Furthermore, it is possible by this technique, called genetic engineering, to introduce bacterial or bacteriophage genes into mammalian cells using a mammalian virus as a vector (*45*).

4) Host range of R plasmids

Although R plasmids have been isolated from all species of the family Enterobacteriaceae, *Vibrio cholerae*, *Pseudomonas aeruginosa*, *Bordetella enterocolitica*, *Aeromonas* group, etc. (see Chapter 2), they are not always freely transmissible to or maintained stably in other species of bacteria different from the original hosts. It was reported that a plasmid R_{100} (TC. CM. SM. SA) of *Shigella* origin was easily lost as a whole after transfer to *V. cholerae* (*92*), or partially lost in *S. typhimurium* to become an R plasmid carrying only TC resistance (*29*), or the abnormally increased (CM. SM. SA) resistance region in *P. mirabilis* (*75*). Abnormal replication as is seen in a part of an R plasmid concerns the loss or amplification of the part, reflecting the composite structure of R plasmids as shown by Clowes (*14*). Such phenomena and the loss of R plasmids as a whole show that their replication is host-dependent.

In another case, the R plasmid DNA introduced into a different host is degradated by a host-specific restriction enzyme. The restriction-modification mechanism by the host bacteria was found in *Salmonella enteritidis* (*4*), in which R plasmids were modified and then became nontransmissible to other species of *Salmonella* probably due to the action of their restriction system. Restriction in different strains was also reported in *Yersinia enterocolitica* (*17*). An R plasmid of *E. coli* was barely transferred to this strain but became transmissible probably due to the damage of restriction enzyme when the recipient *Yersinia* was heated to 50–52°C for 2–3 min before conjugation. A mutant of the *Yersinia* strain to which the R plasmid was transferred at the same frequency as that to *E. coli* was isolated, suggesting that the gene concerning restriction was mutated in this strain.

It has been reported that many R plasmids found in *P. aeruginosa* are nontransmissible to *E. coli* and other species of Enterobacteriaceae (*9, 40, 48*). We classified R plasmids in *P. aeruginosa* into 8 groups according to the incompatibility nature common among R plasmids in other species of bacteria (see Chapter 11). Almost all of *Pseudomonas* R plasmids are classified as members of the group P-2 (*77*). A few plasmids classified in the P-1 or P-3 group are exceptional in their transferability to *E. coli* and to other species of bacteria. The R plasmids of P-1 group are classified in group P in the *E. coli* host in which they also show their characteristic transferability because almost all of the R plasmids isolated in the family Enterobacteriaceae are nontransmissible to *P. aeruginosa*. The R plasmids belonging to P-1 in *P. aeruginosa* system or the P group in the *E. coli* system have a wide host range and are transmissible to other *Pseudomonas* species, including plant pathogenic bacteria, and strains belonging to the family Enterobacteriaceae, including plant pathogenic *Erwinia* species (*12, 50, 71*). Furthermore, they are also transmissible to *Neisseria* species, the photosynthetic *Rhodopseudomonas*, and the nitrogen-fixing *Azotobactor* and *Rhizobium* species (*19, 70*). The wide host range of R plasmids may be interpreted by their two characters, that is, their adaptation ability to escape from the restriction system conferred by a different host, and their ability to make mating pairs with different bacterial cells. When an R plasmid nontransferable to *E. coli* coexisted in a *P. aeruginosa* strain with a P group plasmid RP4, the nontransmissible plasmid became transferable to *E. coli* strains with RP4 (*44;* see Chapter 5). The plasmid thus obtained is still nontransferable between *E. coli* and to *P. aeruginosa* from *E. coli*. But the plasmid becomes transferable to *E. coli* or *P. aeruginosa* only due to the presence of RP4 in the same cell, although the plasmid can replicate in *E. coli* by itself. It appears that they do not have the ability to conjugate with *E. coli* when carried by *E. coli* or *P. aeruginosa* strains and with *P. aeruginosa* when carried by *E. coli* strains. An RP4 and other P group R plasmids will be able to mediate the interspecies transfer of R plasmids which have only a narrow host range, or become vectors of drug resistance genes on such R plasmids by incorporating them by insertion or recombination (*44, 78*).

4. Conclusion

R (or r) plasmids are of particular importance in practical medicine and livestock hygiene because they possess the following genetic properties: (1) an ability to confer drug resistance on the host bacteria by an R (or r) plasmid or by coexistence of various R or r plasmids in a host cell; (2) transferability among various species of bacteria by conjugation, transduction and mobilization; (3) an ability to confer a high level of resistance by increasing their copy number or a part of their drug resistance genes. They can associate with bacterial chromosomes, like the F factor, or with other genetic elements in cytoplasm, and maintain their drug resistance genes on themselves or on other replication units. The genetic flexibility of R (or r) plasmids toward the change of surrounding conditions and the association of drug resistance genes with the genes concerning transferability are responsible for the wide spread of drug resistance genes among various species of bacteria.

REFERENCES

1 Achtman, M. 1973. *In* Current Topics in Microbiology and Immunology, ed. by Basel *et al.*, pp. 79–123, Springer-Verlag, Berlin.
2 Adachi, H., Nakano, M., Inuzuka, M., and Tomoeda, M. 1972. *J. Bacteriol.*, **109**, 1114–1124.
3 Anderson, E. S. 1968. *Annu. Rev. Microbiol.*, **22**, 131–180.
4 Anderson, E. S. and Threlfall, E. J. 1970. *Genet. Res.*, **16**, 207–214.
5 Barth, P. T. and Grinter, N. J. 1974. *J. Bacteriol.*, **120**, 618–630.
6 Bazzicalupo, P. and Tocchini-Valentine, G. P. 1972. *Proc. Natl. Acad. Sci. U.S.*, **69**, 298–300.

7 Beard, J. P. and Connolly, J. C. 1975. *J. Bacteriol.*, **122**, 59–65.
8 Boyer, H. W. 1974. *Fed. Proc.*, **33**, 1125–1127.
9 Bryan, L. E., Semeka, S. D., Van Den Elzen, H. M., Kinnear, J. E., and Whitehouse, R. E. S. 1973. *Antimicrob. Agents Chemother.*, **3**, 625–637.
10 Brinton, C. C. 1971. *Crit. Rev. Microbiol.*, **1**, 105–160.
11 Chang, A. C. Y. and Cohen, S. 1974. *Proc. Natl. Acad. Sci. U.S.*, **71**, 1030–1034.
12 Cho, J. J., Panopoulos, N. J., and Schroth, M. N. 1975. *J. Bacteriol.*, **122**, 192–198.
13 Clewell, D. B. and Franke, A. E. 1974. *Antimicrob. Agents Chemother.*, **5**, 534–537.
14 Clowes, R. C. 1972. *Bacteriol. Rev.*, **36**, 361–405.
15 Clowes, R. C. and Moody, M. 1966. *Genetics*, **53**, 717–726.
16 Cohen, S. N. and Chang, A. C. Y. 1973. *Proc. Natl. Acad. Sci. U.S.*, **70**, 1293–1297.
17 Cornelis, G. and Colson, C. 1975. *J. Gen. Microbiol.*, **87**, 285–291.
18 Courvalin, P. M., Carlier, C., Croissant, O., and Blangy, D. 1974. *Mol. Gen. Genet.*, **132**, 181–192.
19 Datta, N., Hedges, R. W., Shaw, E. J., Sykes, R. B., and Richmond, M. H. 1971. *J. Bacteriol.*, **108**, 1244–1249.
20 Demerec, M., Adelberg, E. A., Clark, A. J., and Hartman, P. E. 1966. *Genetics*, **54**, 61–76.
21 Dempsey, W. B. and Willetts, N. S. 1976. *J. Bacteriol.*, **126**, 166–176.
22 Dijoseph, C. G. and Kaji,A. 1974. *J. Bacteriol.*, **120**, 1364–1369.
23 Hahn, F. E. and Ciak, J. 1971. *Ann. N.Y. Acad. Sci.*, **182**, 295–304.
24 Harada, K., Kameda, M., Suzuki, M., Shigehara, S., and Mitsuhashi, S. 1967. *J. Bacteriol.*, **93**, 1236–1241.
25 Hashimoto, H. and Hirota, Y. 1966. *J. Bacteriol.*, **91**, 51–62.
26 Hashimoto, H. and Mitsuhashi, S. 1966. *J. Bacteriol.*, **92**, 1351–1356.
27 Hashimoto, H., Ike, Y., Odakura, Y., and Mitsuhashi, S. 1975. *In* Microbial Drug Resistance, ed. by S. Mitsuhashi and H. Hashimoto, pp. 93–100, University of Tokyo Press, Tokyo / University Park Press, Baltimore and London.
28 Hashimoto, H., Kono, M., and Mitsuhashi, S. 1964. *J. Bacteriol.*, **88**, 261–262.
29 Hashimoto, H. and Mitsuhashi, S. 1970. *In* Progress in Antimicrobial and Anticancer of Chemotherapy, Tokyo, 1969, ed. by H. Umezawa, pp. 545–551, University of Tokyo Press, Tokyo.
30 Hasuda, K., Krčméry, V., Iyobe, S., and Mitsuhashi, S. 1975. *J. Bacteriol.*, **123**, 329–335.

31 Hedges, R. W. and Jacob, A. E. 1974. *Mol. Gen. Genet.*, **132**, 31–40.
32 Heffron, F., Sublett, R., Hedges, R. W., Jacob, A., and Falkow, S. 1975. *J. Bacteriol.*, **122**, 250–256.
33 Helinski, D. R. 1973. *Annu. Rev. Microbiol.*, **27**, 437–470.
34 Inoue, M., Oshima, H., Okubo, T., and Mitsuhashi, S. 1972. *J. Bacteriol.*, **112**, 1169–1176.
35 Inoue, M., Okubo, T., Oshima, H., and Mitsuhashi, S. 1974. *In* Microbial Drug Resistance, ed. by S. Mitsuhashi and H. Hashimoto, pp. 153–164, University of Tokyo Press, Tokyo / University Park Press, Baltimore and London.
36 Iyobe, S., Hashimoto, H., and Mitsuhashi, S. 1969. *Japan. J. Microbiol.*, **13**, 225–232.
37 Iyobe, S., Hashimoto, H., and Mitsuhashi, S. 1970. *Japan. J. Microbiol.*, **14**, 463–471.
38 Iyobe, S., Hashimoto, H., and Mitsuhashi, S. 1976. In preparation.
39 Iyobe, S., Hashimoto, H., and Mitsuhashi, S. 1976. *J. Bacteriol.*, submitted for publication.
40 Iyobe, S., Hasuda, K., Fuse, A., and Mitsuhashi, S. 1974. *Antimicrob. Agents Chemother.*, **5**, 547–552.
41 Iyobe, S., Kono, M., Ohara, K., Hashimoto, H., and Mitsuhashi, S. 1974. *Antimicrob. Agents Chemother.*, **5**, 68–74.
42 Iyobe, S., Mitsuhashi, S., and Saito, T. 1973. *Antimicrob. Agents Chemother.*, **3**, 614–620.
43 Iyobe, S., Mitsuhashi, S., and Umezawa, H. 1971. *J. Bacteriol.*, **108**, 946–947.
44 Iyobe, S., Sagai, H., Hasuda, K., and Mitsuhashi, S. 1976. *In* Proceedings of the 3rd International Symposium on Infectious Antibiotic Resistance, ed. by S. Mitsuhashi, L. Rosival, and V. Krčméry, Avicenum, Springer-Verlag, Heidelberg, Berlin, and New York, in press.
45 Jackson, D. A., Symons, R. H., and Berg, P. 1972. *Proc. Natl. Acad. Sci. U.S.*, **69**, 2904–2909.
46 Johnston, J. H. and Richmond, M. H. 1970. *J. Gen. Microbiol.*, **60**, 137–139.
47 Katsumata, R., Hashimoto, H., and Mitsuhashi, S. 1975. *J. Bacteriol.*, submitted for publication.
48 Kawakami, Y., Mikoshiba, F., Nagasaki, S., and Matsumoto, H. 1972. *J. Antibiot.*, **25**, 607–609.
49 Kontomicalou, P., Mitani, M., and Clowes, R. C. 1970. *J. Bacteriol.*, **104**, 34–44.
50 Lacy, G. and Leary, J. V. 1975. *J. Gen. Microbiol.*, **88**, 49–57.

51 Meynell, E., Meynell, G. G., and Datta, N. 1968. *Bacteriol. Rev.*, **32**, 55–83.
52 Mitsuhashi, S. 1967. *Japan. J. Microbiol.*, **11**, 49–68.
53 Mitsuhashi, S. 1971. *Ann. N.Y. Acad. Sci.*, **182**, 141–152.
54 Mitsuhashi, S., Harada, K., and Kameda, M. 1961. *Nature*, **189**, 947.
55 Mitsuhashi, S., Hashimoto, H., Tanaka, T., Iyobe, S., and Kawabe, H. 1974. *In* Progress in Chemotherapy, Vol. 1, ed. by G. K. Daikos, pp. 35–47, Hellenic Society of Chemotherapy, Athens.
56 Mitsuhashi, S., Kameda, M., Harada, K., and Suzuki, M. 1969. *J. Bacteriol.*, **97**, 1520–1521.
57 Mitsuhashi, S., Iyobe, S., Hashimoto, H., and Umezawa, H. 1970. *J. Antibiot.*, **23**, 319–323.
58 Mitsuhashi, S., Inoue, M., Kawabe, H., Oshima, H., and Okubo, T. 1973. *In* Contribution to Microbiology and Immunology, Vol. 1, Staphylococci and Staphylococcal Infections, ed. by J. Jeljaszewicz, pp. 144–165, Karger, Basel.
59 Mitsuhashi, S., Inoue, M., Oshima, H., Okubo, T., and Saito, T. 1976. *In* Contribution to Microbiology and Immunology, Vol. 1, Staphylococci and Staphylococcal Infections, ed. by J. Jeljaszewicz, pp. 255–274, Karger, Basel.
59a Mitsuhashi, S. 1975. *In* Drug Action and Drug Resistance in Bacteria, Vol. 2, Aminoglycoside Antibiotics, ed. by S. Mitsuhashi, pp. 269–270, University of Tokyo Press, Tokyo / University Park Press, Baltimore and London.
60 Moody, E. E. M. and Hayes, W. 1972. *J. Bacteriol.*, **111**, 80–85.
61 Moody, E. E. M. and Runge, R. 1972. *Genet. Res.*, **19**, 181–186.
62 Morris, C. F., Hashimoto, H., Mickel, S., and Rownd, R. 1974. *J. Bacteriol.*, **111**, 855–866.
63 Nakae, M., Inoue, M., and Mitsuhashi, S. 1975. *Antimicrob. Agents Chemother.*, **7**, 719–720.
64 Nishimura, Y., Caro, L., Berg, C. M., and Hirota, Y. 1971. *J. Mol. Biol.*, **55**, 441–456.
65 Nishimura, A., Nishimura, Y., and Caro, L. 1973. *J. Bacteriol.*, **116**, 1107–1112.
66 Nordström, K., Ingram, L., and Landbäck, A. 1972. *J. Bacteriol.*, **110**, 562–569.
67 Novick, R. P. 1969. *Bacteriol. Rev.*, **33**, 210–263.
68 Novick, R. P., Clowes, R. C., Cohen, S. N., Curtiss, R., III, Datta, N., and Falkow, S. 1976. *Bacteriol. Rev.*, **40**, 168–189.
69 Ohtsubo, E. 1970. *Genetics*, **64**, 189–197.
70 Olsen, R. H. and Shipley, P. 1973. *J. Bacteriol.*, **113**, 772–780.

71 Panopoulos, N. J., Guimaraes, W. V., Cho, J. J., and Schroth, M. N. 1975. *Phytopathology*, **65**, 380–388.

72 Pearce, L. E. and Meynell, E. 1968. *J. Gen. Microbiol.*, **50**, 159–172.

73 Pinney, R. J. and Smith, J. T. 1971. *Genet. Res.*, **18**, 173–177.

74 Romero, E. and Meynell, E. 1969. *J. Bacteriol.*, **97**, 780–786.

75 Rownd, R. and Mickel, S. 1971. *Nature New Biol.*, **234**, 40–43.

76 Rownd, R. H., Perlman, D., Womble, D. D., Taylor, D. P., and Morris, C. F. 1975. *In* Microbial Drug Resistance, ed. by S. Mitsuhashi and H. Hashimoto, pp. 27–50, University of Tokyo Press, Tokyo / University Park Press, Baltimore and London.

77 Sagai, H., Hasuda, K., Iyobe, S., and Mitsuhashi, S. 1976. *Antimicrob. Agents Chemother.*, **10**, 573–578.

78 Sagai, H., Iyobe, S., and Mitsuhashi, S. 1975. In preparation.

79 Salisbury, V., Hedges, R. W., and Datta, N. 1972. *J. Gen. Microbiol.*, **70**, 443–452.

80 Schnos, M. and Inman, R. B. 1970. *J. Mol. Biol.*, **51**, 61–73.

81 Sharp, P. A., Cohen, S. N., and Davidson, N. 1973. *J. Mol. Biol.*, **75**, 235–255.

82 Smith, H. R., Humphrey, G. O., and Anderson, E. S. 1974. *Mol. Gen. Genet.*, **129**, 229–242.

83 Sugino, Y. and Hirota, Y. 1962. *J. Bacteriol.*, **84**, 902–910.

84 Takano, T. 1966. *Japan. J. Microbiol.*, **10**, 201–210.

85 Takano, T. and Watanabe, T. 1966. *Biochem. Biophys. Res. Commun.*, **25**, 192–198.

86 Tanaka, T., Hashimoto, H., Nagai, Y., and Mitsuhashi, S. 1967. *Japan. J. Microbiol.*, **11**, 155–162.

87 Taylor, A. L. and Trotter, C. D. 1967. *Bacteriol. Rev.*, **31**, 332–353.

88 Terawaki, Y., Kishi, H., and Nakaya, R. 1975. *J. Bacteriol.*, **121**, 857–862.

89 Terawaki, Y., Takayasu, H., and Akiba, T. 1967. *J. Bacteriol.*, **34**, 687–690.

90 Terawaki, Y. and Rownd, R. 1972. *J. Bacteriol.*, **109**, 492–498.

91 Tweats, D. J., Pinney, R. J., and Smith, J. T. 1974. *J. Bacteriol.*, **118**, 790–795.

92 Yokota, T., Kasuga, T., Kaneko, M., and Kuwahara, S. 1972. *J. Bacteriol.*, **109**, 440–442.

93 Yoshida, Y., Terawaki, Y., and Nakaya, R. 1974. *Biochem. Biophys. Res. Commun.*, **59**, 361–369.

94 Yoshikawa, M. 1974. *J. Bacteriol.*, **118**, 1123–1131.

95 Yoshikawa, M. and Akiba, T. 1962. *Japan. J. Microbiol.*, **6**, 121–132.

96 Yoshikawa, M. and Sevag, M. G. 1967. *J. Bacteriol.*, **93**, 245–253.

97 Watanabe, T., Takano, T., Arai, T., Nishida, H., and Sato, S. 1966. *J. Bacteriol.*, **92**, 477–486.

4 TRANSLOCABLE DRUG RESISTANCE DETERMINANTS

Susumu Mitsuhashi

Department of Microbiology, School of Medicine, Gunma University, Maebashi, Japan

It is generally accepted that an R plasmid consists of two major genetic elements, *i.e.*, (1) the element responsible for the autonomous activities of the plasmid, such as replication and conjugal transferability, called transfer factor (T) (*34*), and (2) the element encoding drug resistance.

1. Translocable Drug Resistance Genes

In the transduction of an R plasmid in *Salmonella* strains with bacteriophage epsilon (ε), the drug resistance determinants were consistently segregated between the determinant responsible for tetracycline (TC) resistance and those encoding resistance to chloramphenicol (CM), streptomycin (SM), and sulfanilamide (SA) (*12*). The TC resistance in the transductant was conjugally nontransferable and was not spontaneously or artificially eliminated. The *tet* genes encoding TC resistance were transferred through the F factor to *Escherichia coli* W1177 in which the *tet* genes were found to be located on the *E. coli* chromosome between *pro* and *lac*, near *lac* (*15*). Similarly, the genes

TABLE I. Integration of the Resistance Determinants on R Plasmids into Bacterial Chromosomes

Origin	Resistance determinant		Location	References
	Determinant	Obtained by		
S. newington R$_{ms10}^+$	*tet*	Transduction (ε)	*Salmonella* chromosome	12
S. newington tet	*tet*	F-mating	W1177 chromosome near *lac*	15
S. newington R$_{ms10}^+$	*cml str sul*	Transduction (ε)	*Salmonella* chromosome	14
E. coli R$_{ms10}^+$	*cml str sul*	Transduction (P1)	*E. coli* chromosome	8
E. coli W3630 R$_{9-4}^+$	*cml*	Spontaneous integration	W3630 chromosome near *met*B	21
E. coli W1895 HfrC R$_{9-4}^+$	*cml*	Spontaneous integration	W1895 HfrC chromosome near *lac, ara, gal, mtl,* or *pro*	22

encoding resistance to CM, SM, and SA were found to be integrated into the bacterial chromosome (*8, 25*).

The CM resistance in *E. coli* W3630 R$_{9-4}^+$ is lost at a high frequency during overnight cultivation of the strain at 37°C. We selected the strains possessing stable CM resistance in which the *cml* genes encoding CM resistance were located on the *E. coli* chromosome near *met*B (*21*). We successively obtained various mutant strains in which the *cml* genes of R$_{9-4}$ plasmid are integrated into the *E. coli* chromosome, near *lac, ara, gal, mtl,* or *pro* (*22*) (Table I).

The R plasmid in *E. coli* R$_{ms10}$ (TC. CM. SM. SA)$^+$ was transduced with phage P1. When the transductants were induced by UV irradiation after lysogenization with phage P1, we obtained bacteriophage P1-*cml* which carries all the pertinent phage activities as well as the CM^r character. P1-*cml* multiplies by lytic growth, forming plaques similar to those of normal P1. Transduction of CM^r to the recipient occurs followig lysogenization (*29*).

E. coli F$^+$(P1-*cml*) was obtained by lysogenization of *E. coli* F$^+$ with bacteriophage P1-*cml*. Conjugation of *Salmonella typhi* with *E. coli* F$^+$ (P1-*cml*) gave three types of *S. typhi* CM^r clones: those which carry the entire P1-*cml* phage, those with the P1*d*-*cml* element, and those with nontransferable CM^r. Upon superinfection of *E. coli* carrying P1*d*-*cml* with virulent P1 phage, the lysate was able to transduce the CM^r character at a high frequency, which is considered high frequency of transduction (HFT). Similarly, we obtained the P1d-*cml str sul* element, which is able to transduce resistances to CM, SM, and SA at a high frequency with a helper phage P1 (8). In the transduction of *Salmonella* E group R$^+$ with bacteriophage ε, ε*d-tet* and ε*d-cml str sul* elements were obtained. When *Salmonella* carrying these elements was infected with virulent ε phage, the lysates were able to transduce TC^r or (CM. SM. SA)^r character at a high frequency, called HFT (25).

E. coli (P1-*cml*) was obtained by lysogenization of *E. coli* with active transducing phage P1-*cml* (29). λ-*cml* was obtained when a λ prophage was induced in *E. coli* (P1-*cml*) which carried a gene encoding CM resistance (11). Prophage λ was singly and tandemly inserted into R$_{100}$. Insertions into the transfer genes, insertions into the transfer control gene *fin* 0, and insertions into regions that result in no detectable phenotypic change were found. From the last type, Dempsey and Willets (7) isolated high frequency transducing phage preparations λ-*mer*, λ-*str sul*, and λ-*cml str sul*.

Staphylococcus aureus strains of clinical isolates are multiple-resistant owing to the presence of various types of nonconjugative resistance (r) plasmids, which generally encode single resistance and exist as multiple copies of each plasmid in a cell (19, 36, 37). The TC^r character in *S. aureus* MS3878 carrying nonconjugative plasmid r-ms7(TC) was transduced with bacteriophage S1. Upon infection of the TC-resistant transductants with bacteriophage S1, we obtained bacteriophage S1-*tet* that carries all the pertinent phage activities of S1, as well as the TC^r character. Similarly we obtained S1-*cml* phage as a consequence of transduction of r-ms6(CM) plasmid with S1. Both bacteriophages S1-*tet* and S1-*cml* carry all the pertinent phage activities of S1 and transduce drug resistance to recipient cells following lysogenization, in addition to a genetic region which is responsible for stabilizing lysogeny and in providing all information for replicating themselves (19, 20, 37). The results are summarized in Table II.

The *tet* determinant on an R plasmid was integrated in the *E. coli* W1177 chromosome (5). When *E. coli* W1177 *tet* was infected with F, F-*lac*, R(CM) and T plasmids, we obtained the recombinants between the *tet* determinant and plasmids, i.e., F-*tet*, F-*lac tet* (13, 14), R(CM)-*tet* (24) and T-*tet* (34). We obtained a CM-resistant *E. coli* W3630 strain, in which the *cml* determinant on the R plasmid was integrated

TABLE II. Formation of Recombinants between Resistance Determinants and Bacteriophages

Origin	Bacterio-phage	Resistance determinant	Recombinant	References
E. coli $R_{ms14}{}^+$	P1	*cml*	P1-*cml*	29
E. coli (P1-*cml*)[a]	P1-*cml*	*cml*	P1d-*cml*	30
E.coli $R_{ms10}{}^+$	P1	*cml str sul*	P1d-*cml str sul*	8
E. coli $R_{nr1}{}^+$	P1	*cml tet*	P1-*cml tet*	19
E. coli (P1-*cml*)	λ	*cml*	λ-*cml*	11
E. coli $R_{100}{}^+$	λ	*mer*[b]	λ-*mer*	7
		str sul	λ-*str sul*	
		cml str sul	λ-*cml str sul*	
S. newington $R_{ms10}{}^+$	ε	*tet*	εd-*tet*	25
	ε	*cml str sul*	εd-*cml str sul*	25
S. aureus MS353(TC^r) (S1)[c]	S1	*tet*	S1-*tet*	19, 20, 37
S. aureus MS353(CM^r) (S1)[d]	S1	*cml*	S1-*cml*	19, 37

[a] *E. coli* (P1-*cml*), *E. coli* lysogenized with P1-*cml*.
[b] *mer*, resistance to mercuric chloride.
[c] *S. aureus* MS353(TC^r) was obtained by transduction from MS3878 r-ms7(TC)$^+$ with bacteriophage S1. MS353(TC^r) (S1) carries a nontransferable plasmid encoding TC resistance and is lysogenized with S1.
[d] *S. aureus* MS353(CM^r) was obtained by transduction from MS3878 r-ms6(CM)$^+$ with bacteriophage S1. MS353(CM^r) (S1) carries a nontransferable plasmid encoding CM resistance and is lysogenized with S1.

in the chromosome (*21*). When *E. coli* W3630 *cml* was infected with an R(TC) or F plasmid, we obtained the recombinants F-*cml* and R(TC)-*cml* (*21, 22*). *E. coli* W3110 was lysogenized with an active phage P1-*cml* capable of transducing the CM^r character. When W3110 (P1-*cml*) was infected with an F plasmid, we obtained the recombinant F-*cml*, which possesses both F functions and an ability to confer CM resistance (*29*).

Germ-free pigs were orally contaminated with eight drug-sensitive *E. coli* strains. After confirmation of the establishment of artificial flora, TC (2 mg/kg) was given to the pigs every day in their drinking water. TC-resistant strains were obtained and they were confirmed to be *E. coli* 3002 TC^r according to their biological and immunological properties. Nontransferable TC resistance acquired conjugal transferability by the formation of recombinant Col B-*tet* between the *tet* determinant and Col B plasmid present in one of the eight *E. coli* strains (*35a*).

In vitro-developed resistant mutants were obtained with an *Enterobacter cloacae* on plates containing various concentrations of ampicillin (APC). The nontransferable APC-resistant determinant (*amp*) acquired conjugal transferability by the formation of a recombinant T-*tet amp* between T-*tet* plasmid (*26, 34*) and *amp* determinant (*38*).

The (*str sul*) determinants governing resistance to both SM and SA were obtained from *E. coli* W3110 R_{ms11} (TC. CM. SM. SA)$^+$ by the penicillin (PC)-screening method. The determinants could not be cured by acridine dye and were not transduced to a *rec*$^-$ (recombination deficient) mutant of *E. coli* K12, indicating that the determinants were inserted into the host chromosome. When *E. coli* carrying (*str sul*) determinants was infected with a T-*tet* or T-*tet cml* plasmid, the recombinant T-*tet str sul* or T-*tet cml str sul* plasmid was obtained (*26, 35a*). Table III lists the recombinants between resistance determinants and plasmids.

TABLE III.   Formation of Recombinants between Resistance Determinants and Plasmids

Origin	Infected with plasmid	Recombinants between resistance determinants and plasmids	References
E. coli W1177 *tet*	F	F-*tet*	*13*
	F-*lac*	F-*lac tet*	*14*
	R(CM)	R(CM)-*tet*	*14*
	T	T-*tet*	*26, 34*
E. coli W3110 (*str sul*)	T-*tet*	T-*tet str sul*	*26, 35a*
	T-*tet cml*	T-*tet cml str sul*	
E. coli 3002 *tet*	Col B	Col B-*tet*	*38*
E. coli W3110 (P1-*cml*)	F	F-*cml*	*30*
E. coli W3630 *cml*	F	F-*cml*	*22*
	R(TC)	R(TC)-*cml*	*21*
E. coli JE346 *cml pro*	R_{9-127}(TC)	R(TC)-*cml pro*	*23*
		R(TC)-*pro*	
Ent. cloacae amp	T-*tet*	T-*tet amp*	*35a*

TABLE IV. Pick-up of *cml* and *pro* Genes on the Chromosome by the R_{9-127}(TC) Plasmid

Cross		Selection	Genetic markers of R prime plasmids obtained
Donor	Recipient		
JE346 *cml pro+*	AB2463 *rec− pro−*	Proline	R(TC. CM)-*pro+*
R_{9-127}(TC)+			R(TC)-*pro+*

Donor, *E. coli* JE346; recipient, *E. coli* AB2463 *rec− pro−*. *cml*, chloramphenicol (CM) resistance gene(s).

The *cml* genes on the R_{9-4} plasmid were integrated in various sites of the *E. coli* chromosome, *i.e.*, near *metB*, *lac*, *ara*, *gal*, *mtl*, and *pro* regions (*21–23*). *E. coli* JE346 *cml pro+*, in which the *cml* genes were located near (*proA proB*), was infected with the R_{9-127} (TC) plasmid. When JE346 *cml pro+* R(TC)+ was mated with *E. coli* AB2463 *rec− pro−*, we obtained two types of the transconjugants, *i.e.*, transferable (*tra+ tet cml pro+*), and (*tra+ tet pro+*) with a high conjugal transferability of 10^{-1}.

The (*tra+ tet cml pro+*) and (*tra+ tet pro+*) transconjugants were transduced with bacteriophage P1. When selected on a TC plate, we obtained the (*tra+ tet cml pro+*) and (*tra+ tet pro+*) transductants among various types of the transductants, indicating that the (*proA proB cml*) segment acquired conjugal transferability of 10^{-1} by the formation of R primes, *i.e.*, R (TC. CM)-*pro* and R (TC)-*pro* (Table IV).

An r-ms3(KM) plasmid is a nonconjugative plasmid encoding kanamycin (KM) resistance and is thermosensitive in its own maintenance in host bacteria. When T-*tet* was introduced in W3630 r (KM)+, three types of the transconjugants were formed when selected on the plate containing both TC and KM: (1) the (TC. KM) resistance is conjugally transferred together at a frequency of 10^{-1}, (2) the (TC. KM) resistance is conjugally transferred together at the same transfer frequency as that of the parent T-*tet* plasmid, and (3) the TC resistance is transferable at a low frequency, both resistance determinants existing separately (*24*).

Transduction with phage P1 disclosed the formation of recombinants T-*tet kan*-1 with a high transfer frequency and T-*tet kan*-2 with the same transfer frequency as that of T-*tet* plasmid. The recombinants T-*tet kan*-1 and T-*tet kan*-2 were not thermosensitive in their own maintenance in host bacteria. But most of the KM^r plasmids segregated by transduction resumed the thermosensitivity.

[^{14}C] thymidine-labeled lysates of the strains carrying T-*tet*, r(KM) or T-*tet kan*-1, were ultracentrifuged in ethidium bromide-CsCl density gradients. The fractions of each satellite peak were pooled and dialysed, and the DNAs were examined by electron microscopy after storage at 2°C. The contour lengths of the r(KM) and T-*tet* plasmid DNAs were 11.7±0.3 and 26.4±0.7 μm, respectively. The contour length of a recombinant T-*tet kan*-1 plasmid DNA was 38.6±0.9 μm, indicating that T-*tet kan*-1 plasmid was formed by the cointegration of both r(KM) and T-*tet* plasmids (*24*). The r(KM) plasmid can confer on its host a high level of KM resistance (400 μg/ml) as well as a low level of SM resistance. Biochemical mechanism of KM resistance is due to phosphorylation of the drug but the mechanism of SM resistance by r(KM) plasmid is yet unknown. The high level of KM resistance and the low level of SM resistance were still preserved in all T-*tet kan* recombinants.

While the r(KM) plasmid is temperature-sensitive (*ts*) in its own maintenance, the T-*tet kan* are as stable as the parent T-*tet* plasmid at high temperatures. But a majority of singly KM-resistant transductants segregated from T-*tet kan* plasmids are thermosensitive, indicating that the *ts* gene on an r (KM) plasmid is preserved and masked in both recombinants T-*tet kan*-1 and T-*tet kan*-2.

Kameda *et al.* (*27*) reported that the T-*kan* recombinants become derepressed mutants when an r(KM) plasmid is integrated into T$_{95}$ plasmid, suggesting the homology between the r(KM) plasmid and the regulatory gene(s) of the transfer loci of the T plasmid. In the recombination between T-*tet* and r(KM), one-third of the recombinants were *drd* mutants. The derepression of conjugal transferability in T-*tet kan*-1 was caused by a loss of repressor production for piliation and the site of cointegration in T-*tet kan*-1 was considered to be the regulatory gene of the transfer loci on the T-*tet* plasmid.

R plasmids consist of two major genetic elements, *i.e.*, T factors and resistance determinants. Transfer factors were demonstrated at a high frequency in drug-sensitive clinical isolates (*34*) and consist of two genetic elements responsible for replication and conjugal transferability. Nonconjugative resistance(r) plasmids, as well as R plasmids, are widely distributed among both gram-positive and gram-negative bacteria and are of particular importance in clinical medicine and livestock hygiene. Nonconjugative r plasmids are different from R plasmids according to the lack of a conjugal transferability that is of great importance in plasmid evolution.

A drug resistance determinant is found to be easily translocated from R (or r) plasmids to various sites on the bacterial chromosome, indicating that there are many insertion regions (IS) at various sites on the chromosome. Demonstration of active bacteriophages possessing drug resistance genes such as P1-*cml* (*29*), S1-*tet* (*20*), S1-*cml* (*37*), P1-*tet*, P1-*tet cml* (*33*), P11 *de* (*39*), λ-*cml* (*11*), λ-*str sul*, λ-*cml str sul* (*7*), suggests the presence of IS regions on bacteriophage DNA (*18*). P1 *d-lac* (*32*), P1 *d-pro* (*46*), εd-*tet* (*25*), P1 *d-cml* (*30*), εd-*cml str sul* (*25*) and P1 *d-cml str sul* (*8*) are capable of producing a HFT lysate through a helper phage, and are thought to be the recombinant DNA molecules carrying phage DNA as well as the DNA molecules derived from plasmids.

The author introduced the possibility that r are produced by re-combination between a transducing phage and active phage DNAs, resulting in the loss of phage virulence but in the maintenance of the ability of self-replication and the conferring of drug resistance (*36, 37*). The presence of active phages possessing drug resistance genes strongly supports the possibilities of the evolutionary steps in the for-mation of r plasmids, *i.e.*, the recombination between a transducing phage and active phage DNAs. The resistance determinant translocat-ed from R (or r) plasmids to bacterial chromosome or bacteriophage DNA was picked up by F, F-*lac*, and T, resulting in the formation of resistance plasmids.

2. *Insertion Sequences (IS)*

Recently, a certain DNA segment repeated at multiple sites on an *E. coli* chromosome, in a plasmid and in phages have been shown by electron microscopy to be identical to the insertion sequences (IS region). These IS regions appear to be important to the integration of plasmids into the chromosome and recombination within or among the plasmid DNA itself. IS elements are discrete DNA sequences of a defined length, between 800 and 1,400 base pairs, and they are nor-mal constituents of bacterial chromosome and plasmid DNAs. IS ele-

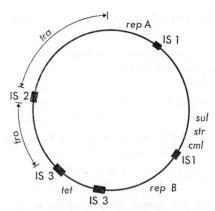

Fig. 1. Genetic map of the IS segments on R_{100}. Abbreviation of drug resistance determinants. *tet*, tetracycline; *cml*, chloramphenicol; *str*, streptomycin; *sul*, sulfanilamide. *tra*, the determinants governing conjugal transferability. Details, see Chapter 3. *rep*A and *rep*B, the genes governing replication of R plasmids.

ments have not been observed to be capable of replicating autonomously. They are detected when transposed to new positions within the same replicon or another replicon within the same cell, causing characteristic genetic effects at their new locations. A genetic map of IS elements on R_{100} is shown in Fig. 1.

As described in this article, drug resistance determinants have been found to translocate as a unit from one site on DNA to others. Moreover, it was found that genetic recombination between these molecular species occurred by *rec*A independent insertion of an entire plasmid genome (or resistance determinants) at a specific DNA locus of another plasmid, and coincident excision of a precisely defined DNA segment originally present at the point of the insertion. Thus, the easy transposition of drug resistance genes to a bacterial chromosome, bacteriophages and sex factors, may be explained by the presence of IS regions on a bacterial chromosome, bacteriophages and transfer factors, resulting in the formation of R (or r) plasmids that have abilities responsible for self-replication and conjugal transferability. Selection force by drugs also plays an important role in the wide spread of R (or r) plasmids among many bacterial strains of various species.

The bacterial chromosome is thought to be rather stable with regard to its gross organization and the genetic maps of various species of bacteria, such as *E. coli, Salmonella, Klebsiella, Pseudomonas, etc.*, are rather similar with respect to the order of functions. By contrast, gross changes in the organization of DNA are more common in bacteriophage and plasmids. DNA molecules of specialized transducing phages are formed by a process termed "illegitimate recombination" (*3, 9*) that takes place between their own DNA and bacterial DNA. The same phenomenon in the F plasmid is known by the formation of F′ plasmids. Drug resistance determinants on R plasmids are known with varying combinations of resistance genes, indicating the largest degree of variability in plasmid DNA organization. In the variability processes, a new genetic element, called the IS element, is found to perform an important role.

When IS elements are transposed singly into bacterial operons, they abolish the function of the gene, into which they are integrated, and they depress the functions of genes located downstream in the direction of transcription and translation (*45*). When an Hfr strain is formed by integration of an F plasmid into the bacterial chromosome,

TABLE V. Some Properties of Transposons

Name	Resistance transposed	R plasmid and phage used for transduction	Transposition observed
TnA(1)	APC	R plasmids	*E. coli* chromosome colE1, pSC101
TnT(1)	TC	R_{ms10}, phage ε	*S. newington* and *E. coli* chromosome, F, F′ and T
		R_6, phage P22	*S. typhimurium* chromosome
TnK(1)	KM	JR67	Phage λ
TnK(2)	KM	JR67	Phage λ
TnK	KM		
(ST)	TP[a] SM	R plasmids	*E. coli* chromosome
TnC(1)	CM	R_{ms10} R_{100}	Phage P1, F, and T Phage λ
		R_{9-4}	*E. coli* chromosome
Tn(S. Su)	SM SA	R_{ms11}	*E. coli* chromosome and T-*tet* plasmid

[a] TP: trimethoprim.

F is found to carry a few defined sequence at a certain region of the chromosome. Further, integration is known to occur at various sites on the bacterial chromosome (6). The variability of R plasmids occurs by the addition or the loss of drug resistance determinants in units called transposons. A transposon consists of one or more drug resistance determinants and is bordered at both ends by DNA sequences that are homologous but inverted with respect to their direction.

Transposons are defined as genetic elements capable of integration into numerous and nonhomologous sequences of DNA. For a given transposon, a specific and nonpermuted sequence is observed regardless of the site it occupies. It is further known that recombination functions of E. coli that are required for promoting of homologus DNAs are not required for transposition. It is suggested that each transposon has an insertion mechanism that is specific for sequences on its own DNA and nonspecific for sequences on the DNA with which it recombines.

Tn9 (42), like other recently described transposons, facilitates its own transposition to diverse replicons in the absence of known re-

Site specificity of integration	Total length (kilobase)	References
Limited number of sites	4.4	Datta et al. (1973) 16, 17, 31, 38, 41, 44
Many sites available, clustering observed	3.8	Harada et al. (1963) 4, 13, 28, 40, 43, 47, 48
Two sites observed in two isolates	5.2	2
Not known	4.1	2
Not known	3.2	43
Very limited number of sites	Not known	1
Two sites observed in two isolates	Not known	Kondo and Mitsuhashi (1964), 10, 11, 18, 30
Various sites	Not known	
Not known	Not known	26, 35

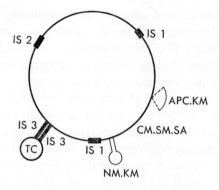

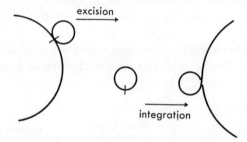

Fig. 2. Transposition of IS elements. The structures are based on heteroduplex studies by Sharp *et al*. (1973).

combination functions. Tn9 carries the *cml* gene which confers upon bacteria high-level resistance to the antibiotic CM. Other transposons encoding drug resistance are listed in Table V. A fictitious figure of IS elements on R_{100} plasmid and transposition of IS elements are shown in Fig. 2.

Genetic and epidemiologic studies of R plasmids offer a new finding that drug resistance genes are easily transposed owing to the presence of IS elements on bacterial chromosomes, bacteriophages, and plasmids. Rapid spread of R plasmids and quick evolution of R plasmids possessing multiple resistances are now accountable for by the presence of transposons and selective influence of drugs used all over the world. It can be assumed that there are three possibilities for the formation of plasmids encoding multiple resistance: (1) recombination between drug resistance plasmids, (2) translocation of a'transposon encoding drug resistance onto a resistance plasmid, and (3) cointegration of a drug resistance transposon (or r plasmid) onto another resistance plasmid.

REFERENCES

1 Barth, P. T., Datta, N., Hedges, R. W., and Grinter, N. J. 1976. *J. Bacteriol.*, **125**, 800–810.

2 Berg, D. E., Davies, J., Allet, B., and Rochaix, J. D. 1975. *Proc. Natl. Acad. Sci. U.S.*, **72**, 3628–3632.

3 Campbell, A. 1962. *Adv. Genet.*, **11**, 101–145.

4 Chan, R. K. and Botstein, D. 1972. *Virology*, **49**, 257–267.

5 Datta, N., Hedges, R. W., Shaw, E. J., Sykes, R. B., and Richmond, M. H. 1971. *J. Bacteriol.*, **108**, 1244–1249.

6 Davidson, N., Deonier, R. C., Hu, S., and Ohtsubo, E. 1975. *Microbiology*, **1**, 56–61.

7 Dempsey, W. B. and Willetts, N. S. 1976. *J. Bacteriol.*, **126**, 166–176.

8 Egawa, R. and Mitsuhashi, S. 1964. *Japan. J. Bacteriol.*, **19**, 237.

9 Franklin, N. 1971. *In* The Bacteriophage Lambda, ed. by A. D. Hershey, pp. 175–194, Cold Spring Harbor Laboratory, New York.

10 Gottesman, M. and Weisberg, R. A. 1971. *In* The Bacteriophage Lambda, ed. by A. D. Hershey, pp. 113–138, Cold Spring Harbor Laboratory, New York.

11 Gottesman, M. M. and Rosner, J. L. 1975. *Proc. Natl. Acad. Sci. U.S.*, **72**, 5041–5045.

12 Harada, K., Kameda, M., Suzuki, M., and Mitsuhashi, S. 1963. *J. Bacteriol.*, **86**, 1332–1338.

13 Harada, K., Kameda, M., Suzuki, M., and Mitsuhashi, S. 1964. *J. Bacteriol.*, **88**, 1257–1265.

14 Harada, K., Kameda, M., Suzuki, M., and Mitsuhashi, S. 1967. *Japan. J. Microbiol.*, **11**, 143–151.

15 Harada, K., Kameda, M., Suzuki, M., Shigehara, S., and Mitsuhashi, S. 1967. *J. Bacteriol.*, **93**, 1236–1241.

16 Heffron, R., Rubens, C., and Falkow, S. 1975. *Proc. Natl. Acad. Sci. U.S.*, **72**, 3623–3627.

17 Hedges, R. W. and Jacob, A. E. 1974. *Mol. Gen. Genet.*, **132**, 31–40.

18 Ikeda, H. and Tomizawa, J. 1965. *J. Mol. Biol.*, **14**, 85–109.

19 Inoue, M., Okubo, T., Oshima, H., and Mitsuhashi, S. 1975. *In* Microbial Drug Resistance, ed. by S. Mitsuhashi and H. Hashimoto, pp. 153–

164, University of Tokyo Press, Tokyo / University Park Press, Baltimore and London.

20 Inoue, M. and Mitsuhashi, S. 1975. *Virology*, **68**, 544–546.

21 Iyobe, S., Hashimoto, H., and Mitsuhashi, S. 1969. *Japan. J. Microbiol.*, **13**, 225–232.

22 Iyobe, S., Hashimoto, H., and Mitsuhashi, S. 1970. *Japan. J. Microbiol.*, **14**, 463–471.

23 Iyobe, S., Hashimoto, H., and Mitsuhashi, S. 1977. *J. Bacteriol.*, submitted for publication.

24 Katsumata, R., Hashimoto, H., and Mitsuhashi, S. 1977. *J. Bacteriol.*, submitted for publication.

25 Kameda, M., Harada, K., Suzuki, M., and Mitsuhashi, S. 1965. *J. Bacteriol.*, **90**, 1174–1181.

26 Kameda, M., Harada, K., Suzuki, M., and Mitsuhashi, S. 1969. *Japan. J. Microbiol.*, **13**, 255–262.

27 Kameda, M., Suzuki, M., Nakajima, T., Harada, K., and Mitsuhashi, S. 1970. *Japan. J. Microbiol.*, **14**, 339–349.

28 Kleckner, N., Chan, R. K., Tye, B. K., and Botstein, D. 1975. *J. Mol. Biol.*, **97**, 561–575.

29 Kondo, E. and Mitsuhashi, S. 1964. *J. Bacteriol.*, **88**, 1266–1276.

30 Kondo, E. and Mitsuhashi, S. 1966. *J. Bacteriol.*, **91**, 1787–1794.

31 Kopecko, D. J. and Cohen, S. N. 1975. *Proc. Natl. Acad. Sci. U.S.*, **72**, 1373–1377.

32 Luria, S. E., Adams, J. N., and Ting, R. C. 1960. *Virology*, **12**, 348–390.

33 Mise, K. and Arber, W. 1975. *In* Microbial Drug Resistance, ed. by S. Mitsuhashi and H. Hashimoto, pp. 165–167, University of Tokyo Press, Tokyo / University Park Press, Baltimore and London.

34 Mitsuhashi, S., Kameda, M., Harada, K., and Suzuki, M. 1969. *J. Bacteriol.*, **97**, 1520–1521.

35 Mitsuhashi, S. 1971. *In* Transferable Drug Resistance Factor R, ed. by S. Mitsuhashi, pp. 1–16, University of Tokyo Press, Tokyo / University Park Press, Baltimore and London.

35a Mitsuhashi, S. 1971. *N.Y. Acad. Sci.*, **182**, 141–152.

36 Mitsuhashi, S., Inoue, M., Kawabe, H., Oshima, H., and Okubo, T. 1973. *In* Contributions to Microbiology and Immunology, Vol. 1, Staphylococci and Staphylococcal Infections, ed. by J. Jeljaszewicz, pp. 144–165, Karger, Basel.

37 Mitsuhashi, S., Inoue, M., Oshima, H., Okubo, T., and Saito, T. 1976. *In* Staphylococci and Staphylococcal Diseases, ed. by J. Jeljaszewicz, pp. 255–274, Gustav Fischer Verlag, Stuttgart and New York.

38 Nakajima, T., Suzuki, M., Kameda, M., Harada, K., and Mitsuhashi, S. 1973. *Japan. J. Microbiol.*, **17**, 251–256.
39 Novick, R. P. 1967. *Virology*, **33**, 155–166.
40 Ptashen, K. and Cohen, S. N. 1975. *J. Bacteriol.*, **122**, 776–781.
41 Richmond, M. H. and Sykes, R. B. 1972. *Genet. Res.*, **20**, 231–238.
42 Rosner, J. L. and Gottesman, M. M. 1976. *In* DNA Insertion, Cold Spring Harbor Laboratory, New York, in press.
43 Sharp, P. A., Cohen, S. N., and Davidson, N. 1973. *J. Mol. Biol.*, **75**, 235–255.
44 So, M., Gill, R., and Falkow, S. 1975. *Mol. Gen. Genet.*, **142**, 239–249.
45 Starlinger, P. and Saedler, H. 1972. *Biochimie*, **54**, 177–182.
46 Stodolsky, M. 1973. *Virology*, **53**, 471–475.
47 Tye, B. K., Chan, R. K., and Botstein, D. 1974. *J. Mol. Biol.*, **85**, 485–500.
48 Watanabe, T., Ogata, Y., Chan, R. K., and Botstein, D. 1972. *Virology*, **50**, 874–882.

5 GENETICS OF CONJUGATION

Neil S. WILLETTS

Department of Molecular Biology, University of Edinburgh, Edinburgh, Scotland

Conjugation is a process for gene transfer between bacteria that requires cell-to-cell contact (*23*), and was originally described in *Escherichia coli* K12 by Lederberg and Tatum (*58*). The genes that encode the proteins required for conjugation are usually carried not by the bacterial chromosome, but by an autonomous plasmid DNA molecule. As a result, such "conjugative" plasmids are able to transfer themselves, and under some circumstances host chromosomal DNA, to a recipient cell. The first conjugative plasmid to be recognized was the *E. coli* K12 sex factor F (*13*, *41*), while more recent observations have shown that other plasmids determining phenotypes, such as colicinogeny (Col factors) and antibiotic resistance (R factors) also frequently possess this property (*34*, *63*, *103*). R factors are of particular importance both because they are numerically by far the largest class of plasmids known, and because the consequent inheritance of antibiotic resistance by pathogenic strains can severely impede the medical treatment of bacterial infections. Conjugative plasmids have now been identified in about 30 different bacterial genera, and many have the ability to transfer intergenerically.

Broadly speaking, the conjugation or transfer systems of bacterial plasmids can all be divided into three interlocking parts: the pilus and other cell surface structures that provide the "machinery" for DNA transfer, the enzymes required for processing the DNA during transfer (together with the specific plasmid DNA sequences that they may recognize), and the surface exclusion product(s) that reduces transfer *into* the cell of the same or a related plasmid. However, there are at least four different types of transfer system, each with these same three basic characteristics; these are called the F, I, N, and P systems. The pili corresponding to these four systems are different both in their structure and in the particular "male-specific" bacteriophages that they adsorb. Furthermore, where investigated, a transfer system of one type will not efficiently transfer a plasmid determining a transfer system of a second type, and there is no surface exclusion between plasmids with different transfer systems. It should be noted that plasmids with the F or I types of transfer system, and perhaps those with the N and P types, can be subdivided into several different incompatibility groups (see Chapters 10, 11).

As yet, the I, N, and P transfer systems have not been extensively studied, and most of our present knowledge of conjugation genetics derives from investigations of plasmids with F-type transfer systems. These will therefore be discussed in detail first.

1. F-type Transfer System

1) The transfer process

Donor cells carrying a conjugative F-type plasmid produce a characteristic external hair-like appendage called a pilus. In the case of the F factor itself, the pilus is about 90 Å across (8, 54), variable in length with a mean of 1 to 2 μm (8, 67, 86), and appears to have an axial groove about 25 Å across (8, 54). It probably has a double-filament structure, consisting of two parallel protein rods (9).

The initial step in conjugation is the formation of a mating pair by interaction between the tip of this pilus and a receptor site on the surface of the recipient cell. Recipient mutants that lack this receptor site have been described (89, 95). Parenthetically, the pilus is also essential for infection of the cell by F-specific isometric RNA phages (which adsorb to the sides of the pilus; 10, 18) and filamentous single-strand DNA phages (which adsorb to the pilus tip; *12*). Thus removal of the pilus from the cell either temporarily by blending (*8, 70*), or permanently by plasmid mutation (*2, 76*, see below) prevents both transfer and F-specific phage adsorption. Mating pair formation is blocked both by filamentous DNA phages (*50, 69, 80*) and by zinc ions (*82*). This indicates that the *tip* of the pilus is involved since this is where filamentous DNA phages adsorb (*12*), and zinc ions also act at the tip since they prevent adsorption of these phages but not of RNA phages that adsorb to the sides of the pilus (*83*).

The pilus may then serve as the conjugation bridge along which the DNA passes (*9*). Alternatively, the pilus may retract by sequential depolymerization of its subunits into the donor cell membrane; this would draw the surfaces of the mating cells together and allow formation of a conjugation bridge not directly involving the pilus. Pilus retraction has been observed on treatment of cells with cyanide ions (*68*) as well as during conjugation (*81*) and infection by an F-specific DNA phage (*52*, but see *72*). However, conclusive evidence that retraction is, or is not, essential for conjugation and F-specific phage infection is still not available.

As a consequence of the formation or further development of the mating pair, a "mating signal" is presumed to be generated, perhaps as a conformational change in the pilus structure. This could trigger retraction, and also synthesis or activation of the enzymes required for plasmid DNA metabolism during transfer. A plasmid-encoded endonuclease may first nick a unique strand of the circular plasmid DNA molecule at a specific site (*108*). The linear single strand is then transferred to the recipient cell with the 5' terminus first (*48a, 74*). Transfer is accompanied by replication of this strand in the recipient cell, and of the remaining strand in the donor cell (*99, 100*). Replication in the donor cell is by a mechanism different from that for vegetative replication (*101*) and in any case is not essential for transfer (*91*). The transferred linear single-stranded plasmid DNA molecule is replicated and recircularized in the recipient cell by processes not yet understood; however, recircularization probably involves recognition of specific DNA sequences since it can occur in a *recA*⁻ recipient (*16*). DNA metabolism during conjugation is discussed in greater detail in Chapter 6.

2) *Genes for transfer*

Many of the genes required for conjugation have been identified by complementation analyses of transfer-deficient (*tra*⁻) plasmid mutants. Such mutants have been isolated by screening mutagenized clones to identify those unable to transfer (*2, 46, 76*), or by taking advantage of the dual role of the pilus and selecting F-specific phage-resistant cells (*76, 98*). One complementation system used the two compatible plasmids F-*gal* and R_{100-1} (*76*); their transfer systems were known to be similar since both determine pili adsorbing F-specific phages, and *tra*⁻ mutants of each could be complemented by the other, wild-type plasmid (*46, 76*). The R_{100-1} *tra*⁻ mutants were transduced with P1 to cells carrying F-*gal tra*⁻ mutants, giving stable heterozygotes for the complementation analysis in which six transfer genes common to both plasmids were identified (*76*). A second complementation system used transient populations of heterozygous cells carrying two different F-*lac tra*⁻ mutants. To construct these, one F-*lac tra*⁻ mutant was transferred into cells carrying a second, either by conjugation from a Su^+ strain carrying an amber-suppressible F-*lac tra*⁻ mutant (*3*) or by P1 transduction (*112*). In these studies, 12 genes required for conjugation were identified (*3, 109, 112*).

All mutants in *tra*A, *tra*B, *tra*C, *tra*E, *tra*F, *tra*H, *tra*K, and *tra*L, and some in *tra*G, were resistant to all F-specific phages (*3, 76, 109, 112*); examination in an electron microscope confirmed that they lacked the pilus (*9, 76*). In contrast to this genetic complexity, the pilus is constructed from a single subunit protein called pilin. In the case of F, pilin has a molecular weight of about 12,000 daltons and carries two phosphate groups and one glucose residue per molecule (*5, 9*). The cell contains a pool of pre-existing pilin molecules (*8, 71*), and these have been located in the outer cell membrane (*5*). F-pilin has a very hydrophobic amino-acid composition, and arginine, cysteine, histidine and proline are absent (*9*). Wild-type F-pilin has two tyrosine residues per molecule, and since suppression of an amber *tra*A⁻ mutant by Su_{III}^+ (which inserts tyrosine), but not by Su_I^+ (which inserts serine), gave pilin with three tyrosine residues per molecule, *tra*A must encode the pilin protein (*65*). Presumably the other eight genes are required for chemical modification of the pilin and its assembly into the pilus structure, although the details of this have not yet been worked out.

All mutants in *tra*I and *tra*D and some in *tra*G still synthesized the pilus. These pili seemed normal since they allowed infection by F-specific phages (except that RNA phages other than Q_β could not infect *tra*D mutants), formed mating pairs (*2*), and retracted on treatment with cyanide ions (*68*). The *tra*I product may be a specific endonuclease required to initiate DNA transfer (*108*, and see below). Mutations in *tra*D did not prevent the adsorption (*2*) or ejection (*85*) stages in RNA phage infection, and the *tra*D product must therefore be required for penetration of the RNA into the cell. By analogy, it may also be required for penetration of the cell surface by plasmid DNA during conjugation. Since only some *tra*G⁻ mutations prevented pilus formation, the *tra*G product may be bifunctional and serve to link DNA metabolism and pilus formation during transfer.

All the nonpiliated and piliated F-*lac tra*⁻ mutants described above retained the property of surface exclusion. This indicates in particular that surface exclusion is not a function of the pilus. Recently, piliated transfer-proficient mutants of F-*lac* that have lost surface exclusion have been obtained (M. Achtman and N. S. Willetts, unpublished data); the *tra*S (surface exclusion) gene product is therefore not required for transfer, and the absence of any relationship between surface exclusion and piliation of the recipient cell is confirmed. Surface exclusion may prevent mating pair formation (and consequently, conjugation) by inactivating the receptor site for the tip of the donor pilus (*2, 115*).

All mutants in a further gene, *tra*J, were transfer-deficient, did not make the pilus, and had lost the property of surface exclusion (*3, 112*). In fact the *tra*J product was required for the synthesis of all the other *tra* gene products (*33*), and *tra*J is therefore a positive control gene.

The operon structure of the F transfer genes has been elucidated by the analysis of polar *tra*⁻ mutations. Initially, polar amber and frameshift mutations (in particular *tra*K4) showed that *tra*B, *tra*C, *tra*F, *tra*G, *tra*H, *tra*K, and *tra*S must lie in a single operon (*3, 112*). More recently, a series of strongly polar *tra*⁻ mutations were generated by inserting the mutator phage Mu into F-*lac* (*45*). Their complementation patterns with representative nonpolar *tra*⁻ mutants indicated that *all* the *tra* genes except *tra*J were in a single operon ("the transfer operon"). Surface exclusion measurements confirmed that *tra*S also belongs to this operon. The *tra*J product is presumably required for expression of the transfer operon, and in accordance with this, "J-independent" regulatory mutants have been isolated which transferred at low levels in the absence of the *tra*J product (*1*).

3) *Mapping transfer genes*
Since plasmids are small, circular DNA molecules, the methods used for mapping bacterial chromosomal genes, by measuring times of entry, recombination frequencies, or co-transduction frequencies, are of little value. Deletion mapping is the preferred method. Deletion mutants of F have been generated by P1 transduction of F-*gal* to *rec*A⁻ strains (*75*) and by co-deletion of λcI857 and a part of F from a transposition Hfr strain that has F-*lac* inserted near *att*ₗ (*51*). A new method involves the abnormal insertion of λcI857 into a plasmid molecule, followed by selection of deletion mutants as temperature-resistant survivors (N. S. Willetts, W. Dempsey, and S. McIntire, unpublished data). This may be the most generally applicable method for mapping plasmid genes, and also for studying control of their expression.

Complementation of the transfer-deficient F-*gal* deletion mutants with R_{100-1} *tra*⁻ point mutants (*75*), and of the Hfr deletion mutants with F-*lac* *tra*⁻ point mutants (*51, 109*), gave the order of the *tra* genes shown in Fig. 1. Surface exclusion measurements located *tra*S between *tra*G and *tra*D, confirming that it is a component of the transfer operon (*110*). Since the deletions entered the transfer region from the *tra*I end, the transfer operon must be transcribed in the direction *tra*A to *tra*I. The pattern of polarity observed with the Mu-induced polar *tra*⁻ mutants mentioned above was consistent with this map order and direction of transcription (*45*).

A locus required in *cis* for transfer, and presumed to be the origin from which this is initiated (*ori*), has also been mapped (Fig. 1; *107*). This transfer origin is not the same as the origin for vegetative replication since F prime deletion mutants that have lost all the *tra* genes and *ori* continue to replicate as autonomous plasmids (S. McIntire and N. S. Willetts; M. Guyer and A. J. Clark, unpublished data).

Electron microscope heteroduplex mapping using F prime deletion mutants has been used to determine the approximate physical locations of the transfer genes and other F loci (*93*) and these are indi-

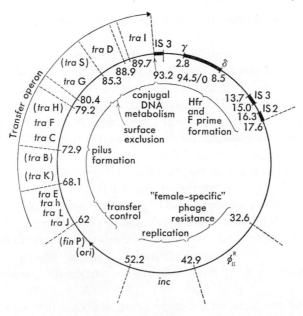

Fig. 1. A map of F. Compiled from data in Refs. *22, 51, 93, 107, 109, 110* and the unpublished data of M. Guyer and N. Davidson, and of N. S. Willetts. IS3, $\gamma\delta$, and IS2 are insertion sequences, *inc* is a gene required for incompatibility, and ϕ_{II}^R is a locus giving resistance to female-specific phages; other symbols are explained in the text. The numbers are kilobase coordinates. The radial dotted lines represent the physical bounds of the markers shown between them; the genetic, but not physical, locations are known for markers shown in parentheses.

cated in Fig. 1. The *tra* genes all lie between coordinates 62 and 93.2 kilobase (kb) (*22*), and the transfer operon therefore comprises 23 to 31 kb pairs (15 to 20×10^6 daltons), with an expected transcription time of 6 min (*45*).

4) Transfer control
Most F-type plasmids express only a small fraction of their full potential for transfer, pilus production and surface exclusion; this is due to a plasmid-determined system that inhibits expression of the transfer genes (*21, 27, 47, 63, 104, 113*). Plasmids with such transfer inhibition systems have the advantage of reduced levels of unnecessary *tra* protein synthesis and of protection against F-specific phages

in the natural environment, whilst they retain the potential for transfer.

Plasmid mutants with expression of the conjugation system increased 100- to 1,000-fold have been isolated (*27, 31, 38, 48, 61, 94*), and genetic analysis of these has shown that two structural genes are required for inhibition (*31, 38, 94*). These are designated *finO* (formerly *i*, *fi*, or *fin*) and *finP* (formerly *traP*), and together form the "FinOP" system. These two genes are located near to *traJ* (Fig. 1; N.S. Willetts and W. Dempsey, unpublished data).

The *finO* products of the majority of F-type plasmids are interchangeable (*32*), and in particular can all inhibit the transfer of F which is a naturally occurring *finO⁻* plasmid. Fertility inhibition was first recognized by this effect (*104*). *finO⁻* plasmid mutants inhibit neither their own transfer nor that of F. Curiously, several non-F-type plasmids, such as the N group plasmid R_{128} and an otherwise cryptic plasmid present in many *Salmonella* strains, carry *finO⁺* genes (*35, 37, 96*).

The *finP* products, on the other hand, are often not interchangeable between plasmids, and several different specificities have been recognized (*32, 35, 38*; see Table I below). *finP⁻* mutants of F (*31*), R_6 (*94*), R_{136} (*38*), Col B2 (*35, 40*) and R_{124} (*35, 62*) have been isolated, and like *finO⁻* mutants, transfer at high frequencies and carry recessive mutations (*31, 35, 38*). Unlike *finO⁻* mutants, however, they still inhibit F transfer (*35, 38, 40, 62, 94*). The mechanism of interaction between the *finO* and *finP* proteins and their site of action has not yet been elucidated.

Dominant mutations in this site of action (*traO*), which prevent transfer inhibition by the FinOP system, have been described for F and for R_{136} (*31, 38*). Full expression of transfer, pilus formation and surface exclusion was restored, indicating that the FinOP system has a single site of action (*31*). Genetic assay of *tra* gene products during transfer inhibition showed that the FinOP system prevents transcription (the repressor model; *63*) or translation of *traJ* (*33, 111*). Since the *traJ* product is required for expression of the transfer operon (*33*), this explains why transfer, pilus formation and surface exclusion are all decreased during transfer inhibition. It also explains why transfer of J-independent F-*lac* mutants is not inhibited by the FinOP system (*1*). As expected, *traO* is very tightly linked to *traJ* (*33*).

Transfer inhibition is temporarily relieved after transfer of a FinOP+ plasmid to a plasmid-free cell, resulting in the phenomenon of HFT (high frequency of transfer) cultures (21, 102). The HFT is probably due to transient synthesis of the traJ product before transfer inhibition is established. Expression of the transfer operon can thereby continue for about 4 hr, and only after this are the transfer proteins diluted out by cell growth (111). This phenomenon allows efficient "infections spread" of the plasmid to all the cells of a population.

Although the transfer inhibition systems of most F-type plasmids are FinOP systems, other systems inhibiting transfer of F-type plasmids but carried by non-F-type plasmids, have been identified and partially characterized (35, 36, 60, 116).

5) Plasmid specificity

Although all F-type plasmids probably encode totally analogous sets of genes for transfer and its control, the products of these genes are not always interchangeable between plasmids. F-type plasmids can be arranged into groups on this basis for each of the plasmid-specific genes, and Table I summarizes some of the correlations observed. There seems to be no obligatory association of particular plasmid-

TABLE I. Specificity among F-type Plasmids

Plasmid	F incompatibility group	traI and ori	traS	traA	finP
F	I	I	I	Ia	I
Col V2	I	I	II	Ia	I
R_1	II	III	III	III	III
R_{100}	II	IV	IV	IV	IV
R_{136}	II	IV	IV	IV	IV
R_{538-1}	II	III	II	Ib	V
Col B2	II	I	II	II	II
Col B4	II or III	III	II	II	V
Col VBtrp	IV	I	III	I	II
R_{124}	IV	I	II	Ib	II

Data used in constructing this table were taken from Refs. 4, 26, 32, 35, 38, 59, 88, 106, 114, 115 and the unpublished data of N.S. Willetts. Labeling as group I, II, etc., is on a separate arbitrary basis for each column.

specific alleles either with one another or with a particular incompatibility group. Assortment could have resulted from recombination between alleles in different genes, after their generation by mutation, during plasmid evolution. Observations in an electron microscope of heteroduplexes between single-stranded DNA molecules of the F-type plasmids F, R_{100}, R_1, and R_6 showed that about 90% of their transfer regions were homologous (*92*). Discontinuities cannot be seen in at least some of the regions where plasmid-specific alleles should be located, indicating that relatively minor changes in DNA sequence may be involved.

Perhaps the most important plasmid-specific genes are *tra*I and *tra*J; for example, the *fin*O⁻ F-type plasmid R_{100-1} did not complement *tra*I⁻ or *tra*J⁻ mutants of F-*lac* (*106*), and F-*lac* did not complement analogous mutants of R_{100-1} (N. S. Willetts, unpublished data). Similarily R_{1-19} did not complement the *tra*I⁻ and *tra*J⁻ F-*lac* mutants, whilst Col V2 and Col VB*trp* both did so (*4*).

The *tra*I product is not required for pilus formation, and, furthermore, it shows the same specificity pattern as the origin of transfer (*88*). This has lead to the hypothesis that it is a specific endonuclease that recognizes the corresponding plasmid origin sequence during the initiation of DNA transfer (*88, 108*). This hypothesis also explains why the F transfer system synthesized by cells carrying both the *fin*O⁺ plasmid R_{100} and an F-*lac* *tra*O⁻ mutant can transfer F-*lac* DNA but not R_{100} DNA (*31, 33*): the requisite R_{100} *tra*I product that recognizes the R_{100} transfer origin is not made because expression of the R_{100} transfer system is inhibited, and the F *tra*I product does not recognize the R_{100} transfer origin. In contrast, since the *fin*O⁺ plasmid R_{124} is transferred at a high frequency by cells carrying F-*lac* *tra*O⁻, the *tra*I products of R_{124} and of F must be interchangeable (*35*).

Although the *tra*J product controls synthesis of the *tra*I product, its plasmid specificity is not due simply to this; the failure of R_{100-1} or R_{1-19} to complement F-*lac* *tra*J⁻ (*4, 106*) proves that the *tra*J product is itself plasmid-specific. However, little additional information is presently available.

The plasmid specificity of the transfer control gene *fin*P was described above, and contrasted to the relative nonspecificity of the other transfer control gene, *fin*O (*32, 35*).

The fourth gene with major specificity variants is *tra*S. Four different F-type surface exclusion systems have been identified so far; plasmids within each group exclude themselves and members of the same group, but not members of other groups (*4, 114, 115*). It is emphasized that surface exclusion is not related to incompatibility; the two phenomena have entirely different bases, and plasmids with the same surface exclusion system may fall into different incompatibility groups and *vice versa*.

Although F-type pili made by different F-type plasmids are closely related in adsorbing the same F-specific phages and in their morphological (*54*) and serological (*55, 57*) properties, small differences have been found. Thus the efficiency of plating of F-specific phages varies from plasmid to plasmid (*4, 26, 66, 106*); this at least partially reflects varying efficiencies of adsorption (*85*), and is due to variations in the pilin gene, *tra*A (*4, 106*). The difference in density between F and R_{1-19} pili (*6*) is probably also due to variations in *tra*A, as are the minor serological differences between different F-type pili (*55*). Despite these differences, the overall similarity of F-type pili is emphasized by the formation of "mixed pili" by cells containing two F-type plasmids, with subunits of each type assembled together (*6, 56*). Also, some of the differences are reproduced in *tra*A$^-$ point mutants of F that (unlike the original *tra*A$^-$ mutants) are *tra*$^+$ but show reduced levels of adsorption and plating of F-specific RNA phages (R. Weppelman, K. Ippen-Ihler, and C. C. Brinton, personal communication; W. Paranchych and N. S. Willetts, unpublished data). Finally, it seems likely that all F-type pilin subunits are modified in the same way as F pilin (*i.e.*, two phosphate groups and one glucose residue per molecule). This has been directly demonstrated for R_{1-19} (*5*), and full complementation of all pililess F-*lac tra*$^-$ mutants (except, of course, for F-*lac tra*J$^-$), by the F-type plasmids Col V2, Col VB*trp*, R_{100-1}, R_{1-19}, and R_{538-1} *fin*$^-$ (*4, 106;* N. S. Willetts, unpublished data) leads to the same conclusion.

2. *I, N, and P Transfer Systems*

As described in the Introduction, the I, N, and P transfer systems seem to be similar in overall biochemical characteristics to the F-type system. However, the four systems do not interact, and they are apparently unrelated genetically. The dissimilarities are emphasized by hybridization (*28*, *39*, *49*) and electron microscope heteroduplex (*92*) studies that show little if any sequence homology between the DNA molecules of plasmids with different types of transfer system. The available data for the I, N, and P transfer systems will be briefly presented.

1) The I transfer system

Plasmids belonging to the several I incompatibility groups synthesize a pilus that does not adsorb F-specific phages, but instead adsorbs the I-specific filamentous single-stranded DNA phage If1 (*64*). Conversely, F-type pili do not adsorb If1. I-specific RNA phages have not yet been described. F-type and I-type pili are also different in their structure (*57*) and immunological reactions (*55*), and cells carrying both an I-type and an F-type plasmid form separate pili of each type rather than mixed pili (*56*). Two classes of I-type pili have been distinguished serologically (*55*).

Transfer-deficient mutants of the I-type plasmid R_{64-11} have been described only cursorily (*105*). These were not complemented by F-*lac*, and F-*tra*⁻ mutants were not complemented by I-type plasmids (*17*, *105*).

As in the case of the F-type plasmids F and R_{538-1} *drd*, a unique strand of R_{64-11} DNA was transferred during mating, and in each case this was the denser of the two strands separated in poly (U, G)-CsCl gradients (*99*). Transfer of R_{64-11} DNA from *dna*B⁻ donor cells to minicells has been extensively investigated (*29*, *30;* see Chapter 6); as in the case of F, the *dna*B product was not required for transfer replication in the donor cell. Furthermore, *de novo* synthesis of RNA but not of protein was apparently necessary for the initiation of R_{64-11} transfer (*30*). Surface exclusion by R_{64-11} was also demonstrated (*29*).

All naturally-occurring I-type plasmids show only low levels of transfer and pilus formation since like F-type plasmids they encode transfer inhibition systems; numerous mutants transferring and synthesizing pili at high levels have been obtained (*63*, *73*). However, these have not yet been subjected to genetic analysis and the mechanism of transfer inhibition is unknown. Although the I-type transfer inhibition system does not inhibit transfer of Fin⁻ F-type plasmids (*57*, *90*), the delayed kinetics for establishment of inhibition by a newly-transferred I-type plasmid are similar to those of FinOP⁺ F-type plasmids (*84*), and an analogous two-stage control system may be in operation.

2) *The N transfer system*

Cells carrying a plasmid belonging to incompatibility group N are sensitive to the N-specific filamentous DNA phage IKe, which represents a third group of male-specific phages (*53*). However, examination of cells carrying N group plasmids in an electron microscope has failed to reveal pili (*11*); the surface structure responsible for IKe adsorption must therefore be either a very short pilus, or located entirely within the cell surface. The same surface structure is probably also involved in transfer, since mutants have been described that have become simultaneously IKe-resistant and transfer-deficient (*24*).

The N transfer system is also unusual in that it is not found in association with a transfer inhibition system: cells carrying wild-type N group plasmids are thus fully sensitive to IKe, and the apparently inefficient transfer of N group plasmids (*24, 25*) may be due instead to the inefficiency of mating pair formation (or of some other step in conjugation) under the mating conditions normally used. Curiously, the incompatibility group X plasmid R_{6K} appears to inhibit the N transfer system (*87*).

3) *The P transfer system*

R factors belonging to the P incompatibility group(s) determine a transfer system that includes a pilus (*7*) and a surface exclusion system (*44*). Cells carrying such R factors are sensitive to a fourth group of male-specific phages that includes the RNA phage PRR1 (*77, 79*), the filamentous DNA phage Pf3 (*97*), and the icosahedral DNA phages PRD1 (*78*), PR3 and PR4 (*97*). PRR1 adsorbs to the short pili present on cells carrying P group plasmids, but Pf3, PR3, and PR4 may adsorb to other plasmid-determined surface structures (*7*). However, most transfer-deficient mutants of the P group plasmid RP1 were simultaneously resistant to PRR1, Pf3, PR3, and PR4 (*97*). Two further transfer-deficient mutants retained sensitivity to all four phages.

Interestingly, PRD1, PR3, and PR4 can also infect cells carrying an N group plasmid (*7, 78*), indicating some relationship between the P and N transfer systems. Partial homology between the DNA of a P and of an N group plasmid has been reported in one case (*49*) but not another (*28*). A further similarity to N group plasmids is that wild-type P group plasmids do not determine a transfer inhibition system. Cells carrying P group plasmids are thus fully sensitive to P-specific phages, although again, they are rather poor donors (*14, 20, 77*).

Although P group R factors were originally identified in *Pseudomonas aeruginosa*, they have since been found in other genera, such as *Proteus* (*43*) and *Providencia* (*42*). They are notable for their extremely broad host range, including *Pseudomonas*, the Enterobacteriaceae, *Proteus* and *Rhizobium* (*14, 19, 20, 77*). It is not yet clear whether the more restricted host range of other plasmids is due to absence of the appropriate conjugational receptor site from the recipient cell surface, or to inability of transferred plasmid DNA to replicate.

Other *Pseudomonas* R factors such as R_{P1-1} and R_{91} are also P-type in that they render the host cell sensitive to the P-specific phages PRR1, PR3, and PR4, although not to Pf3 (*14, 15, 97*). However, these plasmids belong to a different incompatibility group, and have a narrower host range (*14, 15*). They also differ in encoding a transfer inhibition system that reduces their own transfer and pilus formation, although not that of a co-existing R_{P1} plasmid (*15*). Mutants lacking this transfer inhibition system have been isolated (*15, 97*).

Yet other *Pseudomonas* plasmids such as FP5 and R_{38} do not themselves make the host cell sensitive to P-specific phages, but do determine systems preventing transfer and pilus formation by R_{P1} (*97*).

3. Conclusion

In this chapter, I have tried to present some of the salient features of conjugation and its genetics, especially for the F-type transfer system where investigation has been most extensive. However, this emphasis on the F-type system is merely a historical accident and hopefully a compensatory effort will be made in future to understand to an equal degree the I, N, and P transfer systems, and others as yet totally obscure. Only then will it be possible to appreciate the general features of conjugation, and to understand the possible evolutionary relationship between the different transfer systems. There is an increasing realization of the importance of bacterial plasmids in ecology and epidemiology, bacterial evolution and inheritance, and the techniques of genetic engineering, as witnessed by the increasing numbers of known plasmids, of genera recognized to carry plasmids, and of publications relating to plasmids. Efforts to analyze the underlying genetics of conjugation should be stimulated by these factors, as well as by the intrinsically interesting features of conjugation itself that range from the structural components required and their connection to the processing of DNA during transfer, to the intricate systems for the regulation of conjugation.

REFERENCES*

1 Achtman, M. 1973. *Genet. Res.*, **21**, 67–77.
2 Achtman, M., Willetts, N. S., and Clark, A. J. 1971. *J. Bacteriol.*, **106**, 529–538.
3 Achtman, M., Willetts, N. S., and Clark, A. J. 1972. *J. Bacteriol.*, **110**, 831–842.
4 Alfaro, G. and Willetts, N. S. 1972. *Genet. Res.*, **20**, 279–289.
5 Beard, J. P. and Connolly, J. C. 1975. *J. Bacteriol.*, **122**, 59–65.
6 Beard, J. P., Howe, T. G. B., and Richmond, M. H. 1972. *J. Mol. Biol.*, **66**, 311–313.
7 Bradley, D. E. 1974. *Biochem. Biophys. Res. Commun.*, **57**, 893–900.
8 Brinton, C. C. 1965. *Trans. N.Y. Acad. Sci.*, *Ser. II*, **27**, 1003–1054.
9 Brinton, C. C. 1971. *Crit. Rev. Microbiol.*, **1**, 105–160.
10 Brinton, C. C., Gemski, P., and Carnahan, J. 1964. *Proc. Natl. Acad. Sci. U.S.*, **52**, 776–783.
11 Brodt, P., Leggett, F., and Iyer, R. 1974. *Nature*, **249**, 856–858.
12 Cavalli, L. L., Lederberg, J., and Lederberg, E. M. 1953. *J. Gen. Microbiol.*, **8**, 89–103.
13 Chandler, P. M. and Krishnapillai, V. 1974. *Genet. Res.*, **23**, 239–250.
14 Chandler, P. M. and Krishnapillai, V. 1974. *Genet. Res.*, **23**, 251–257.
15 Caro, L. G. and Schnös, M. 1966. *Proc. Natl. Acad. Sci. U.S.*, **56**, 126–132.
16 Clark, A. J. and Margulies, A. D. 1965. *Proc. Natl. Acad. Sci. U.S.*, **53**, 451–459.
17 Cooke, M., Meynell, E., and Lawn, A. M. 1970. *Genet. Res.*, **16**, 101–112.
18 Crawford, E. M. and Gesteland, R. F. 1964. *Virology*, **22**, 165–167.
19 Datta, N. and Hedges, R. W. 1972. *J. Gen. Microbiol.*, **70**, 453–460.
20 Datta, N., Hedges, R. W., Shaw, E. J., Sykes, R. B., and Richmond, M. H. 1971. *J. Bacteriol.*, **108**, 1244–1249.

* The literature survey for this chapter was completed in February 1975.

21 Datta, N., Lawn, A. M., and Meynell, E. 1966. *J. Gen. Microbiol.*, **45**, 365–376.

22 Davidson, N., Deonier, R. C., Hu, S., and Ohtsubo, E. 1974. *Microbiology*, 56–65.

23 Davis, B. D. 1950. *J. Bacteriol.*, **60**, 507–508.

24 Dennison, S. and Baumberg, S. 1973. *Proc. Soc. Gen. Microbiol.*, **1**, 10.

25 Datta, N. and Hedges, R. W. 1971. *Nature*, **234**, 222–223.

26 Dennison, S. and Hedges, R. W. 1972. *J. Hyg.*, **70**, 55–61.

27 Egawa, R. and Hirota, Y. 1962. *Japan. J. Genet.*, **37**, 66–69.

28 Falkow, S., Guerry, P., Hedges, R. W., and Datta, N. 1974. *J. Gen. Microbiol.*, **85**, 65–76.

29 Fenwick, R. G. and Curtiss, R. 1973. *J. Bacteriol.*, **116**, 1212–1223.

30 Fenwick, R. G. and Curtiss, R. 1973. *J. Bacteriol.*, **116**, 1224–1235.

31 Finnegan, D. J. and Willetts, N. S. 1971. *Mol. Gen. Genet.*, **111**, 256–264.

32 Finnegan, D. J. and Willetts, N. S. 1972. *Mol. Gen. Genet.*, **119**, 57–66.

33 Finnegan, D. J. and Willetts, N. S. 1973. *Mol. Gen. Genet.*, **127**, 307–316.

34 Fredericq, P. 1969. *In* Ciba Foundation Symposium on Bacterial Episomes and Plasmids, ed. by G. E. W. Wolstenholme and M. O'Connor, Churchill, London, pp. 163–174.

35 Gasson, M. J. and Willetts, N. S. 1975. *J. Bacteriol.*, **122**, 518–525.

36 Grindley, J. N. and Anderson, E. S. 1971. *Genet. Res.*, **17**, 267–271.

37 Grindley, N. D. F., Grindley, J. N., and Anderson, E. S. 1972. *Mol. Gen. Genet.*, **119**, 287–297.

38 Grindley, N. D. F., Grindley, J. N., Smith, H. R., and Anderson, E. S. 1973. *Mol. Gen. Genet.*, **120**, 27–34.

39 Guerry, P. and Falkow, S. 1971. *J. Bacteriol.*, **107**, 372–374.

40 Hausmann, C. and Clowes, R. C. 1971. *J. Bacteriol.*, **107**, 900–906.

41 Hayes, W. 1953. *J. Gen. Microbiol.*, **8**, 72–88.

42 Hedges, R. W. 1974. *J. Gen. Microbiol.*, **81**, 171–181.

43 Hedges, R. W., Datta, N., Coetzee, J. N., and Dennison, S. 1973. *J. Gen. Microbiol.*, **77**, 249–259.

44 Hedges, R. W. and Jacob, A. E. 1974. *Mol. Gen. Genet.*, **132**, 31–40.

45 Helmuth, R. and Achtman, M. 1975. *Nature*, **257**, 652–656.

46 Hirota, Y., Fujii, T., and Nishimura, Y. 1966. *J. Bacteriol.*, **91**, 1298–1304.

47 Hirota, Y., Nishimura, Y., Ørskov, F., and Ørskov, I. 1964. *J. Bacteriol.*, **87**, 341–351.

48 Hoar, D. I. 1970. *J. Bacteriol.*, **101**, 916–920.

48a Ihler, G. and Rupp, W. D. 1969. *Proc. Natl. Acad. Sci. U.S.*, **63**, 138–143.

49 Ingram, L. C. 1973. *J. Bacteriol.*, **115**, 1130–1134.

50 Ippen, K. A. and Valentine, R. C. 1967. *Biochem. Biophys. Res. Commun.*, **27**, 674–680.

51 Ippen-Ihler, K., Achtman, M., and Willetts, N. S. 1972. *J. Bacteriol.*, **110**, 857–863.

52 Jacobson, A. 1972. *J. Virol.*, **10**, 835–843.

53 Khatoon, H., Iyer, R. V., and Iyer, V. N. 1972. *Virology*, **48**, 145–155.

54 Lawn, A. M. 1966. *J. Gen. Microbiol.*, **45**, 377–383.

55 Lawn, A. M. and Meynell, E. 1970. *J. Hyg.*, **68**, 683–694.

56 Lawn, A. M., Meynell, E., and Cooke, M. 1971. *Ann. Inst. Pasteur*, **120**, 3–8.

57 Lawn, A. M., Meynell, E., Meynell, G. G., and Datta, N. 1967. *Nature*, **216**, 343–346.

58 Lederberg, J. and Tatum, E. L. 1946. *Cold Spring Harbor Symp. Quant. Biol.*, **11**, 113–114.

59 MacFarren, A. C. and Clowes, R. C. 1967. *J. Bacteriol.*, **94**, 365–377.

60 Meynell, E. 1973. *J. Bacteriol.*, **113**, 502–503.

61 Meynell, E. and Datta, N. 1967. *Nature*, **214**, 885–887.

62 Meynell, E. and Lawn, A. M. 1973. *Proc. Soc. Gen. Microbiol.*, **1**, 2.

63 Meynell, E., Meynell, G. G., and Datta, N. 1968. *Bacteriol. Rev.*, **32**, 55–83.

64 Meynell, G. G. and Lawn, A. M. 1968. *Nature*, **217**, 1184–1186.

65 Minkley, E. G., Polen, S., Brinton, C. C., and Ippen-Ihler, K. 1976. *J. Mol. Biol.*, **108**, 111–121.

66 Nishimura, Y., Ishibashi, M., Meynell, E., and Hirota, Y. 1967. *J. Gen. Microbiol.*, **49**, 89–98.

67 Novotny, C., Carnahan, J., and Brinton, C. C. 1969. *J. Bacteriol.*, **98**, 1294–1306.

68 Novotny, C. P. and Fives-Taylor, P. 1974. *J. Bacteriol.*, **117**, 1306–1311.

69 Novotny, C., Knight, W. S., and Brinton, C. C. 1968. *J. Bacteriol.*, **95**, 314–326.

70 Novotny, C., Raizen, E., Knight, W. S., and Brinton, C. C. 1969. *J. Bacteriol.*, **98**, 1307–1319.

71 Novotny, C. P., Taylor, P. F., and Lavin, K. 1972. *J. Bacteriol.*, **112**, 1083–1089.

72 O'Callaghan, R., Bradley, R., and Paranchych, W. 1973. *Virology*, **54**, 220–229.

73 Ohki, M. and Ozeki, H. 1968. *Mol. Gen. Genet.*, **103**, 37–41.

74 Ohki, M. and Tomizawa, J. 1968. *Cold Spring Harbor Symp. Quant. Biol.*, **33**, 651–657.

75 Ohtsubo, E. 1970. *Genetics*, **64**, 189–197.

76 Ohtsubo, E., Nishimura, Y., and Hirota, Y. 1970. *Genetics*, **64**, 173–188.

77 Olsen, R. H. and Shipley, P. 1973. *J. Bacteriol.*, **113**, 772–780.

78 Olsen, R. H., Siak, J., and Gray, R. H. 1974. *J. Virol.*, **14**, 689–699.

79 Olsen, R. H. and Thomas, D. D. 1973. *J. Virol.*, **12**, 1560–1567.

80 Ou, J. T. 1973. *J. Bacteriol.*, **114**, 1108–1115.

81 Ou, J. T. and Anderson, T. F. 1970. *J. Bacteriol.*, **102**, 648–654.

82 Ou, J. T. and Anderson, T. F. 1972. *J. Bacteriol.*, **111**, 177–185.

83 Ou, J. T. and Anderson, T. F. 1972. *J. Virol.*, **10**, 869–871.

84 Ozeki, H. 1965. *Zentralbl. Bakteriol. Parasitenk., Abt. 1*, **196**, 160–173.

85 Paranchych, W. 1975. *In* The RNA Phages, ed. by N. Zinder, Cold Spring Harbor Laboratory, New York, pp. 85–111.

86 Paranchych, W., Ainsworth, S. K., Dick, A. J., and Krahn, P. M. 1971. *Virology*, **45**, 615–628.

87 Pinney, R. J. and Smith, J. T. 1974. *J. Gen. Microbiol.*, **82**, 415–418.

88 Reeves, P. and Willetts, N. S. 1974. *J. Bacteriol.*, **120**, 125–130.

89 Reiner, A. M. 1974. *J. Bacteriol.*, **119**, 183–191.

90 Romero, E. and Meynell, E. 1969. *J. Bacteriol.*, **97**, 780–786.

91 Sarathy, P. V. and Siddiqi, O. 1973. *J. Mol. Biol.*, **78**, 443–451.

92 Sharp, P. A., Cohen, S. N., and Davidson, N. 1973. *J. Mol. Biol.*, **75**, 235–255.

93 Sharp, P. A., Hsu, M., Ohtsubo, E., and Davidson, N. 1972. *J. Mol. Biol.*, **71**, 471–497.

94 Silver, R. P. and Cohen, S. N. 1972. *J. Bacteriol.*, **110**, 1082–1088.

95 Skurray, R. A., Hancock, R. E. W., and Reeves, P. 1974. *J. Bacteriol.*, **119**, 726–735.

96 Smith, H. R., Humphreys, G. O., Grindley, N. D. F., Grindley, J. N., and Anderson, E. S. 1973. *Mol. Gen. Genet.*, **126**, 143–151.

97 Stanisich, V. A. 1974. *J. Gen. Microbiol.*, **84**, 332–342.

98 Tomoeda, M., Shuta, A., and Inuzuka, M. 1972. *J. Bacteriol.*, **112**, 1358–1363.

99 Vapnek, D., Lipman, M. B., and Rupp, W. D. 1971. *J. Bacteriol.*, **108**, 508–514.

100 Vapnek, D. and Rupp, W. D. 1970. *J. Mol. Biol.*, **53**, 287–303.

101 Vapnek, D. and Rupp, W. D. 1971. *J. Mol. Biol.*, **60**, 413–424.

102 Watanabe, T. 1963. *J. Bacteriol.*, **85**, 788–794.

103 Watanabe, T. 1963. *Bacteriol. Rev.*, **27**, 87–115.

104 Watanabe, T. and Fukasawa, T. 1962. *J. Bacteriol.*, **83**, 727–735.

105 Willetts, N. S. 1970. *Mol. Gen. Genet.*, **108**, 365–373.

106 Willetts, N. S. 1971. *Nature New Biol.*, **230**, 183–185.
107 Willetts, N. S. 1972. *J. Bacteriol.*, **112**, 773–778.
108 Willetts, N. S. 1972. *Annu. Rev. Genet.*, **6**, 257–268.
109 Willetts, N. S. 1973. *Genet. Res.*, **21**, 205–213.
110 Willetts, N. S. 1974. *J. Bacteriol.*, **118**, 778–782.
111 Willetts, N. S. 1974. *Mol. Gen. Genet.*, **129**, 123–130.
112 Willetts, N. S. and Achtman, M. 1972. *J. Bacteriol.*, **110**, 843–851.
113 Willetts, N. S. and Finnegan, D. J. 1970. *Genet. Res.*, **16**, 113–122.
114 Willetts, N. S. and Maule, J. 1973. *Genet. Res.*, **21**, 297–299.
115 Willetts, N. S. and Maule, J. 1974. *Genet. Res.*, **124**, 81–89.
116 Willetts, N. S. and Paranchych, W. 1974. *J. Bacteriol.*, **120**, 101–105.

6 MECHANISM OF CONJUGATION

Roy CURTISS III,* Raymond G. FENWICK, Jr.,** Raul
GOLDSCHMIDT,* and Joseph O. FALKINHAM III***
*Department of Microbiology, Institute of Dental Research and
Cancer Research and Training Center, University of Alabama
in Birmingham, Birmingham, U.S.A.,* Robert J. Kleberg, Jr.
Center for Human Genetics, Department of Medicine, Baylor
College of Medicine, Houston, U.S.A.,** and Department of
Biology, Virginia Polytechnic Institute, Blacksburg, U.S.A.****

Conjugation was discovered in *Escherichia coli* K12 by Lederberg and
Tatum (*72*) as a type of genetic transfer requiring cell-to-cell contact
(*37*). It was subsequently learned that donor and recipient strains ex-
isted and that donor ability was due to the presence of a conjugative
plasmid termed F (*21, 51*). Conjugative plasmids, especially those conferring resistance to antibiotics, are now ubiquitous among gram-negative organisms in nature and conjugation has become an important
factor in the evolution of new microbial types better able to adapt to
changing environments, more capable of causing bacterial disease and/
or with greater facility to survive during antimicrobial therapy.

In reviewing recent contributions to our understanding of the
mechanism of conjugational plasmid transfer it has become obvious to
us that the diversity of plasmid systems studied by different methods
and investigators makes generalization difficult if not often invalid.
Hopefully real and/or apparent discrepancies will be reinvestigated to
determine their bases. Until then our conclusions and inferences must
be considered as provisional. When not otherwise indicated the studies
cited have been performed with plasmids in *E. coli* K-12.

1.   Early Stages

1)   Union between donor and recipient cells

Soon after mixing donor and recipient cell populations together there is a concentration, medium viscosity and temperature-dependent rate for the formation of donor: recipient cell unions. This process has been referred to as pair formation in the "old" literature, but Achtman (2) has recently provided substantial data to indicate that mating cells very rapidly form aggregates containing as many as 13 mating cells. He also noted that the mating efficiency of donor and recipient cells was independent of the aggregate size. Mating aggregates have been routinely observed by conjugation researchers but their presence has not altered our choice of vocabulary. We thus propose to abandon the use of the term "pair formation" and substitute in its place the more correct term "union formation." (The word union seems preferable to aggregate since the latter is rather nonspecific whereas the former at least has some connotation of sexuality. We also disfavor the term "mate formation" since the word mate in its usual sense implies a pairwise coupling.)

We therefore redefine specific and effective pair formation (29) as specific and effective union formation; the former being those events that occur in the absence of energy metabolism in either parent (33) to permit formation of unions that are stable during gentle dilution (48) and the latter being those events that convert a specific union to a state in which cellular connections are established between donor and recipient cells through which DNA can pass. Donor cells possessing homologous or closely related conjugative plasmids do not exchange either plasmid or chromosomal genetic information except at low frequency (21) and there is evidence to suggest that this is due to interference with specific union formation. This process has variously been termed entry exclusion (82), surface exclusion (4), exit exclusion (8), or just plain exclusion (78).

Union formation was first studied by Lederberg (71) using phase contrast microscopy and this procedure is still being used to advantage in studying these events (2, 15, 87). Electron microscopy has also been used (7, 15, 35, 47) although the different procedures for specimen preparation have given different results. Indeed, serial thin section studies are now known to give artifacts since the same structures are seen for donor: donor and recipient: recipient "matings" as are observed for donor: recipient matings (*66, 113*). The experimental investigation of union formation was greatly facilitated by deHaan and Gross (*48*) who provided an operational definition for specific unions as those that were stable during gentle dilution. This gentle dilution procedure was used by them and subsequently by others to investigate many aspects of the union formation process. More recently, particle counters, often with multichannel analyzers, have been used to good advantage in studies on union formation (*2, 86, 110*).

2) Role of donor pili

In 1964, Brinton *et al.* (*17*) observed that donor cells but not recipient cells possessed hair-like appendages termed donor pili that acted as the receptor sites for attachment of donor-specific RNA phages along their lengths. It was subsequently learned that the donor-specific DNA phages attached to the tips of donor pili (*20*). Based on the pioneer work of Brinton and his colleagues (*15, 16*) as well as contributions by others (*29, 104, 106*; see Chapter 5) it is considered that donor pili play an essential role during bacterial conjugation as well as for donor-specific phage infection. Most conjugative plasmids, including those in the F, I, and P incompatibility groups, specify the synthesis of donor pili whose antigenic properties and abilities to attach given donor-specific phages are generally correlated with the plasmid incompatibility group or subgroup to which they belong. Plasmids in the N group, however, do not specify detectable pili (*19*) although cells with N plasmids are sensitive to the donor-specific phage Ike (*63*). Donor-specific phages have not yet been isolated for cells harboring plasmids of the many less well-studied incompatibility groups. Thus it would be premature to conclude that donor phage receptors either are or are not universally essential for bacterial conjugation.

Although numerous studies indicated that donor pili are necessary for specific union formation and it could be inferred that the tip of the donor pilus interacted in some specific way with the recipient cell surface (*16, 29*), some of the more compelling evidence in support of these ideas has been recently provided by Ou and Anderson (*86, 88, 89*). They found that 10^{-3} M Zn^{2+} inhibited specific union formation but not later stages of conjugation (*88*) and, in confirmation of Tzagoloff and Pratt (*105*), demonstrated that 10^{-3} M Zn^{2+} inhibited attachment of donor-specific DNA phages which attach to the tips of donor pili but not of donor-specific RNA phages which attach to the sides of donor pili (*89*). Ou (*86*) very convincingly demonstrated by using a Coulter counter that addition of high multiplicities of donor-specific DNA phages to donor cells prior to mixing with recipient cells could completely abolish specific union formation whereas the addition of comparable multiplicities of donor-specific RNA phages had a much less dramatic effect. Thus, it now seems certain that the mechanism of involvement of donor pili in specific union formation includes a prerequisite interaction between the donor pilus tip and the recipient cell surface.

3) Roles of cell surface layers

Although the only antigenic difference so far detected between isogenic donor and recipient cells is due to the presence of donor pili on the donor (*49*), there is substantial evidence that the production of donor pili is not required for the expression of entry exclusion (*4, 85*; see Chapter 5) but is due to the activity of the *traS* gene which has nothing to do with pilus synthesis and function (*3, 120*). It would thus seem likely that donor and recipient cells differ by at least one other structural entity due to the *traS* gene. The product of this gene could either be incorporated directly into the donor cell surface or cause an enzymatic alteration of some structural element in the donor cell surface. In either case, the effect of inhibiting exchange of genetic information between donor cells would be the same.

In terms of the murein rigid layer of the cell envelope, its absence in donor cells (by treatment with penicillin in hypertonic medium) does not affect the synthesis of donor pili (*15*) and its absence in donor and recipient cells does not impair mating ability (*8*). Beard and Bishop (*8*) have found, however, that the absence of the murein layer in R^+ donor spheroplasts permits them to mate with R^+ donor cells as recipients at frequencies that are similar to those obtained when using R^- cells as recipients. Thus, removal of the murein layer of the donor parent abolishes entry exclusion whereas removal of the murein layer of the R^+ recipient permits normal expression of entry exclusion. Beard and Bishop therefore conclude that the product of the *traS* gene in the R^+ recipient is not part of the murein layer but must either interact with or be dependent upon the integrity of the murein layer of the donor parent.

The outer membrane of the donor cell surface is very much involved in the conjugational process since this is the location for the pool of pilus subunit proteins (9) and thus is probably the site for pilus assembly. A high percentage of Hfr and F+ mutants resistant to the phages T_3, T_4, T_7, and λ were found to be defective in conjugation (28) and since these phages have receptors in the outer membrane (103), these results suggested an involvement of the donor cell's outer membrane in conjugation. Recipients with similar phage resistance phenotypes were conjugation proficient, however (28). Subsequent studies demonstrated that some of these phage-resistant donor mutants, although defective as donors, possessed donor pili (Curtiss, unpublished). Watanabe et al. (111), in studies with rough mutants of *Salmonella typhimurium*, noted some impairment of donor ability when most carbohydrates were missing from the outer membrane lipopolysaccharide (LPS). Recipient ability of these same mutants, however, depended on the donor plasmid used and sometimes increased with loss of some carbohydrate moieties from the LPS and then decreased when the mutant lacked most of the LPS carbohydrate. Similar results on recipient ability of *E. coli* mutants lacking LPS carbohydrate moieties were obtained by Wiedemann and Schmidt (115). Monner et al. (80) found that mutations conferring high-level resistance to ampicillin (APC) were associated with changes in sensitivity to the "recipient-specific" phage ϕW, alterations in the carbohydrate composition of the LPS and reduced mating abilities of both Hfr donor and F⁻ recipient strains. The defects were associated with reduced union-forming ability which in the case of the Hfr mutants could be ascribed in part to the reduced plating efficiency of the donor-specific phage MS-2 although the attachment rate of MS-2 was only reduced twofold. Thus, it would appear that these mutations, like those described by Curtiss (28, unpublished), affected the function rather than the presence of donor pili.

Further insight into the involvement of recipient cell surface components in conjugation has been obtained by the isolation and characterization of conjugation-deficient (*con*⁻) mutants. Reiner (93) found that about 5% of the mutants resistant to the single-stranded DNA phage ST-1 were *con*⁻ and these were divided into two groups.

Group A mutants gave 10^4- to 10^6-fold reductions in recipient ability, were nonflagellated and gave rough colonies. Group B mutants gave 10- to 10^2-fold reductions in recipient ability, were temperature-sensitive, had increased sensitivity to deoxycholate and gave smooth colonies. Achtman (*2*) found by use of a Coulter counter that group B mutants did not form detectable frequencies of mating unions whereas group A mutants formed 30% as many unions as the *con⁺* parent. Skurray *et al.* (*102*) isolated *con⁻* recipients that were resistant to phage K3 and lacked outer membrane protein 3a (*99*). Although they found no pair formation with these mutants by using a modification of the de Haan and Gross (*48*) dilution procedure, Achtman (*2*) found a 70% reduction in union-forming ability by use of the Coulter counter; a result similar to that obtained with Reiner's group A mutants which are also resistant to phage K3. Manning and Reeves (*74*) have screened a large number of phage-resistant recipient mutants and found that several groups, presumably with alterations in LPS composition, were *con⁻*.

We (*31, 39, 40*; Falkinham and Curtiss, unpublished; Curtiss and Moody, unpublished) have isolated a large number of *con⁻* recipient mutants that possess a great diversity of phenotypes relative to phage, APC, fosfomycin, and sodium dodecylsulfate sensitivity, utilization of carbohydrate energy sources, ability to synthesize alanine and rates of growth. Among the mutants isolated were some similar in properties to those isolated by Monner *et al.* (*80*), Reiner (*93*) and Skurray *et al.* (*102*). One class is APC-resistant, phage K3-resistant and does not form specific unions as measured microscopically or by use of a Coulter counter; these are analogous to Reiner's group B mutants. Some of these mutants are defective in matings with donors possessing either F or I group conjugative plasmids whereas others are only defective in matings with F group donors. A second group is analogous to the K3-resistant group A mutants of Reiner and the *con⁻* mutants of Skurray *et al.*; they form specific unions which are very unstable. The more interesting and novel group of *con⁻* mutants, however, have defects which cause impairments in effective union formation, DNA transfer and stable inheritance of plasmid DNA. Many of these mutants have secondary phenotypic defects that are associated with lesions of the inner cell membrane.

Taken collectively, all these results indicate that the recipient and donor outer membrane and the recipient inner membrane are very important for conjugational DNA transfer and that the donor cell murein layer is necessary for the manifestation of the entry exclusion phenotype that is expressed by a donor strain when used as a recipient.

4)   Consequences of specific union formation

In Brinton's (15) pilus-conduction model for conjugational DNA transfer, the establishment of a specific union would be sufficient to permit DNA transfer. In the absence of positive evidence to support the pilus-conduction model and of circumstantial evidence against it, Curtiss (29) proposed the pilus-withdrawal model to provide a mechanism to bring donor and recipient cells into direct wall-to-wall contact to enable establishment of a conjugation tube or bridge through which DNA could be transferred. In this model, specific union formation as defined by deHaan and Gross (48) would be followed by effective union formation to yield wall-to-wall unions as first visualized by Anderson et al. (7).

Ou and Anderson (87), by use of micromanipulation techniques, have provided convincing evidence in support of the pilus-conduction model but noted that close mating pairs were twice as effective as loose mating pairs (those not in cell-to-cell contact and presumably connected by a donor pilus) in yielding genetic recombinants. They did not, however, indicate the relative frequencies with which loose and close pairs were observed nor the frequency of aggregates of donor and recipient cells although the observation of the latter class of mating unions was noted. It is thus not possible to calculate from their data an approximate value for the contribution of loose mating unions to the total recombinant yield.

Evidence compatible with but not proving the pilus-withdrawal model has been reviewed by Curtiss (29). Marvin and Hohn (76) independently proposed a pilus-withdrawal model to account for infection of donor cells by the filamentous donor-specific DNA phages and Jacobson (60) has provided evidence in support of this hypothesis. Bradley (11, 12) has also presented evidence for pilus withdrawal during RNA phage infection of Pseudomonas aeruginosa. Lawn and Meynell (69) found that addition of pilus-specific antibodies to donor cultures caused a marked increase in the number of donor pili per cell. They interpreted their data to indicate that pilus antibodies either prevented normal retraction of pili, therefore leading to an accumulation of extended pili or upset the normal equilibrium between pilus subunit proteins and assembled pili to cause an increase in assembled pili. Novotny and Fivest-Taylor (*83*) also presented evidence to indicate that donor pili retract into the donor cell by treatment of cells with 10^{-2} M CN^- and that low temperature, pilus-specific antiserum and attachment of donor-specific RNA phages blocked retraction.

Evidence for the occurrence of close mating unions has been obtained by Goldschmidt and Curtiss (unpublished) who demonstrated bidirectional exchange of sensitivity to bacteriophage λ between Hfr and F^- cells as a consequence of conjugation. Such exchange only occurred under conditions in which conjugation could take place and was manifested by the ability of λ to inhibit growth of nearly all cells of the λ-resistant minority parent after conjugation with the λ-sensitive majority parent. Their data therefore suggests that the *E. coli* outer membrane has some fluidity and plays an important role during bacterial conjugation. This latter conclusion is supported by the data described in the preceding section.

In summary, there is evidence that indicates that donor pili can act to transport DNA from donor to recipient cells and a much larger mass of data that indicates that the more common and efficient means for DNA transfer involves the formation of close cell-to-cell contact for effective unions. That *E. coli*, and presumably other conjugationally proficient organisms, should have two means to accomplish genetic transfer should not be too surprising since backup and/or alternate mechanisms for accomplishing a necessary objective are standard fare in biological organisms, even with regard to sexuality (*27*).

5) Nature of the mating signal relative to initiation of DNA transfer
Many individuals have postulated that initiation of the events leading to transfer of plasmid or chromosomal DNA in the donor parent occurs after and as a consequence of specific union formation. Thus it has been thought that such events are a result of an interaction between the tip of the donor pilus and a specific pilus tip receptor on the recipient cell surface (now believed to be composed of carbohydrate sidechains on the LPS and specific outer membrane proteins). Curtiss and Fenwick (*32*) have described the initial steps leading to transfer of the R_{64-11} plasmid as binding of cytoplasmic circular DNA molecules

to the donor cell inner membrane, action of an initiator protein (presumably an endonuclease encoded by the *traI* gene) to yield a structure capable of transferring a unique single strand of DNA to the recipient and the synthesis of a rifampin-sensitive product (presumably an RNA primer necessary to initiate conjugational DNA synthesis). In studies on the genetic transfer of the R_{64-11} plasmid in the presence or absence of rifampin, Curtiss (*30*) noted that development of resistance of R_{64-11} transfer to inhibition by rifampin commenced within 15 sec after mixing donor and recipient cells and was complete within 5 min. Parallel studies revealed that this resistance to rifampin developed about 5 min before comparable frequencies of specific unions were formed (as measured either by the dilution procedure of deHaan and Gross (*48*) or by use of a Coulter counter). Since rifampin completely inhibited RNA synthesis within 2 min after its addition in the R_{64-11} donor strain, it was concluded that initiation of events leading to conjugational transfer preceded the formation of specific unions. Attempts to detect a soluble factor produced by recipient cells were unsuccessful (Curtiss, unpublished). It was also observed that the frequency of R_{64-11} transfer decreased as the square of the dilution of the donor and recipient populations prior to mating and thus there was no indication of a chemotactic response leading to higher than expected frequencies of conjugation in dilute mating populations. It would thus appear that initiation of events leading to R_{64-11} transfer is caused by some type of unstable physical interaction between donor and recipient cells that does not immediately lead to a specific union.

2. Transfer

1) Products of conjugation

Early efforts to discern the mechanism of conjugational DNA transfer between cells of *E. coli* or other Enterobacteriaceae centered around the description of the molecular products of the process. To do this a variety of systems and techniques were utilized to identify donor cell DNA that had been transferred to a recipient. Analysis of DNA transferred from Hfr (*59*) or F' (*92*) cells grown in the presence of density isotopes prior to mating revealed that the transferred DNA was replicated at some time during the mating. Autoradiographic localization of radioactively labeled F (*53*) and Hfr chromosomal (*47*) DNA in re-

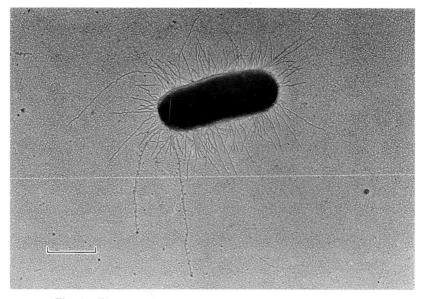

Fig. 1.   Electron micrograph of sex pili from *E. coli* ML3674 Hfr. Small particles are the male phages f_2 attached to the pili. Bar represents 1 μm. (Photographed by H. Hashimoto)

cipient cells suggested that recipients contained only a single strand of donor DNA synthesized prior to mating. Ohki and Tomizawa (*84*) showed that the strand complementary to the transferred donor DNA is synthesized in the recipient cell. Cohen *et al.* (*25, 26*) also found that F, F', and Hfr DNA isolated from DNA-deficient recipient minicells is single-stranded. To determine whether both strands of DNA in donor cells have equal probabilities of being transferred, Ohki and Tomizawa (*84*) and Rupp and Ihler (*96*) examined λ prophage DNA transferred to recipients from F' and Hfr donors. They found that each donor transferred a specific λ strand and that the strand transferred was dependent on the direction or polarity of F' or Hfr chromosome transfer to the recipient cell. From their data and available information about the orientation of λ prophage within the *E. coli* chromosome, they were able to conclude that the unique strand being transferred enters the recipient with its 5' terminus as the leading extremity. Vapnek and Rupp (*107*) ruled out the possibility that both strands of

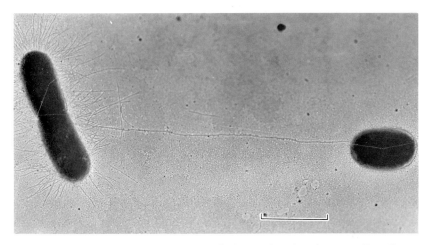

Fig. 2. Electron micrograph of the conjugation between *E. coli* ML3674 Hfr and *E. coli* JE2217 *pil⁻ fla⁻*. Bar represents 1 μm. (Photographed by H. Hashimoto)

donor DNA are transferred to recipient cells with a subsequent degradation of one unique strand when they confirmed that a unique strand of F DNA is transferred to recipients and demonstrated that its complement was conserved in the donor cells where it acted as a template for synthesis of a strand to replace the one transferred to recipients. Vapnek *et al.* (*109*) extended these findings by showing that both F-like and I-like R plasmids have the same pattern of asymmetric transfer and replication.

2) Kinetics of transfer

Donor cells which carry some temperature-sensitive mutations (*dnaB* (*ts*) and *dnaG(ts)*) that inhibit vegetative replication of both plasmid and chromosomal DNA at 42°C (*112*) are still able to carry out genetic transfer at restrictive temperatures (*10, 75*). Rather than transferring DNA in the absence of any DNA synthesis, such donors do synthesize DNA during matings at 42°C (*13, 14, 42, 75, 108*) and the majority of the replicated DNA is that synthesized to replace the strand being transferred to the recipient cells (*42, 108*). These findings not only show that there are differences between vegetative and conjugational

DNA replication but they reveal a method that can be used to study conjugation mechanisms within donor cells because *dnaB(ts)* donor cells can be used to specifically label the DNA synthesized to replace the strand being conjugationally transferred to a recipient (*108*). Fenwick and Curtiss (*42*) studied conjugational replication and transfer using R_{64-11}^+ *dnaB(ts)* donor cells and DNA-deficient recipient minicells. Minicells were utilized as recipients so that donors and recipients could be rapidly and efficiently separated when the matings were terminated. They found that all plasmids in all donor cells transferred the DNA single strand synthesized in the donors prior to mating to recipient minicells within the first 20 min of mating. Furthermore, R_{64-11} DNA synthesized in the donor during this first round of plasmid transfer (to replace the transferred strand) began to appear in the recipients 8 to 10 min after the matings started and after 30 min all plasmids had transferred on the average two single-stranded copies to the recipients. They calculated that R_{64-11} should only take 3 min to be transferred and from their data concluded that, although the plasmids were capable of transferring multiple copies of single-stranded DNA, the transfer must be discontinuous with a delay between the transfer of one copy and the next. Furthermore, the DNA they isolated from the recipient minicells was single-stranded and the length of monomeric R_{64-11} molecules or smaller, which was also taken as evidence that the unit of transfer was a single copy of the plasmid and thus that transfer was discontinuous. After 5 min of mating, 70 to 80% of the conjugationally replicated R_{64-11} DNA in the donor cells was associated with the inner cell membrane implicating this as the site of conjugational replication (Fenwick and Curtiss, unpublished). After 15 to 20 min, when all plasmids had undergone at least one round of transfer and replication, the fraction of conjugationally replicated R_{64-11} DNA attached to the inner cell membrane decreased to about 35% and the remainder was present as unattached open and closed circular plasmid molecules. Furthermore, when nalidixic acid, an antibiotic that stops both conjugational replication and transfer (*13, 26, 57*), was added to such a mating, it caused a dramatic increase in the amount of conjugationally replicated plasmid DNA that was membrane bound in the donor cells (*44*). This was taken as additional evidence that the site of conjugational DNA replication is the inner cell membrane. Another implication of these findings is that part of the discontinuous mode of R_{64-11} plasmid tranfer might involve the release of the plasmid from the membrane between rounds of conjugation replication and transfer.

Although data obtained for F and both F-like and I-like R plasmids (*41, 107–109*) are compatible with or support Fenwick and Curtiss' (*32, 42–44*) conclusions on the discontinuous transfer mechanism for R_{64-11}, data obtained by both Matsubara (*77*) and Ohki and Tomizawa (*84*) on F' transfer are not. Matsubara and Ohki and Tomizawa obtained evidence for the transfer of plasmid molecules to recipients that were several times the molecular weight of the F' plasmid isolated from the donor parent. Their data were therefore compatible with the rolling circle model of plasmid transfer proposed by Gilbert and Dressler (*46*). At this time it is not known whether these differences between transfer mechanisms for R and F' plasmids are real or are due to methodological differences.

3) Macromolecular requirements
As discussed above, there is a close relationship between DNA synthesis and DNA transfer during conjugation. There is evidence that donor cells must be able to initiate DNA synthesis to conjugationally transfer DNA (*94*) but that continued DNA synthesis is not necessary for the completion of conjugational chromosome transfer (*36, 58, 91, 98*). This initiation of conjugational DNA replication is thought to be controlled by the conjugative plasmid (*1*). The initiation of vegetative DNA replication in *E. coli* is dependent on the synthesis of proteins (*67*) and untranslated RNA (*68*). Fenwick and Curtiss (*43*) found that the addition of chloramphenicol to $R_{64-11}{}^{+}$ *dnaB(ts)* donors 5 min before they were mixed with recipient minicells did not impair their capacity to initiate conjugational transfer and replication. However, under these conditions only one round of plasmid transfer occurred. Thus the donor cells apparently contained all proteins necessary for conjugational transfer but one or more of them was consumed during the transfer of a single copy of the plasmid. This finding also confirms the discontinuous mode of transfer of this plasmid as proposed by Fenwick and Curtiss (*42*). Since the transfer genes of F are organized into a very large operon (*3*) and the time necessary to transcribe and translate such an operon should be much longer than those times observed for the initiation of conjugational transfer and replication, it is

not surprising to find that donor cells maintain a sufficient quantity of these gene products to initiate the process.

When Fenwick and Curtiss (*42*) exposed R_{64-11}^+ *dnaB* (*ts*) donors to rifampin 5 min before the addition of minicell recipients at 42°C, conjugational transfer and replication was blocked. However, a similar addition after the mating had begun did not inhibit the round of plasmid transfer that was underway but did prevent subsequent rounds of plasmid transfer. They therefore concluded that the initiation of conjugational transfer and replication requires the synthesis of an untranslated RNA which possibly serves as a primer for the initiation of DNA synthesis. However, Wilkins and Hollom (*118*) did not find that the initiation of F'-*lac* and Col I transfer from *dna*+ cells at 37°C was sensitive to rifampin. Unfortunately, neither Fenwick and Curtiss (*43*) or Curtiss (*30*) tested the effect of rifampin on inhibiting R_{64-11} plasmid transfer by *dnaB(ts)* donors mated at 37°C nor did Wilkins and Hollom (*118*) test the effects of rifampin on inhibiting F'-*lac* and Col I transfer either by *dnaB*+ donors at 42°C or by *dnaB* (*ts*) donors at 37 or 42°C. Thus these differences could be due to the plasmids studied, the chromosomal genotype of the plasmid donor or to differences in the experimental methodologies. In this regard, it should be mentioned that rifampin blocks RNA synthesis much more efficiently in strains with I group R plasmids than in strains with either F group R plasmids or no plasmids (*95*). Also, the *dnaB*+ gene product is thought to be involved in the initiation of DNA synthesis possibly by promoting the synthesis of an RNA primer (*50, 114*) but, as discussed above, conjugational DNA replication is not inhibited in *dnaB(ts)* donors under conditions which block the vegetative replication of conjugative plasmids and the chromosome. Since rifampin will block the initiation of conjugational replication of R_{64-11} in *dnaB(ts)* donors at 42°C (*43*) but not of F'-*lac* or Col I at 37°C in *dnaB*+ donors (*118*), it follows that RNA polymerase might be able to substitute for the *dnaB(ts)* gene product to promote the initiation of conjugational replication at 42°C but not of vegetative replication. If this is true, it would be expected that rifampin would not inhibit plasmid transfer by either *dnaB*+ donors or by *dnaB(ts)* donors mated at permissive temperatures.

Little is known about the DNA polymerase activity that is responsible for conjugational replication. Wilkins and Hollom (*118*) found that the presence of the *polA1* mutation in *dnaB(ts)* donors did not affect the conjugational replication of F'-*lac* or Col I so conjugational replication is not dependent on DNA polymerase I. In addition, Hirota and Nishimura (personal communication) found that an F'-*lac/polA1 polB1 dnaE(ts)* donor transfers F'-*lac* in matings at 42°C, although it loses its donor capabilities with prolonged incubations at 42°C. However, there are no data on either the amount of residual DNA synthesis by polymerases I, II, and III under these conditions or whether F'-*lac* transfer is accompanied by conjugational replication.

4) Driving forces for transfer
Cohen *et al.* (*26*) observed that different donor types transferred about the same amount of DNA to DNA-deficient minicells and subsequent research (*42, 62, 100, 101*) has confirmed this and demonstrated that the maximum length of single-stranded DNA transferred is about 50×10^6 daltons. This is about the maximum amount of DNA that can be forcefully transmitted to a recipient before it is necessary for effective homologous pairing between transmitted Hfr and long F' DNA and the comparable portion of the recipient chromosome to permit continuation of DNA transfer with an expenditure of energy on the part of the recipient (*36, 90*). Thus it would appear that the donor cell supplies the force to transfer short conjugative plasmids and the lead regions of long F' plasmids and of Hr chromosomes. Jacob *et al.* (*59*) proposed that the conjugational repplication of DNA in the donor cell is the driving force for transfer. Although it has been possible to demonstrate a very close correlation between the amount of DNA transferred to recipients and the amount of conjugational replication in donors (*42–44*), it is difficult to unambiguously show that transfer is dependent on replication. In fact, Sarathy and Siddiqi (*98*) have shown that Hfr chromosomal transfer can occur in the absence of any detectable DNA synthesis in *thyA dnaB(ts)* donor cells mated at 42°C in the presence of high concentrations of uracil. This, along with the requirement that donor cells be able to initiate DNA replication in order to commence conjugational transfer, might mean that the initiation event or, more specifically, the synthesis of an RNA primer could provide the force required to transfer DNA to a recipient cell (*30, 32*).

5) *Mobilization of other DNAs*

Conjugative plasmids can promote the transfer of nonconjugative plasmid and chromosome DNA. One way for this to occur is by formation of stable covalent linkages between the conjugative plasmid and chromosome to form Hfr donors (*18, 34, 61*) or between the conjugative and nonconjugative plasmids to form cointegrates (*23*). Although only 10 to 20% of the observed fertility of F+ cultures is the result of the formation of stable Hfr donors (*18, 34*), the majority of chromosome transfer from donors carrying most conjugative plasmids requires a functional *recA* gene product (*24, 81*). However, the *recA+* promoted recombination event might not have to be completed because chromosome mobilization due to recombination between homologous regions of F'-*lac* and the chromosome is only reduced slightly when the donors are *recB⁻* or *recC⁻* (*116*). The persistent but low levels of chromosome transfer from *recA⁻* donors and the *recA⁻* independent mobilization of the chromosome in donors carrying Col Ib*drd* and R₁*drd19* (*81*) demonstrate that mobilization can be promoted by host activities that are independent of *recA+* or by plasmid-determined mechanisms.

Nonconjugative plasmids and *tra⁻* conjugative plasmid mutants are often mobilized very efficiently by conjugative plasmids (*119*). In some instances this is due to stable integration of one plasmid into the other such as the fusion of a tetracycline resistance plasmid into the transfer factor *Δ* (*6, 79*). In other situations, however, efficient transfer of a nonconjugative plasmid such as Col E1 can be promoted by F without covalent linkage since Clowes (*22*) has demonstrated that donor strains carrying both plasmids can transfer either one or the other. In addition, Col E1 can be efficiently transferred by an F-*lac traI* mutant without transfer of the F-*lac* plasmid (*5*). The *traI* locus of F produces a plasmid-specific product which might have endonuclease activity to open the strand of F DNA to be transferred (see Chapter 5). Thus, the host cell or the Col E1 plasmid itself might provide a comparable activity. It is tempting to speculate that one of the three proteins in the Col E1 relaxation complex, which can cause a strand-specific nick in Col E1 DNA (*52*), might be necessary for Col E1 transfer. In this regard, it is also interesting to note that Col E1, which requires DNA polymerase I for vegetative replication, also requires that activity in the donor cell when it is being mobilized by

Col V but Col V is transferred in the absence of this polymerase (*65*). Nevertheless, there is still a paucity of information on the mechanism of nonconjugative plasmid transfer by conjugative plasmids since nothing is known about the conformation of mobilized plasmid DNA during transfer, whether it is double or single stranded and if single stranded, whether the single strand is unique or not. Until these questions are resolved, it is difficult to interpret the requirement for the *polA* gene product and to determine whether there is a relationship between vegetative replication of the nonconjugative plasmid and its mobilization and transfer by a conjugative plasmid.

3. Establishment

1) Fate of conjugationally transferred DNA

Since, as described above, conjugationally transferred plasmids enter recipient cells as linear single strands of DNA but exist in donor cells as double-stranded and covalently closed circular (CCC) molecules (*23*), they must undergo several processes in order to become established in the recipient transconjugant. Conjugationally transferred plasmid and chromosomal DNA initially attaches to the inner cell membrane of DNA-deficient recipient minicells (*101*). Since F, R, and short F′ DNA is partially converted to double-stranded DNA in minicells (*25, 26*; Curtiss, unpublished) but Hfr chromosomal and long F′ DNA are not (*26*) the attachment must precede the synthesis of the complement to the transferred strand of DNA. Falkow *et al.* (*41*) have followed conjugational DNA replication in recipient cells by measuring incorporation of radioactive thymine during matings between R_1drd19 donors unable to utilize thymine and UV-irradiated recipients unable to replicate their own DNA, a technique originally developed by Freifelder and Freifelder (*45*). They found that linear double-stranded molecules are synthesized while ·the plasmid DNA is associated with the inner cell membrane of the recipient. Later these molecules are converted to open circular molecules and finally they are released from the membrane as CCC plasmid DNA molecules. Dowman and Meynell (*38*) have shown that plasmids which are present in 1 to 2 copies per chromosome exist as CCC DNA molecules unattached to membrane structures except when they are vegetatively replicated. Thus the release of the conjugationally transferred and newly replicated DNA from the inner cell membrane probably represents the final unique step in the conjugational process.

Falkinham and Curtiss (unpublished) have isolated a number of *con⁻* recipient mutants which give nearly normal yields of recombinants in matings with Hfr donors but much reduced frequencies of inheritance of F′ and/or R_{64-11} plasmids. Some of these mutants must be defective in the initial establishment of plasmid DNA since the rare transconjugants inheriting a plasmid maintain stably (*39*). Others are defective in plasmid maintenance as well since they lose inherited plasmids at appreciable frequencies. Since some of these *con⁻* mutants that are defective in plasmid establishment and/or maintenance are fosfomycin resistant and/or are defective in utilizing numerous carbohydrates, it seems logical to believe that the primary lesions may be associated with defects in the inner cell membrane.

Since, under rapid growth conditions, recipient cells can have 3 to 4 chromosome equivalents per cell, multiple copies of a newly transferred plasmid must be generated if all progeny of that cell are to inherit the plasmid. This could be achieved by the transfer of multiple copies of plasmid DNA to a recipient or by the rapid replication of a plasmid within the recipient. Ohki and Tomizawa (*84*) and Matsubara (*77*) examined specifically labeled F′ and F DNA isolated from recipient cells and found DNA that sedimented more rapidly through sucrose gradients than linear monomers of the plasmid DNA molecules. They proposed that the donor cells transferred longer than unit length molecules by a continuous rolling circle type of mechanism. However, Fenwick and Curtiss (*42*) and Falkow *et al.* (*41*) only detected monomeric lengths of R_{64-11} and R_1drd19 DNA molecules in recipients and only one copy of R_{64-11} is conjugationally transferred in the absence of RNA or protein synthesis which indicates that R_{64-11} transfer is discontinuous (*43*). Hershfield (*54*) has suggested, based on measurements of R_1drd19-directed DNA, RNA and protein syntheses, that the plasmid replicates within a recipient cell to give 2 to 3 plasmids for each one transferred. Thus, the available data indicate that both I-like and F-like R plasmids are transferred in a discontinuous fashion as opposed to the continuous mechanism proposed for F and F′ transfer. In either case, however, all progeny of the transconjugant cell would be likely to inherit a plasmid copy.

2) Macromolecular requirements

Since the first step in the establishment of a plasmid in a recipient cell is its replication to a double-stranded form, several investigators have attempted to determine what cellular functions are required for that process. Wilkins and Hollom (*118*) have shown that conjugational replication of F'-*lac* and Col I in recipients is unaffected in *polA1* strains but is eliminated in *dnaE*(ts) mutants at 43°C. Thus it would appear that DNA polymerase III and not I or II is required to synthesize the complement to a transferred DNA strand. Kingsbury and Helinski (*65*) demonstrated that a functional DNA polymerase I is required for the establishment of Col E1 when it is conjugationally transferred by mobilization with ColV to a *polA*(ts) recipient at 43°C. However, as opposed to the conjugative plasmids being discussed, DNA polymerase I is also required for the vegetative replication of Col E1. There are conflicting reports about the effects of *dnaB*(ts) mutations on conjugational DNA synthesis in recipients. Bresler *et al.* (*14*) have shown that the *dnaB266* mutation has no effect on conjugational replication of Hfr chromosomal, or F', DNA in either donor or recipient cells but that the *dnaB43* mutation will inhibit conjugational replication of both types of donor DNA in the recipients and have no effect in the donors. However, Kielland-Brandt (*64*) has demonstrated the synthesis of β-galactosidase after the transfer of F' 13 to *dnaB43* recipient cells at the restrictive temperature and that would imply that the plasmid had become double-stranded. Furthermore, Vapnek and Rupp (*108*) have shown that F will form CCC molecules in *dnaB43* recipients at 43°C. The conjugational replication of F'-*lac* and Col I is also not restricted in *dnaB70* recipients (*118*). The inconsistencies cited might be reflections of the different genetic backgrounds within which the *dnaB*(ts) alleles were being studied, the different plasmids used and/or the variety of experimental procedures used.

There does not seem to be a requirement for protein synthesis directed by a conjugative plasmid for at least the early steps in its establishment. This is reasonable because the incoming DNA must have its complementary strand synthesized before it can be transcribed. The formation of double-stranded and CCC molecules of F is not inhibited in recipients by several antibiotics that inhibit RNA or protein synthesis (*56*). Conjugational DNA synthesis of F'-*lac* and Col I in *dna*+ recipients mated at 37°C is not inhibited by rifampin and in fact might be stimulated, whereas in *dnaB70* recipients mated at 42°C, rifampin inhibited the conjugational replication of F'-*lac* but stimulated that of Col I (*118*). As discussed above, the initiation of DNA synthesis might become sensitive to rifampin and thus dependent on RNA polymerase when the *dnaB* gene product cannot facilitate the synthesis of RNA primers for DNA synthesis. Col I replication may be insensitive to rifampin because it does not require or might provide its own priming activity. Wilkins (*117*) has demonstrated that derepressed I-like plasmids can suppress a *dnaG*(*ts*) mutant's inability to replicate DNA at 42°C even when they are conjugatively transferred to such recipients at restrictive temperatures. The *dnaG* gene product also plays a role in the initiation of DNA synthesis (*68*, *73*) and thus the Col I plasmid might not be dependent on the *dnaB* gene product or RNA polymerase because it provides it own activities for the initiation of DNA synthesis. Alternatively, some but not all conjugative plasmids may be transferred with an attached RNA primer from the donor as proposed by Curtiss and Fenwick (*32*) in one model for the mechanism of plasmid transfer. Such results point out the danger of drawing firm conclusions about the requirements for establishment from the results of any one experimental system when conjugative plasmids have such a diversity of properties.

3) *Incompatibility*
Conjugative plasmids can be grouped into incompatibility groups within which members of the same group will not stably coexist in the same host cell. As a part of the replicon hypothesis, Jacob *et al.* (*59*) suggested that closely related plasmids compete for the same replication or maintenance sites which because of their limited numbers do not allow stable coexistence of related plasmids. LeBlanc and Falkow (*70*) have shown that the conjugative replication of R_1drd19 in a UV-irradiated recipient possessing an incompatible plasmid does not go to completion but that a normal replicative intermediate of R_1drd19 accumulates in such cells. Hershfield *et al.* (*55*) demonstrated that this intermediate is associated with the inner cell membrane and thus the release of R_1drd19 DNA into the cytoplasm as CCC DNA is inhibited. Saitoh and Hiraga (*97*), however, found normal production of CCC molecules of F in phenocopies of recipient cells possessing incompatible plasmids but found that subsequent replication of the entering

plasmid was blocked. Such differences might reflect different responses of F and R₁*drd19* to the situation or of the neutralization of a cellular function required for the expression of incompatibility by UV irradiation or when phenocopies of cells carrying an incompatible plasmid are used as recipients.

4. Conclusion

In previous reviews on the mechanism of conjugation there has been an emphasis on the genetic aspects of the process and on DNA and DNA metabolism. We have therefore focused our attention on the increasing information that implicates the involvement of membrane structures and functions in all steps of conjugation. In our view the most notable observations are as follows: a) cytoplasmic plasmid DNA attaches to the donor cell inner membrane where it undergoes conjugational replication to replace the single strand of plasmid DNA being transferred to the recipient, b) the outer membranes of donor and recipient cells may fuse and exchange proteins as a consequence of effective union formation, c) mutational alteration of the donor cell outer membrane impairs donor pilus assembly or function and/or inhibits effective union formation, d) mutational alteration of the recipient cell outer membrane inhibits specific and/or effective union formation, e) mutational alteration of the recipient cell inner membrane inhibits specific and/or effective union formation or DNA transfer or plasmid establishment, and f) conjugationally transferred single-stranded DNA is initially found attached to the recipient cell inner membrane where a complementary strand is synthesized before it becomes a circular plasmid molecule in the cytoplasm. Thus, DNA transfer during conjugation may involve the unidirectional transport of a DNA-membrane complex from the donor to the recipient.

REFERENCES

1 Achtman, M. 1973. *Curr. Top. Microbiol. Immunol.*, **60**, 79–123.
2 Achtman, M. 1975. *J. Bacteriol.*, **123**, 505–515.
3 Achtman, M. and Helmuth, R. 1975. *In* Microbiology—1974, ed. by D. Schlessinger, pp. 95–103, American Society for Microbiology, Washington, D.C.

4 Achtman, M., Willetts, N., and Clark, A. J. 1971. *J. Bacteriol.*, **106**, 529–538.

5 Alfaro, G. and Willetts, N. S. 1972. *Genet. Res.*, **20**, 297–289.

6 Anderson, E. S. and Natkin, E. 1972. *Mol. Gen. Genet.*, **114**, 261–265.

7 Anderson, T. F., Wollman, E. L., and Jacob, F. 1957. *Ann. Inst. Pasteur*, **93**, 450–455.

8 Beard, J. P. and Bishop, S. F. 1975. *J. Bacteriol.*, **123**, 916–920.

9 Beard, J. P. and Connolly, J. C. 1975. *J. Bacteriol.*, **122**, 59–65.

10 Bonhoeffer, F. 1966. *Z. Vererbungsl.*, **98**, 141–149.

11 Bradley, D. E. 1972. *Biochem. Biophys. Res. Commun.*, **47**, 142–149.

12 Bradley, D. E. 1972. *J. Gen. Microbiol.*, **72**, 303–319.

13 Bresler, S. E., Lanzov, V. A., and Lukjaniec-Blinkova, A. A. 1968. *Mol. Gen. Genet.*, **102**, 269–284.

14 Bresler, S. E., Lanzov, V. A., and Likhachev, V. T. 1973. *Mol. Gen. Genet.*, **120**, 125–131.

15 Brinton, C. C., Jr. 1965. *Trans. N. Y. Acad. Sci.*, Ser II, **27**, 1003–1054.

16 Brinton, C. C., Jr. 1971. *CRC Crit. Rev. Microbiol.*, **1**, 105–160.

17 Brinton, C. C., Jr., Gemski, P., Jr., and Carnahan, J. 1964. *Proc. Natl. Acad. Sci. U.S.*, **52**, 776–783.

18 Broda, P. 1967. *Genet. Res.*, **9**, 35–47.

19 Brodt, P., Leggett, F., and Iyer, R. V. 1974. *Nature*, **249**, 856–858.

20 Caro, L. G. and Schnös, M. 1966. *Proc. Natl. Acad. Sci. U.S.*, **56**, 126–132.

21 Cavalli, L. L., Lederberg, J., and Lederberg, E. M. 1953. *J. Gen. Microbiol.*, **8**, 89–103.

22 Clowes, R. C. 1963. *Genet. Res.*, **4**, 162–165.

23 Clowes, R. C. 1972. *Bacteriol. Rev.*, **36**, 361–405.

24 Clowes, R. C. and Moody, E. E. M. 1966. *Genetics*, **53**, 717–726.

25 Cohen, A., Fisher, W. D., Curtiss, R., III, and Adler, H. I. 1968. *Proc. Natl. Acad. Sci. U.S.*, **61**, 61–68.

26 Cohen, A., Fisher, W. D., Curtiss, R., III, and Adler, H. I. 1968. *Cold Spring Harbor Symp. Quant. Biol.*, **33**, 635–641.

27 Comfort, A. 1972. The Joy of Sex. Crown Publishing Co., New York.

28 Curtiss, R., III. 1965. *J. Bacteriol.*, **89**, 28–40.

29 Curtiss, R., III. 1969. *Annu. Rev. Microbiol.*, **23**, 69–136.

30 Curtiss, R., III. 1975. *In* Microbial Drug Resistance, ed. by S. Mitsuhashi and H. Hashimoto, pp. 169–183, University of Tokyo Press, Tokyo / University Park Press, Baltimore and London.

31 Curtiss, R., III and Falkinham, J. O., III. 1974. Am. Soc. Microbiol. Annu. Meet. Abstr., p. 40.

32 Curtiss, R., III and Fenwick, R. G., Jr. 1975. *In* Microbiology—1974,

ed. by D. Schlessinger, pp. 156–165, American Society for Microbiology, Washington, D.C.

33 Curtiss, R., III and Stallions, D. R. 1967. *J. Bacteriol.*, **94**, 490–492.

34 Curtiss, R., III and Stallions, D. R. 1969. *Genetics*, **63**, 27–38.

35 Curtiss, R., III, Caro, L. G., Allison, D. P., and Stallions, D. R. 1969. *J. Bacteriol.*, **100**, 1091–1104.

36 Curtiss, R., III, Charamella, L. J., Stallions, D. R., and Mays, J. A. 1968. *Bacteriol. Rev.*, **32**, 320–348.

37 Davis, B. D. 1950. *J. Bacteriol.*, **60**, 507–508.

38 Dowman, J. E. and Meynell, G. G. 1973. *Biochim. Biophys. Acta*, **299**, 218–230.

39 Falkinham, J. O., III. 1975. *Genetics*, **80**, 529.

40 Falkinham, J. O., III and Curtiss, R., III. 1976. *J. Bacteriol.*, **126**, 1194–1206.

41 Falkow, S., Tompkins, L. S., Silver, R. P., Guerry, P., and LeBlanc, D. J. 1971. *Ann. N.Y. Acad. Sci.*, **182**, 153–171.

42 Fenwick, R. G., Jr. and Curtiss, R., III. 1973. *J. Bacteriol.*, **116**, 1212–1223.

43 Fenwick, R. G., Jr. and Curtiss, R., III. 1973. *J. Bacteriol.*, **116**, 1224–1235.

44 Fenwick, R. G., Jr. and Curtiss, R., III. 1973. *J. Bacteriol.*, **116**, 1236–1246.

45 Freifelder, D. R. and Freifelder, D. 1968. *J. Mol. Biol.*, **32**, 15–24.

46 Gilbert, W. and Dressler, D. 1968. *Cold Spring Harbor Symp. Quant. Biol.*, **33**, 473–484.

47 Gross, J. D. and Caro, L. G. 1966. *J. Mol. Biol.*, **16**, 269–284.

48 deHaan, P. and Gross, J. D. 1962. *Genet. Res.*, **3**, 251–272.

49 Harden, V. and Meynell, E. 1972. *J. Bacteriol.*, **109**, 1067–1074.

50 Hayes, S. and Szybalski, W. 1973. *In* Molecular Cytogenetics, ed. by B. A. Hamkalo and J. Papaconstantinou, pp. 277–283, Plenum Press, New York.

51 Hayes, W. 1953. *J. Gen. Microbiol.*, **8**, 72–88.

52 Helinski, D. R., Lovett, M. A., Williams, P. H., Katz, L., Kupersztoch-Portnoy, Y. M., Guiney, D. G., and Blair, D. G. 1975. *In* Microbiology —1974, ed. by D. Schlessinger, pp. 104–114, American Society for Microbiology, Washington, D.C.

53 Herman, R. K. and Forro, F. 1964. *Biophys. J.*, **4**, 335–353.

54 Hershfield, M. V. 1972. Ph. D. Dissertation. Georgetown University, Washington, D.C.

55 Hershfield, V., LeBlanc, D. J., and Falkow, S. 1973. *J. Bacteriol.*, **115**, 1208–1211.

56 Hiraga, S. and Saitoh, T. 1975. *J. Bacteriol.*, **121**, 1000–1006.
57 Hollom, S. and Pritchard, R. H. 1965. *Genet. Res.*, **6**, 479–483.
58 Ishibashi, M. 1966. *Japan. J. Genet.*, **41**, 75–89.
59 Jacob, F., Brenner, S., and Cuzin, F. 1963. *Cold Spring Harbor Symp. Quant. Biol.*, **28**, 329–348.
60 Jacobson, A. 1972. *J. Virol.*, **10**, 835–843.
61 Kahn, P. L. 1968. *J. Bacteriol.*, **96**, 205–214.
62 Khachatourians, G. G., Sheehy, R. J., and Curtiss, R., III. 1974. *Mol. Gen. Genet.*, **128**, 23–42.
63 Khatoon, H., Iyer, R. V., and Iyer, V. N. 1972. *Virology*, **48**, 145–155.
64 Kielland-Brandt, M. C. 1972. *Mol. Gen. Genet.*, **116**, 360–364.
65 Kingsbury, D.T. and Helinski, D.R. 1973. *J. Bacteriol.*, **114**, 1116–1124.
66 Lancaster, J. H. and Skvarla, J. J. 1970. *Nature*, **226**, 556–557.
67 Lark, K. G. 1969. *Annu. Rev. Biochem.*, **38**, 569–604.
68 Lark, K. G. 1972. *Nature New Biol.*, **240**, 237–240.
69 Lawn, A. M. and Meynell, E. 1972. *Nature*, **235**, 441–442.
70 LeBlanc, D. J. and Falkow, S. 1973. *J. Mol. Biol.*, **74**, 689–701.
71 Lederberg, J. 1956. *J. Bacteriol.*, **71**, 497–498.
72 Lederberg, J. and Tatum, E. L. 1946. *Cold Spring Harbor Symp. Quant. Biol.*, **11**, 113–114.
73 Louarn, J.-M. 1974. *Mol. Gen. Genet.*, **113**, 193–200.
74 Manning, P. A. and Reeves, P. 1975. *J. Bacteriol.*, **124**, 576–577.
75 Marinus, M. G. and Adelberg, E. A. 1970. *J. Bacteriol.*, **104**, 1266–1272.
76 Marvin, D. A. and Hohn, B. 1969. *Bacteriol. Rev.*, **33**, 172–209.
77 Matsubara, K. 1968. *J. Mol. Biol.*, **38**, 89–108.
78 Meynell, G. G. 1969. *Genet. Res.*, **13**, 113–115.
79 Milliken, C. E. and Clowes, R. C. 1973. *J. Bacteriol.*, **113**, 1026–1033.
80 Monner, D. A., Jonsson, S., and Boman, H. G. 1971. *J. Bacteriol.*, **107**, 420–432.
81 Moody, E. E. M. and Hayes, W. 1972. *J. Bacteriol.*, **111**, 80–85.
82 Novick, R. P. 1969. *Bacteriol. Rev.*, **33**, 210–235.
83 Novotny, C. P. and Fives-Taylor, P. 1974. *J. Bacteriol.*, **117**, 1306–1311.
84 Ohki, M. and Tomizawa, J. 1968. *Cold Spring Harbor Symp. Quant. Biol.*, **33**, 651–658.
85 Ohtsubo, E., Nishimura, Y., and Hirota, Y. 1970. *Genetics*, **64**, 173–188.
86 Ou, J. T. 1973. *J. Bacteriol.*, **114**, 1108–1115.
87 Ou, J. T. and Anderson, T. F. 1970. *J. Bacteriol.*, **102**, 648–654.
88 Ou, J. T. and Anderson, T. F. 1972. *J. Bacteriol.*, **111**, 177–185.
89 Ou, J. T. and Anderson, T. F. 1972. *J. Virol.*, **10**, 869–871.
90 Paul, A. V. and Riley, M. 1974. *J. Mol. Biol.*, **82**, 35–56.

91 Pritchard, R. H. 1965. *In* Genetics Today (Proc. XI Int. Congr. Genet.), pp. 55–78, Pergamon Press, London.

92 Ptashne, M. 1965. *J. Mol. Biol.*, **11**, 829–838.

93 Reiner, A. M. 1974. *J. Bacteriol.*, **119**, 183–191.

94 Roeser, J. and Konetzka, W. A. 1964. *Biochem. Biophys. Res. Commun.*, **16**, 326–331.

95 Romero, E., Riva, S., Fietta, A. M., and Silvestri, L. G. 1971. *Nature New Biol.*, **234**, 56–58.

96 Rupp, W. D. and Ihler, G. 1968. *Cold Spring Harbor Symp. Quant. Biol.*, **33**, 647–650.

97 Saitoh, T. and Hiraga, S. 1975. *J. Bacteriol.*, **121**, 1007–1013.

98 Sarathy, P. V. and Siddiqi, O. 1973. *J. Mol. Biol.*, **78**, 443–451.

99 Schnaitman, C. A. 1974. *J. Bacteriol.*, **118**, 442–453.

100 Sheehy, R. J., Orr, C., and Curtiss, R., III. 1972. *J. Bacteriol.*, **112**, 861–869.

101 Shull, F. W., Jr., Fralick, J. A., Stratton, L. P., and Fisher, W. D. 1971. *J. Bacteriol.*, **106**, 626–633.

102 Skurray, R. A., Hancock, R. E. W., and Reeves, P. 1974. *J. Bacteriol.*, **119**, 726–735.

103 Tamaki, S., Sato, T., and Matsuhashi, M. 1971. *J. Bacteriol.*, **105**, 968–975.

104 Tomoeda, M., Inuzuka, M., and Date, T. 1975. *Prog. Biophys. Mol. Biol.*, **30**, 23–56.

105 Tzagoloff, H. and Pratt, D. 1964. *Virology*, **24**, 373–380.

106 Valentine, R. C., Silverman, P. M., Ippen, K. A., and Mobach, H. 1969. *Adv. Microb. Physiol.*, **3**, 1–52.

107 Vapnek, D. and Rupp, W. D. 1970. *J. Mol. Biol.*, **53**, 287–303.

108 Vapnek, D. and Rupp, W. D. 1971. *J. Mol. Biol.*, **60**, 413–424.

109 Vapnek, D., Lipman, M. B., and Rupp, D. W. 1971. *J. Bacteriol.*, **108**, 508–514.

110 Walmsley, R. H. 1973. *J. Bacteriol.*, **114**, 144–151.

111 Watanabe, T., Arai, T., and Hattori, T. 1970. *Nature*, **225**, 70–71.

112 Wechsler, J. A. and Gross, J. D. 1971. *Mol. Gen. Genet.*, **113**, 273–284.

113 Werquin, M., Martin, G., and Guillanme, J. B. 1970. *Ann. Inst. Pasteur-Lille*, **21**, 25–32.

114 Wickner, S., Wright, M., and Hurwitz, J. 1974. *Proc. Natl. Acad. Sci. U.S.*, **71**, 783–787.

115 Wiedemann, B. and Schmidt, G. 1971. *Ann. N.Y. Acad. Sci.*, **182**, 123–125.

116 Wilkins, B. M. 1969. *J. Bacteriol.*, **98**, 599–604.

117 Wilkins, B. M. 1975. *J. Bacteriol.*, **122**, 899–904.
118 Wilkins, B. M. and Hollom, S. E. 1974. *Mol. Gen. Genet.*, **134**, 143–156.
119 Willetts, N. S. 1972. *Annu. Rev. Genet.*, **6**, 257–268.
120 Willetts, N. S. 1974. *J. Bacteriol.*, **118**, 778–782.

7 PHYSIOLOGY OF R FACTORS

Kenji HARADA and Susumu MITSUHASHI
Department of Microbiology, School of Medicine, Gunma University, Maebashi, Japan

The R plasmid consists of the two main genetic elements governing both the autonomous activities of plasmid and the determinants responsible for drug resistance. The fascinating properties of plasmid autonomy are the replication, self-regulation and the conjugal transferability of itself. The host bacteria carrying R plasmid acquire an ability to promote the chromosome transfer, called maleness, although bacteria themselves have no genetic determinants responsible for maleness on their chromosome. An ability of R plasmid to confer drug resistance on its host has become a big problem in medical and pharmaceutical fields because of the rapid spread of drug-resistant strains and of the repealing drug effectiveness against bacteria. The appearance of R plasmid has also offered us the following problems: the origin of the drug resistance determinants and the association of plasmid with the determinants governing drug resistance. The physiological studies of R plasmid, in addition to the molecular and genetic studies of R plasmid, tell us the most important biological properties of R plasmid and give us the materials to solve the plasmid problems in practical and fundamental research fields.

1. *Conjugal Transfer of R Plasmids*

The most important properties of R plasmids are their conjugal transmissibility, autonomous replication, and wide host range (*17, 37*). Conjugal transfer of R factor is demonstrated by the following facts: (a) transmission of resistance is not mediated by transduction, transformation, or filtrable agents (*3, 18, 19, 43*); (b) the transmission of drug resistance between *Escherichia coli* strains or between *Shigella* and *E. coli* strains, takes place regardless of the polarity of the F factor, indicating that this type of drug resistance is transferred without any relation to the transfer of the host chromosome and that the genes on the transmissible agent are not located on the host chromosome (*43*); (c) the transmission of drug resistance is interrupted by treatment of the mixed culture in a blender (*69*).

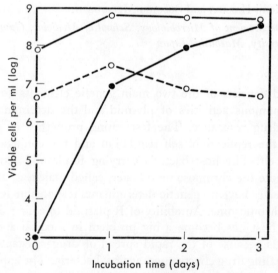

Fig. 1. Conjugal transfer of R factor. Donor, *S. flexneri* 3a R₁₁ (TC. CM. SM. SA)⁺; recipient, *E. coli* 0-26. Exponential phase of cultures of both donor and recipient in broth was mixed. At appropriate time of incubation in static culture the number of each donor and recipient cells was counted on agar plates and recipient cells which acquired drug resistance by infection with R factor were counted on the selection plate containing CM. —O— recipient; --O-- donor; —●— R⁺ recipient.

Mixed incubation of a small number of R+ cells with a large number of sensitive recipient cells results in the rapid acquisition of the R factor by a majority of the recipient cells (Fig. 1).

The R plasmids are transferable from the donor cells at higher frequencies during the early stationary phase than from those in the late stationary growth phase. Transfer frequency of R factors is decreased by aging the donor cells in liquid culture at the stationary phase of growth, but the transferability at high frequency is regained when the donor cells are inoculated into fresh culture medium. It

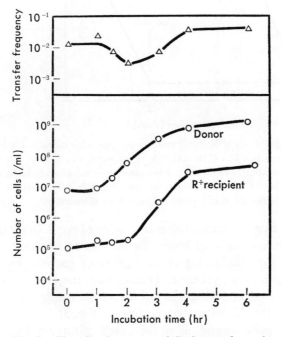

Fig. 2. Transfer frequency of R factors from donors at various growth phase. Donor, W4861 *pur⁻ lac⁻* R_{10}^+; recipient, 58-161 *met⁻*F⁻. Both donor and recipient were inoculated in brain heart infusion (BHI) broth and incubated at 37°C. Each donor and recipient culture was diluted 100-fold with fresh BHI broth and incubated at 37°C with shaking. Each donor culture at various growth phase times was mixed with 3.5-hr culture of the recipient, and incubated at 37°C with shaking. After 1 hr of mixed culture, R+ recipient cells were selected on minimal agar plate containing CM (25 μg/ml), lactose (1%), and methionine (50 μg/ml).

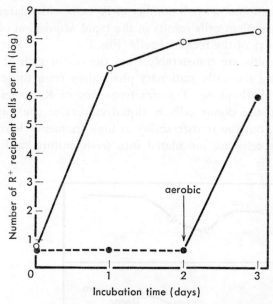

Fig. 3. Inhibition of R factor transfer by anaerobic culture. Donor, *S. flexneri* 3a R_{11}(TC. CM. SM. SA)+; recipient, *E. coli* 0-26. Overnight broth cultures of donor and recipient were mixed and incubated at 37°C. One of the mating mixtures was placed in a Thunberg tube from which the air was removed. ○ aerobic; ● anaerobic.

should be noted that the transmission frequency of the R factor during the early logarithmic phase of host cells is three to five times lower than at the late (or middle) logarithmic phase of growth (Fig. 2), a phenomenon which is not yet clear. Transmission frequency of R factors is also decreased when a mixed culture of both donor and recipient cells is placed under anaerobic conditions (Fig. 3).

Effect of temperature and pH of the mixed culture on the transfer of R factors was reported by Akiba and Iwahara (4), who indicated that the optimal temperature for R transfer is between 37 and 42°C and optimal pH for R transfer is 7.2. According to results reported from our laboratory (48), the optimal pH for the transmission of R factors is 7.5 and the optimal temperature is 37°C. Changes in both incubation temperature and pH greatly affect the transmission of R factors (Figs. 4 and 5).

Observing that the genetic structure of the *E. coli* chromosome is

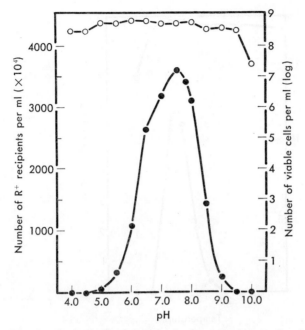

Fig. 4. Optimal pH of the mixed culture for the transfer of R factor. ● R⁺ conjugants which acquired R factor; ○ total number of bacterial cells in the mixed culture. See legend at Fig. 1.

circular, the first step of conjugal transfer of chromosomal DNA involves a breakage of the circular structure. Subsequently, the resulting linear structure is transferred (33). It was later discovered that the chromosome of *E. coli* K12 strain is physically circular and that the breakage of this structure is a necessary step for transfer. Two models have been presented for the conjugal transfer of DNA: (a) transfer of the DNA after completion of its replication in a donor cell (2), and (b) transfer of the DNA during replication (35) (see also reviews; 15, 59). Recent findings strongly suggested that single-stranded DNA is transferred during mating (10, 52, 58, 67).

One can distinguish three main stages in the transfer of an R factor. The first stage, the formation of specific pairing, extends from the moment when both donor and recipient cells meet to the time a mating bridge is formed for the transfer of the R factor genetic material. The second stage, or the transfer of the genetic material of the R

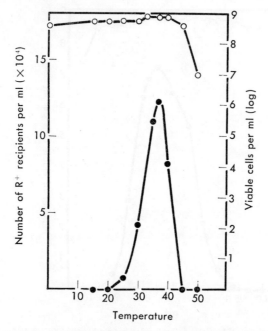

Fig. 5. Optimal temperature of mixed culture for the transfer of R factor. ● R⁺ conjugants which acquired R factor; ○ total number of bacterial cells in the mixed culture. See legend at Fig. 1.

factor, takes place through the mating bridge. The third, or pheno-typic expression of genetic material, takes place inside the recipient bacterium, to which the genetic material has been transferred. Replication and transfer of R plasmids are described in Chapters 5, 6, 8.

A cross *E. coli* W4861 R⁺ × *E. coli* 58-161 was carried out under usual conditions. As shown in Fig. 6, a linear relationship was observed between the number of donor cells in the mixed culture and that of R⁺ conjugants which acquired R factors with a wide range of from 10^5 to 10^9 of the donor cells, under conditions in which the number of recipient cells was kept nearly constant (5×10^8 to 10^9 organisms per ml). These data show that the transmission frequency of an R_{10} factor under such conditions is nearly constant (2×10^{-2}). These facts can be accounted for by postulating that the transfer of an R plasmid takes place as a single event and an epidemic spread of R plasmids does not take place within 60 min of mixing the cultures under these

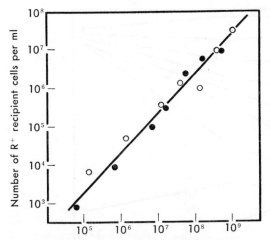

Fig. 6. Effect of the number of donor cells in mixed culture on the transmission frequency of an R factor. Donor, *E. coli* W4861 *pur⁻* R_{10}(TC. CM. SM. SA)⁺; recipient, *E. coli* 58-161 *met⁻*. Each overnight donor and recipient culture was diluted 100-fold with broth and incubated at 37°C with shaking. After 3.5 hr of incubation, a donor culture was serially diluted with a recipient culture (1×10^9 organisms/ml) and the mixed cultures were incubated at 37°C with gentle shaking. After 1 hr of incubation, R⁺ recipient cells were selected by plating on ALGa agar plate containing methionine and CM. Two experiments (● and ○) are shown in the figure.

conditions. Consequently, it may be concluded that one cell out of 50 $R_{10}{}^+$ donor cells is a competent donor for such conjugal process.

The effect of the number of donor cells in mixed culture on the transmission frequency was then investigated. As shown in Fig. 7, the transmission of the R factor did not take place when the donor of the R factor was diluted out below 10^3 per ml out of a total of 10^9 cells in mixed culture.

In the studies of the transmissibility of drug resistance, we have noticed that the transmission frequency of resistance is manifold; some donors have high frequency of transmission and some very low. The frequencies of conjugal transfer of R factor are generally lower than those of F factor in *E. coli* K12, which range from 10^{-2} to 10^{-5} per donor cell at 37°C for 1 hr in the *E. coli* K12 strain system. Similarly,

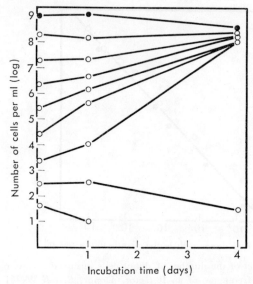

Incubation time (days)

Fig. 7. Dilution effect of donor cells on the transfer frequency of R factor. Donor, *E. coli* 0-26R$_{10}^+$; recipient, *E. coli* 0-26. Overnight culture of R$^+$ cells was diluted serially with overnight culture of R$^-$ cells and incubated at 37°C. Number of R$^+$ cells were examined at indicated days. ● number of the total cells; ○ number of the R-factor resistant cells.

TABLE I. Donor and Recipient Ability of R Factor

Donor	Recipient		
	S. flexneri 2a	*E. coli* K12 F$^-$	*S. newington*
S. flexneri 2a	1.2×10^{-3}	3.6×10^{-2}	2.0×10^{-9}
E. coli K12 F$^-$	4.6×10^{-3}	7.4×10^{-2}	1.0×10^{-9}
S. newington	5.4×10^{-4}	1.2×10^{-4}	1.5×10^{-4}

R$_{10}$(TC. CM. SM. SA) was used. Conditions for conjugal transfer, see legend at Fig. 1. Number indicates the transmission frequency of R factor and is expressed as the number of the R$^+$ conjugants per number of donor cells.

the recipient ability to accept R factors is manifold in the various recipient strains used. A representative result is shown in Table I.

The ability to donate an R factor is presently explained as the ability to form sex-pilus (*40, 41*). Ozeki *et al.* (*54, 62*) found that Col factors can be transferred with very high frequency by cells which have just received the factors, whereas cells carrying the factors are normally poor donors. They obtained a population which contained a high ratio of competent donor cells by growing a small number of Col$^+$ cells with a large number of sensitive cells overnight, then diluting the mixed cells culture in fresh medium and incubating for 2 hr. Similarly, the frequency of R-factor transfer can be as high as approximately 100% in these cells which have newly acquired the R factors. Such populations are called HFRT (high frequency resistance transfer) (75, 76) in analogy with the term of HFCT (high frequency colicin transfer) (54, 62). The competent cells contained in HFRT lose their donor competence after several generations, although they still retain the R factors and the drug resistance phenotype.

To investigate the kinetics of R transfer, *i.e.*, specific pairing between donor and recipient cells, transfer of genetic material, and phenotypic expression of the R factor, a time course experiment on R-factor transfer was carried out (48). It is well known that blender treatment breaks the specific pairing, or effective contact (34), between bacteria of donor and recipient types (Fig. 8).

The line L_1 intersects the abscissa at a and does not pass through the origin. The time t_1, an interval between a and the origin, means the minimal time to form an effective contact between donor and recipient cells. Under the conditions described in the text, the time t_1 for the transfer of R factor was 2 min in both crosses, *E. coli* W4861 R$^+$ × *E. coli* 58-161 and *Shigella flexneri* 2a R$^+$ × *E. coli* 58-161. The line L_2, time course for the transfer of R factor after blending, intersects the abscissa at b and the time t_2, an interval between b and the origin, means the minimal time to transfer genetic material of the R factor after contact has been established. The time t_2 in the two crosses described above was 4 and 12 min, respectively, after the cells were placed in contact. The line L_1 intersects the line L_2 at 15 min after mixing.

This indicates that the transfer of the genetic material of the R factor, in a cross *E. coli* W4861 R$^+$ × *E. coli* 58-161, is completed within 15 min after the cells were placed in contact and since the blender treatment does not interrupt its transfer despite the break in pairing between bacteria of donor and recipient types.

Finally, the third step of R transfer, *i.e.*, the phenotypic expres-

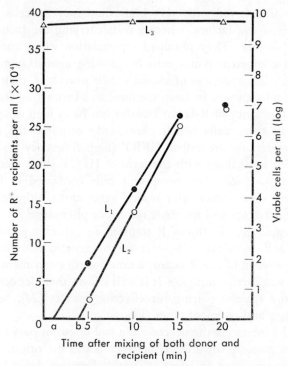

Fig. 8. The kinetics of R factor transfer. Donor, *E. coli* W4861 *pur*-R_{10}(TC. CM. SM. SA)+; recipient, *E. coli* 58-161 *met*-. Each overnight broth culture of the donor and recipient was diluted 100-fold with fresh BHI broth and incubated at 37°C with shaking. After 3.5 hr of incubation, both donor (5.5×10^9 organisms/ml) and recipient (6.1×10^9 organisms/ml) at exponential phase were mixed in equal parts and incubated at 37°C with gentle shaking. At appropriate time intervals, the sample was withdrawn and plated on ALGa agar containing methionine (10 μgs/ml) and CM (12.5 μg/ml) to select the R+ conjugants (line L_1). A line L_2 indicates the time course of R+ conjugants when plated on selective media after blender treatment for 30 sec at 15,000 rpm. A line L_3 indicates the number of total cells.

sion of the transferred R factor was investigated. The strains of donor (*S. flexneri* 2a R+) and recipient (*E. coli* 58-161 *met*-) were inoculated into brain heart infusion (BHI) broth. After overnight incubation at 37°C, each of the donor and recipient cultures was diluted 100-fold with BHI broth and again incubated at 37°C for 3.5 hr with shaking.

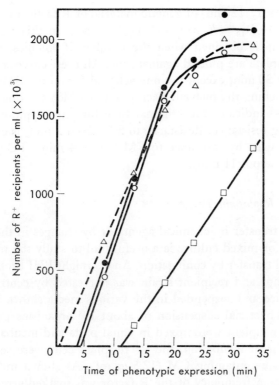

Fig. 9.   The kinetics of phenotypic expression of drug resistance following infection with R factor. Donor, *S. flexneri* 2a 1144 R_{10} (TC. CM. SM. SA)$^+$; recipient, *E. coli* 58-161.   △ SA;   ● CM;   ○ TC;   □ SM.

The donor (1.4×10^9 organisms/ml) and the recipient (2.7×10^9 organisms/ml) cultures in exponential phase of growth were mixed in equal parts. After shaking for 10 min at 37°C, the mixture was diluted 1,000-fold with the medium ALGa (medium A containing lactose and glutamic acid, *11*) containing methionine (10 μg/ml) to prevent and recipient cells. At appropriate time intervals thereafter, samples were withdrawn and plated on ALGa agar medium containing methionine (10 μg/ml) and each of four drugs: tetracycline (TC) (12.5 μg/ml), chloramphenicol (CM) (12.5 μg/ml), streptomycin (SM) (25 μg/ml), and sulfanilamide (SA) (50 μg/ml). The results are shown in Fig. 9.

The time 0 in the figure indicates, as stated earlier, the minimal transmission time (t_2, 12 min) of genetic material of R factor in a cross *S. flexneri* 2a 1144 $R_{10}{}^+ \times E.$ *coli* 58-161. As is seen in this figure, a linear relationship is obtained when the number of colonies formed on the selective plate are plotted against time. All these curves reach a plateau at about 30 min, except the one selected for on the SM plate, which delays reaching the plateau. Each point at which the line intersects the abscissa indicates the minimal time for phenotypic expression of each drug resistance. Resistance to SA (about 2 min) is expressed earliest, followed by resistance to CM (about 4 min), TC (about 5 min) and SM (about 11 min).

2.   Inhibition of R-plasmid Transfer

Inhibition of R transfer by chemical agents or by changes in the various conditions for mixed culture is a useful tool to study the mechanisms of plasmid transfer by conjugation. An overnight BHI broth culture of each donor and recipient strain was harvested by centrifugation, washed twice and suspended in the various media shown in the table to make a bacterial suspension of about 10^8 organisms per ml. The donor and recipient were mixed in equal parts and incubated at 37°C. After 24 hr of incubation, the R^+ recipient cells were selected on an ALGa plate containing CM (12.5 μg/ml). As shown in Table II, the transmission frequency of the R factor was markedly reduced in saline with or without glucose and in a synthetic medium lacking glucose, whereas its transfer was restored in a synthetic medium with

TABLE II.   Transfer Frequency of R Factor in the Various Media for Mixed Culture

Media for mixed culture	Transfer frequency[a]
BHI broth	1
Medium A +0.1% glucose	0.19
Medium A	$< 10^{-5.4}$
Saline +0.1% glucose	$< 10^{-5.4}$
Saline	$< 10^{-5.4}$

Donor, *S. flexneri* 3a R_{11}(TC. CM. SM. SA)$^+$; recipient, *E. coli* 0-26. BHI, brain heart infusion broth; medium A (*11*) consists of 0.8% $Na_2HPO_4 \cdot 12H_2O$, 0.2% KH_2PO_4, 0.05% sodium citrate$\cdot 3H_2O$, 0.01% $MgSO_4 \cdot 7H_2O$, and 1.0% $(NH_4)_2SO_4$.
[a] Relative value.

TABLE III. Inhibition of R Factor Transfer by Various Metabolic Inhibitors

Inhibitor	Concentration of inhibitor (M)	Inhibition of transfer (in percent of control)
KCN	10^{-3}	99
Na malonate	10^{-3}	91
Dinitrophenol	10^{-3}	93
NaAsO$_2$	10^{-3}	91
NaF	5×10^{-3}	73
Monoiodoacetate	10^{-4}	63
Control	—	0

Donor, *S. flexneri* 3a R$_{11}$(TC. CM. SM. SA)$^+$; recipient, *E. coli* 0-26. Overnight BHI broth cultures of donor and recipient were mixed and incubated at 37°C with addition of inhibitors. After overnight incubation, R$^+$ recipient cells were selected on ALGa agar containing CM (12.5 μg/ml).

glucose as well as in BHI broth (*48*). When the mixed culture in BHI broth was placed in a Thunberg tube, from which air was removed with a vacuum pump, the transfer of the R factor did not take place. It was, however, rapidly restored when brought back to aerobic conditions (Fig. 3).

To know the mechanism of R-factor transfer, various metabolic inhibitors were added to the mating mixture of donor and recipient (*12, 48*). The concentration of inhibitors used in this experiment allowed the growth of donor and recipient cells. As shown in Table III, potassium cyanide markedly inhibited the transfer of R factors. Also, malonate, 2, 4-dinitrophenol, and sodium azide, *i.e.*, all inhibitors of oxidative phosphorylation, reduced the transfer to about one-tenth of that of the control.

The inhibitors of glycolysis, such as sodium fluoride and mono-iodoacetate, did not inhibit the R-factor transfer to any appreciable extent. From these results it is concluded that the transfer of R factor requires the energy supplied by oxidative phosphorylation; but it still remains to be investigated as to which process in conjugal transfer is inhibited, *i.e.*, effective contact, transfer of genetic materials, or expression of the transferred genetic material.

It was reported by Goss *et al.* (*16*) that nalidixic acid (NA) (1-ethyl-1,4-dihydro-7-methyl-4-oxo-1,8-naphthyridine-3-carboxylic acid) inhibits specifically the synthesis of DNA in *E. coli* but has little

TABLE IV. Inhibition of R Factor Transfer by Nalidixic Acid (NA)

Concentration of NA (μg/ml)	Inhibition of transfer (in percent of control)
0 (control)	0
6.25	27
12.5	26
25.0	44
50.0	53
100.0	82

Donor, *E. coli* W4861 *pur*⁻ R_{10}(TC. CM. SM. SA)⁺; recipient, *E. coli* 58-161 *met*⁻. Overnight BHI broth cultures of donor and recipient were mixed in equal parts with or without addition of NA, and incubated at 37°C. After 1 hr of incubation, R⁺ recipient cells were selected on ALGa agar containing methionine (10 μg/ml) and CM (12.5 μg/ml).

effect on protein and ribonucleic acid synthesis. The inhibition of DNA synthesis in *E. coli* was observed after exposure to NA for 10 min. It was also found that NA was shown to stop chromosomal transfer in F-mating by the inhibition of DNA synthesis even when the transfer of chromosome has already begun before NA was added (*1, 30*).

From these results we examined the effects of NA on the transfer of R factors. NA was added to the mating mixture when the donor and recipient cells were placed in contact. As seen in Table IV, NA had only a slight effect on the transfer of the R factor even at high concentrations. In contrast, a marked effect on the transfer of the R factor was observed when the donor strain was preliminarily treated with NA before being placed in the mating mixture, and, successively, the mating mixture was treated with the same concentration of the drug (Table V).

The marked inhibition of transfer was observed after exposure of the donor strain to NA at 10 μg/ml for 10 min, whereas to only 3% inhibition was seen in the control (*48, 49*).

It is noted, however, that even under the above-mentioned conditions, that is when NA at a high concentration (10 μg/ml) is applied for 10 min or more before mating and successively thereafter, the transfer of R factor still proceeds though at a rate of less than 1/1,000 of that of the control. This may be accounted for by the assumption that there are two types of R factor in the cell: one is incompetent for

TABLE V. Transfer Inhibition of R Factor by Pretreatment of Donor Cells with Nalidixic Acid (NA)

Time of NA treatment before mixing (min)	R^+ recipients obtained per donor cell	Transfer frequency (relative rate)
Control	1.5×10^{-2}	1
0	4.9×10^{-4}	3.3×10^{-2}
10	3.2×10^{-5}	2.1×10^{-3}
20	2.4×10^{-5}	1.6×10^{-3}
30	4.3×10^{-5}	2.9×10^{-3}
60	1.0×10^{-5}	6.7×10^{-4}

Donor, *E. coli* W4861 *pur*$^-$ R_{10}(TC. CM. SM. SA)$^+$; recipient, *E. coli* 58-161 *met*$^-$. Before mixing both donor and recipient cells, donor cells were pretreated with NA (10 μg/ml) for various time intervals shown in the table. The same concentration of NA as in the pretreatment was added to the mixed culture. After 1 hr of incubation with gentle shaking at 37°C, R^+ recipient cells were selected on ALGa agar containing methionine and CM.

transfer but becomes transferable when its replication takes place, and the other is competent for transfer because of the incompletion of its ring closure. The former takes the major part of the R factor in the cell and its transfer is inhibited by NA or by the inhibition of DNA synthesis, while the latter is not. Mitomycin C, an inhibitor of DNA synthesis, also inhibited the transfer of R factor and markedly reduced the number of viable cells of both donor and recipient in the mating mixture. The effect of adenine or tryptophan starvation on the transfer of R factor was investigated. The transfer of the R factor does not change when the rate of protein synthesis in the donor cells of *E. coli* JE346 *ade*$^-$*trp*$^-$B$_1$$^-R^+$ is lowered by tryptophan starvation. However, the rate of R-factor transfer is reduced to about 5% of the control when the rate of DNA synthesis in the donor cell population is lowered by adenine starvation. These facts show that the inhibition of DNA synthesis affects the transfer of R factor but the inhibition of protein synthesis does not (*48*). It was reported that R-factor transfer was inhibited by cholic acid derivatives which do not show any antibacterial activities on the both donor and recipient cells (*5*).

3. Formation of Pili by R Factors

Bacterial cells harboring F(or F′) factors are distinguished from F$^-$

cells by their ability to conjugate and donate chromosomal material to female cells. Bacteria carrying F factors produce a specific antigen absent from F⁻ cells (53) and are sensitive to a group of F-specific RNA phages (38, 60). These genetic properties indicate that F(or F') factor determines the formation of a surface structure responsible for (a) conjugation, (b) serological specificity, and (c) absorption of specific male phages. The phage receptor was later identified as a specific pilus (8, 9).

It has been reported that F and R factors differ in many genetic properties: (a) wider host range of the R factor than that of F(17, 37), (b) chromosomal transfer with R occurs at a very low frequency (63), (c) the F antigen is apparently absent from R⁺ cultures that are insensitive to the F-specific phage (29). Moreover, some R factors inhibit the ability of the F factor: when R factor is transferred to a cell carrying F factor, the properties of the cell dependent on the F factor disappear, and only reappear when the R factor is lost (50).

On the other hand, the two factors R and F are recognized as really identical in many respects. The apparent distinctions between both factors are accounted for by the fact that the fertility functions of the R factors are normally expressed in the minority of R⁺ bacteria, whereas those of the F are normally expressed in the majority of an F⁺ population. Furthermore, it was postulated that this restriction of R function is due to a repressor, made by R but not by F factor. This repressor can also act on the F factor when both factors are present in a cell. As stated before, cells which have recently acquired an R factor are capable of transmitting the factor with higher frequencies than the cells which had previously acquired an R factor and had passed it on for many generations. These facts can be accounted for by postulating that there is a lag between the cell acquiring the R factor and the development of its repressor (40, 41, 75). The disappearance of F function in cells harboring both F and R factors was consequently attributed to alterations of the F-specific surface structure through an epistatic effect of the R factor which suppresses the expression of F (29).

On the other hand, it was suggested (40, 41) that the surface structure produced by the R factor is simply the F-specific structure. It was also found that the cells newly infected with R factor, in which repression has evidently not established, were infected with an F-phage with a much higher frequency. But the unexpressed state of the

R factor in newly infected cells is only transient, and the bacteria become phenotypically F⁻ and the plaques are not formed when such cells are plated with the F-phage, because the normal repressed state of the R factor appears with the time it takes for the formation of the indicator lawn of R⁺ cells. This view is strengthened by the finding that the cultures carrying R factors contain only a few cells with pili which cannot be distinguished from F pili (*40, 41*) to which male-specific RNA phages are adsorbed (*38*). Practically, HFRT populations contain a much greater proportion of the cells carrying such pili (*40, 41*). It seems more likely that the expression of donor competence in HFRT cells is due to the absence of repressors for the formation of F pili in the newly infected cells, and after several generations of donor cells the cells become those of poor donor ability due to the accumulation of the repressor.

4. Plasmid Interference

It was reported by Nakaya *et al.* (*50*) that R factors present in F⁺ and Hfr strains reduce the frequencies of recombination to about 10^{-2} of those without R factor. This fact was confirmed by our laboratory; the frequencies of recombination between Hfr × F-R⁺, Hfr R⁺ × F⁻ and Hfr R⁺ × F-R⁺, being reduced to about 10^{-1}, 10^{-2}, to 10^{-5} of those in such crosses without R factor, respectively (*20*). Similarly, the presence of R factor in Hfr strains was found to reduce the frequencies of recombination to about 10^{-2} of those in Hfr strains (*74, 80*). It was also reported that R factors present in F⁺ and F′⁺ strains suppress the transfer of F and F′ factors (*74*).

The bacterial cells carrying two types of R factor as a result of superinfection segregate at high frequency losing either one of the two R factors or both (*21, 24, 25*). These facts may be interpreted to show that there exists superinfection immunity and mutual exclusion (*25*). Superinfection immunity is a phenomenon in which the transfer of plasmids is suppressed by the presence of homologous or heterologous plasmids in the recipients. It is known that the bacterial cells harboring two homologous or heterologous plasmids in the cytoplasm as a result of superinfection segregate at high frequency to either one of the two plasmids or lose both. This phenomenon is called the mutual exclusion of plasmids (*25, 77*).

In contrast, it was found by chance that an R_{ms15} (SM. SA) factor isolated from a naturally occurring strain does not show any superinfection immunity or mutual exclusion against R factors, indicating that naturally occurring R factors can be classified into two types, irs^+ and irs^-. The term irs is an abbreviation for interaction between R factors. Most R factors carrying (SM) or (SM. SA) resistance, isolated from natural sources, were found to show neither superinfection immunity nor mutual exclusion of R factors. Thus, they are probably irs^- (47).

Similarly, some R factors including R_{ms15} (SM. SA) do not suppress the functions of F of *E. coli* K12, called fi^-, whereas fi^+ R factors do suppress them (77). Most R factors are capable of converting male bacteria of *E. coli* K12 to resistance to male-specific f phages, but fi^- R factors do not (73). These facts can be interpreted according to the theory that the formation of F pili by an F factor is repressed by the presence of fi^+ R factors and that the mechanism of formation of F pili by F is sensitive to the repressor produced by fi^+ R factors (41). Egawa and Hirota (13) isolated a mutant R_{100-1} factor from R_{100}. This mutant R factor obtained by single-step mutation partly lost the inhibitory function of the transfer of the host chromosome by F factor, was in cytoplasmid state, capable of multiplying autonomously and was of conjugal infectivity, just as R_{ms15} (SM. SA). *E. coli* K12 strain carrying an R_{100-1} factor lost its resistance to phage f_1. From these findings, they concluded that R factor carries a genetic site which governs the inhibition of fertility of *E. coli* K12 donated by F factor and of the formation of male substance on the surface of host cells. This genetic site on the R factor was referred to as i, similar to the *ifm*. It was reported that a specific substance essential to the infection by an R factor seems to exist on R+ cells, and may contain polysaccharides (31). But the formation of this surface substance may be independent of the inhibition of the mating substance formation by F factor, since R_{ms15} and R_{100-1} do not inhibit the fertility of the F factor which still possesses conjugal transmissibility.

Yoshikawa and Akiba (81) found that some R factors suppress plaque formation of phages λ and P1kc, and they classified these naturally occurring R factors into two types, spp^+ and spp^-. The term spp is an abbreviation for suppression of plaque formation. This fact was confirmed by Watanabe *et al.*, who reported that fi^- R factors restricted and modified phages λ, T_1, and T_7 (*78*). Similar to the findings of Arber (*7*), this indicated that ^{32}P incorporated into phage DNA was easily detected in the TCA (trichloroacetic acid)-soluble fraction after infection. But an *fi⁻* R factor, which restricts phages T_1 and T_7 without modifying them, was found to restrict and not to modify F-specific phage, W31, in *E. coli* K12, but not to restrict phage P-22 in *Salmonella typhimurium* LT-2 (*78*). Interference between R plasmids is now used in classifying them as incompatibility groups, and is described in Chapters 10, 11.

5.   *The Molecular Nature and Control of the Replication of Plasmids*

Since R factors replicate autonomously, are conjugally transferable, and capable of conferring genetic characters on their host, it is most likely that they are composed of nucleic acid. According to the finding or spontaneous loss of R factor from the host bacteria (*42, 44, 46, 68*), we examined the effect of acriflavin on the loss or segregation of R factors, indicating that the loss frequency of R factors from *Salmonella*, *Shigella*, and from *E. coli* was about 50, 5, and 1%, respectively (*44–46*). Artificial elimination of R factors by acridine dyes was also reported by Watanabe and Fukasawa (*71*), and they concluded that acriflavin inhibits the replication of R factors in donor bacteria (*6*). These facts also indicated that the replication of R factors is controlled by a different replicon from that of the host chromosome. By contrast, Yoshikawa and Sevag (*82*) reported that the R⁺ cells were killed when grown in the presence of atabrine, whereas R⁻ cells were not. Comparative studies of the inhibitory effect of atabrine on R⁻ and R⁺ strains of *E. coli* concluded that the "curing" effect of acridine dyes as well as atabrine on R factor was accountable for by the killing of R⁺ cells and the increase in the number of R⁻ cells which appear by spontaneous loss of the R factor in a population.

We studied the effect of base analogues such as 5-bromouracil and 5-fluorouracil on the R_{11} (TC. CM. SM. SA) factor in either *E. coli* K12 *thy⁻* (thymineless) or *E. coli* K12 *ura⁻* (uracilless). When *E. coli* K12 *thy⁻* R_{11}^+ was inoculated into a medium containing 5-bromouracil, the R factor was lost at high frequency from the host cell and segregated at high frequency between the resistance markers. Transmission frequency of the R factor cultivated in the broth containing 5-

bromouracil was decreased markedly compared to that in normal broth. Similarly, elimination and segregation of the R factor increased when *E. coli* K12 *ura⁻* R_{11}^{+} was inoculated into a broth containing 5-fluorouracil instead of uracil, and the transfer of R_{11} factor was completely inhibited. These facts strongly suggest that the component of R factor is deoxyribonucleic acid (*32*).

Previous studies of the molecular nature and size of the R factor have shown that the R factor is inactivated by ^{32}P decay after transfer to an R⁻ recipient (*55, 72*) and by UV irradiation when transduced by phage P1*kc* with a sensitive cross-section which is similar in size to that of bacteriophage (*51*). Painter and Ginoza (*55*) reported the inactivation of R factor by ^{60}Co gamma radiation, by incorporated ^{32}P, and by incorporated tritium as tritium-labeled thymine. Assuming the efficiency of inactivation by ^{32}P is 10%, the phosphorus content of the R factor was estimated to be about 2×10^5 P atoms per plasmid, and they suggested that the R factor contains double-stranded DNA with a molecular weight of the order of 3 to 8×10^7.

It is known that F⁺ cells have a shoulder in equilibrium density containing 50% GC (guanine-cytosine) content. This satellite DNA disappears upon acridine curing of the F-merogenote (*14, 39*). According to a similar experiment of equilibrium density gradient analysis of DNA isolated from *Proteus mirabilis* R⁺, it was found that the naturally occurring R factors, R_{100} (NR1) and R_{11}, consisted of two regions: DNA of 58% GC and of 52% GC content (*56*), the plasmid DNA being eliminated from the cells treated with acridine dyes or UV light (*14, 56*) (see Chapter 3).

6. Number of R Plasmids in a Host Cell

According to the technique of CsCl density gradient centrifugation, it was reported that the 58% GC component was detected in *E. coli* R⁺ but it was impossible to resolve the 52% GC component since its base composition, and hence its buoyant density, is too similar to that of the *E. coli* host chromosomal DNA. The proportion of the 58% GC component relative to the *E. coli* chromosomal DNA suggested that there is only one copy of the R factor per host chromosome in the *E. coli* strain (*56*). However, Hashimoto and Hirota (*26*) reported that the isolation frequency of unselected markers appearing in R factor recombinants was much higher in markers of recipient R factors than those of the donor R factor. This finding "recipient effect" was found to be quite similar to the majority effect, which was reported by Streisinger and Bruce (*61*) in the recombination of two types of bacteriophage. Consequently, they suggested that the number of R factors in *E. coli* strain was not one copy per host chromosome but two or more in this genus (*26*). It was also found that in *E. coli* K12 *ara⁻* strain carrying R(*tet*-s, *str*-r, *sul*-r, *cml*-s), the rate of mutation *cml*-r/*ara⁺* or *tet*-r/*ara⁺* caused by treatment with nitrosoguanidine was about four times higher at the early logarithmic phase of growth than that at either the late logarithmic or stationary phase. This fact indicated that the reversion frequency of point mutant *cml*-s (or *tet*-s) on R factor to *cml*-r (or *tet*-r) was four times higher at early logarithmic phase than that from the marker *ara⁻* to *ara⁺* on *E. coli* chromosome. Accordingly, these results implied that there would be four copies of the R factor per host chromosome at the early logarithmic phase of *E. coli* strain or that an R factor would harbor larger numbers of copies of resistance determinants. If an R factor harbors two copies of resistance determinants, there would be two copies of the R factor per host chromosome (*79*). Recent findings of the plasmid number are described in Chapter 8.

It was reported that the number of R factors in strains of both *E. coli* and *Serratia marcescens* was one per host chromosome (*56, 57*). Accordingly, plasmid replication in *E. coli* and *S. marcescens* appears to be under stringent control, in contrast to the relaxed control of *P. mirabilis* (*57*). However, this conclusion in *E. coli* strain does not coincide with our own which was derived from the "recipient effect" in R factor recombination (*26*) and from a mutation rate derived by using a mutagenic agent (*79*).

As described above, R(TC. CM. SM. SA) factors are isolated most frequently in Japan from both *E. coli* and *Shigella* strains. R_{100} (TC. CM. SM. SA) (the same as R-factor R_{NR1}) and R_{11} (TC. CM. SM. SA) factors have been extensively investigated in Japan as well as in the United States and Europe. The R(TC. CM. SM. SA) factors as well as the R factors carrying triple, double, and single resistance with reference to TC, CM, SM, and SA, were found to be quite stable in the *E. coli* K12 strain, indicating that these R factors replicate autonomously and are capable of conjugal transfer as a whole and that the segregant forms of R factors in their resistance determinants can be obtained, but their frequency is less than 10^{-5}.

In the transduction of R(TC. CM. SM. SA) factor with phage P1, most of the transductants carried four-drug resistance and were capable of both conjugal transfer and autonomous replication, indicating that the R factor was transduced with P1 as a whole plasmid. In contrast, the transductants obtained in the systems of *Salmonella* E group and epsilon phages (ε_{15} and ε_{34}) or *S. typhimurium* and phage P22, were found to be incapable of transferring their resistance by conjugation, and their R factors were not eliminated by treatment with acridine dyes, the R(TC. CM. SM. SA) factor being consistently segregated between TC and (CM. SM. SA) (*22, 70*). These facts strongly suggested that the R factor consists of resistance determinants and transfer factors (RTF, T). The latter is the genetic element responsible for episomality such as autonomous replication and conjugal transferability. The former is the genetic element responsible for conferring drug resistance. In the transduction of R(TC. CM. SM. SA) factor with ε_{15}, a lysate capable of transducing the markers for TC or (CM. SM. SA) resistance at high frequency was obtained and called the HFT (high frequency transduction) lysate. The transducing element is a defective element which lacks certain functions of phage ε_{15} (*36*). The resistance determinant, *i.e.*, defective transducing element, was transferred to *E. coli* K12 strain from *Salmonella* with a cooperation by the F factor and was found to be integrated into the *E. coli* chromosome between *lac* and *pro*, near *lac* (*23*). From these results, we considered that the resistance determinant obtained by transduction with ε is likely to be integrated into the *Salmonella* chromosome and a small segment from the R factor. Therefore, we referred to the resistance determinant of the R factor as a small segment that has lost the episomic abilities responsible for autonomous replication and conjugal transferability.

When R(TC. CM. SM. SA) factor was transferred to *Salmonella* E group by conjugation, a high frequency (about 10%) of R factor segregation was found to take place and segregation consistently occurred between TC and the other remaining resistance markers (CM. SM. SA). The R(TC) factor was segregated ordinarily from the R(TC. CM. SM. SA) factors and the R(CM. SM. SA) factor was not (*22, 45*). This fact can be accounted for by the genetic structure of R factor

(27), in which the genetic determinants responsible for both conjugal transferability *(tra)* and autonomous replication *(rep)* located closely to the TC-resistance determinant(s) *(tet)*. These results coincided with those of transduction experiments. Such a type of R(TC. CM. SM. SA) factor was referred to as the TC type. By contrast, there is another type of R(TC. CM. SM. SA) factor, from which the R(CM. SM. SA) factor segregated spontaneously in *Salmonella* B group or by transduction with bacteriophage, called CM type of R(TC. CM. SM. SA) *(28)*. Accordingly, the resistance determinants which do not carry the genes, *rep*, *tra*, and *stb* (see Chapter 3), cannot exist as plasmids except for integration into other replicons such as the host chromosome, bacteriophage, or plasmid.

According to epidemiological surveys involving some 10,000 *Shigella* and *E. coli* strains, we found that among the strains carrying R factors, 85% harbored a single type of R factor and 15% carried two types of R factor in a cell, the latter being called the hetero-R state. Among the strains in the hetero-R state, isolation of strains harboring both R(SM. SA) and R(TC. CM. SM. SA) factors was most frequent and the R(SM. SA) factors were all *irs⁻* *(64–66)*. Our idea of the hetero-R state is quite different from the notion that R factor easily dissociates into T(or RTF) and resistance determinant, and R plasmid is a composite structure that consists of T and the element governing drug resistance.

REFERENCES

1 Adelberg, E. A. 1965. U.S.-Japan Scientific Seminar, Molecular Basis of Heredity, Hawaii, May.
2 Adelberg, E. A. and Pittard, J. 1965. *Bacteriol. Rev.*, **29**, 161–172.
3 Akiba, T., Koyama, T., Isshiki, S., Kimura, S., and Fukushima, T. 1960. *Nihon Iji Shimpo*, **1886**, 45–50 (in Japanese).
4 Akiba, T. and Iwahara, S. 1961. *Medicine and Biology*, **60**, 42–44 (in Japanese).
5 Akiba, T. and Koyama, T. 1961. *Medicine and Biology*, **61**, 35–38 (in Japanese).
6 Arai, T. and Watanabe, T. 1967. *Genet. Res., Camb.*, **10**, 241–249.
7 Arber, W. 1965. *Annu. Rev. Microbiol.*, **10**, 365–378.
8 Brington, C. C., Gemski, P., and Carnahan, J. 1964. *Proc. Natl. Acad. Sci. U.S.*, **52**, 776–783.

9 Brington, C. C. 1965. *Trans. N.Y. Acad. Sci.*, **27**, 1003–1054.

10 Cohen, A. W. D., Fisher, R., Curtiss, R., III, and Adler, H. I. 1968. *Proc. Natl. Acad. Sci. U.S.*, **61**, 61–68.

11 Davis, B. D. and Mingioli, E. S. 1950. *J. Bacteriol.*, **60**, 17–28.

12 Egawa, R., Hashimoto, H., and Mitsuhashi, S. 1961. *Japan. J. Bacteriol.*, **16**, 703–704 (in Japanese).

13 Egawa, R. and Hirota, Y. 1962. *Japan. J. Genet.*, **37**, 66–69.

14 Falkow, S., Wohlhieter, J. A., Citarella, R. V., and Baron, L. S. 1964. *J. Bacteriol.*, **88**, 1598–1601.

15 Falkow, S., Johnson, E. M., and Baron, L. S. 1967. *Annu. Rev. Genet.*, **1**, 87–116.

16 Goss, S., Deitz, W. H., and Cook, T. M. 1964. *J. Bacteriol.*, **88**, 1112–1118.

17 Harada, K., Suzuki, M., Kameda, M., and Mitsuhashi, S. 1960. *Japan. J. Exp. Med.*, **30**, 289–299.

18 Harada, K., Kameda, M., Suzuki, M., and Mitsuhashi, S. 1960. *Tokyo Iji Shinshi*, **77**, 22 (in Japanese).

19 Harada, K., Kameda, M., and Mitsuhashi, S. 1961. *Japan. J. Bacteriol.*, **16**, 6–16 (in Japanese).

20 Harada, K., Kameda, M., Suzuki, M., Egawa, R., and Mitsuhashi, S. 1961. *Japan. J. Exp. Med.*, **31**, 291–299.

21 Harada, K., Kameda, M., Suzuki, M., Kakinuma, Y., and Mitsuhashi, S. 1961. *Gunma J. Med. Sci.*, **10**, 201–205.

22 Harada, K., Kameda, M., Suzuki, M., and Mitsuhashi, S. 1963. *J. Bacteriol.*, **86**, 1332–1338.

23 Harada, K., Kameda, M., Suzuki, M., Shigehara, S., and Mitsuhashi, S. 1967. *J. Bacteriol.*, **93**, 1236–1241.

24 Hashimoto, H., Honda, T., Morimura, M., Tanaka, T., Nakano, T., and Mitsuhashi, S. 1961. *Gunma J. Med. Sci.*, **10**, 206–208.

25 Hashimoto, H. 1962. *Japan. J. Bacteriol.*, **17**, 942–951 (in Japanese).

26 Hashimoto, H. and Hirota, Y. 1966. *J. Bacteriol.*, **91**, 51–62.

27 Hashimoto, H. and Mitsuhashi, S. 1966. *J. Bacteriol.*, **92**, 1351–1356.

28 Hashimoto, H. and Mitsuhashi, S. 1970. *Prog. Antimicrob. Anticancer Chemother.*, **2**, 545–551.

29 Hirota, Y., Nishimura, Y., Ørskov, F., and Ørskov, I. 1964. *J. Bacteriol.*, **87**, 341–351.

30 Hollom, S. and Pritchard, R. H. 1965. *Genet. Res., Camb.*, **6**, 479–483.

31 Iijima, T. 1961. *Japan. J. Genet.*, **36**, 381.

32 Iyobe, S., Kondo, E., and Mitsuhashi, S. 1963. *Gunma J. Med. Sci.*, **12**, 89–94.

33 Jacob, F. and Wollman, E. L. 1958. *Compt. Rend.*, **247**, 154–156.

34 Jacob, F. and Wollman, E. L. 1961. *In* Sexuality and the Genetics of Bacteria, Academic Press, New York.

35 Jacob, F., Brenner, S., and Cuzin, F. 1963. *Cold Spring Harbor Symp. Quant. Biol.*, **28**, 329–348.

36 Kameda, M., Harada, K., Suzuki, M., and Mitsuhashi, S. 1965. *J. Bacteriol.*, **90**, 1174–1179.

37 Kuwabara, S., Koyama, T., Akiba, T., and Arai, T. 1963. *Med. Biol.*, **66**, 38–41 (in Japanese).

38 Loeb, T. and Zinder, N. D. 1961. *Proc. Natl. Acad. Sci. U.S.*, **47**, 282–289.

39 Marmur, J., Rownd, R., Falkow, S., Baron, L. S., Schildkraut, C., and Doty, P. 1961. *Proc. Natl. Acad. Sci. U.S.*, **47**, 972–979.

40 Meynell, E. and Datta, N. 1965. *Nature*, **207**, 884–885.

41 Meynell, E. and Datta, N. 1966. *Genet. Res., Camb.*, **7**, 134–140.

42 Mitsuhashi, S., Harada, K., and Kameda, M. 1960. *Tokyo Iji Shinshi*, **77**, 462 (in Japanese).

43 Mitsuhashi, S., Harada, K., and Hashimoto, H. 1960. *Japan. J. Exp. Med.*, **30**, 179–184.

44 Mitsuhashi, S., Hashimoto, H., Harada, K., Kameda, M., and Matsuyama, T. 1960. *Japan. J. Bacteriol.*, **15**, 844–848 (in Japanese).

45 Mitsuhashi, S., Harada, K., and Kameda, M. 1961. *Japan. J. Exp. Med.*, **31**, 119–123.

46 Mitsuhashi, S., Harada, K., and Kameda, M. 1961. *Nature*, **189**, 947.

47 Mitsuhashi, S. 1963. *Protein, Nucleic Acid, Enzyme*, **8**, 216–236 (in Japanese).

48 Mitsuhashi, S. 1965. *Gunma J. Med. Sci.*, **14**, 169–209.

49 Mitsuhashi, S., Egawa, R., and Hashimoto, H. 1966. Abstr. IX Int. Congr. Microbiol., Moscow, p. 549.

50 Nakaya, R., Nakamura, H., and Murata, Y. 1960. *Biochem. Biophys. Res. Commun.*, **3**, 654–659.

51 Nakamura, A. and Nakaya, R. 1962. *Japan. J. Bacteriol.*, **17**, 556–557 (in Japanese).

52 Ohki, M. and Tomizawa, J. 1968. *Cold Spring Harbor Symp. Quant. Biol.*, **33**, 651–658.

53 Ørskov, I. and Ørskov, F. 1960. *Acta Pathol. Microbiol. Scand.*, **48**, 37–46.

54 Ozeki, H., Howarth, S., and Clowes, R. C. 1961. *Nature*, **190**, 986–989.

55 Painter, R. B. and Ginoza, H. 1966. *Biophys. J.*, **6**, 153–162.

56 Rownd, R., Nakaya, R., and Nakamura, A. 1966. *J. Mol. Biol.*, **17**, 376–393.

57 Rownd, R., Watanabe, H., Mickel, S., Nakaya, R., and Gargan, B. 1969. *Prog. Antimicrob. Anticancer Chemother.*, **2**, 535–544, 1970.
58 Rupp, W. D. and Ihler, C. 1968. *Cold Spring Harbor Symp. Quant. Biol.*, **33**, 647–650.
59 Scaife, J. 1967. *Annu. Rev. Microbiol.*, **21**, 601–638.
60 Sekijima, Y. and Iseki, S. 1966. *Japan. Acad. Sci.*, **42**, 980–983.
61 Streisinger, G. and Bruce, V. 1960. *Genetics*, **45**, 1289–1296.
62 Stocker, B. A. D., Smith, S. M., and Ozeki, H. 1963. *J. Gen. Microbiol.*, **30**, 201–221.
63 Sugino, Y. and Hirota, Y. 1962. *J. Bacteriol.*, **84**, 902–910.
64 Tanaka, T., Hashimoto, H., Nagai, Y., and Mitsuhashi, S. 1967. *Japan. J. Microbiol.*, **11**, 155–162.
65 Tanaka, T., Nagai, Y., Hashimoto, H., and Mitsuhashi, S. 1969. *Japan. J. Microbiol.*, **13**, 187–191.
66 Tanaka, T., Tsunoda, M., and Mitsuhashi, S. 1975. *In* Microbial Drug Resistance, ed. by S. Mitsuhashi and H. Hashimoto, pp. 187–199, University of Tokyo Press, Tokyo / University Park Press, Baltimore and London.
67 Vielemeter, W., Bonhoeffer, F., and Scuette, A. 1968. *J. Mol. Biol.*, **37**, 81–86.
68 Watanabe, T. and Lyang, K. W. 1962. *J. Bacteriol.*, **84**, 422–430.
69 Watanabe, T. and Fukasawa, Y. 1960. *Biochem. Biophys. Res. Commun.*, **3**, 660–665.
70 Watanabe, T. and Fukasawa, T. 1961. *J. Bacteriol.*, **82**, 202–209.
71 Watanabe, T. and Fukasawa, T. 1961. *J. Bacteriol.*, **81**, 679–683.
72 Watanabe, T. and Takano, T. 1962. *Med. Biol.*, **65**, 111–114 (in Japanese).
73 Watanabe, T., Fukasawa, T., and Takano, T. 1962. *Virology*, **17**, 218–219.
74 Watanabe, T. and Fukasawa, T. 1962. *J. Bacteriol.*, **83**, 727–735.
75 Watanabe, T. 1963. *J. Bacteriol.*, **85**, 788–794.
76 Watanabe, T. 1963. *J. Bacteriol.*, **27**, 87–115.
77 Watanabe, T., Nishida, H., Ogata, C., Arai, T., and Sato, S. 1964. *J. Bacteriol.*, **88**, 716–726.
78 Watanabe, T., Takano, T., Nishida, H., and Sato, S. 1966. *J. Bacteriol.*, **92**, 477–486.
79 Yabe, Y., Hashimoto, H., and Mitsuhashi, S. 1969. Abstr. 41st Congr. Soc. Japan. Geneticists.
80 Yoshikawa, M. and Akiba, T. 1961. *Japan. J. Microbiol.*, **5**, 375–381.
81 Yoshikawa, M. and Akiba, T. 1962. *Japan. J. Microbiol.*, **6**, 121–132.
82 Yoshikawa, M. and Sevag, M. G. 1967. *J. Bacteriol.*, **93**, 245–253.

8 MOLECULAR NATURE AND REPLICATION OF R FACTORS

Robert H. Rownd and David D. Womble

Laboratory of Molecular Biology and Department of Biochemistry, University of Wisconsin, Madison, U.S.A.

The mechanism which coordinates the replication and the segregation of the genetic material with cellular division is one of the most fundamental examples of a system of metabolic regulation. Studies on bacterial plasmids have revealed many interesting features of the control and the mechanism of DNA replication in bacteria (*15, 22, 35, 36, 71*). Owing to their relatively small size, plasmids can be isolated as intact DNA molecules in both the resting (*15, 36*) and the replicating states (*20, 37, 56, 57, 75, 91*), thus allowing a more definitive characterization of the structure of the DNA. This is of considerable advantage in comparison with the study of the replication and the structure of bacterial or eucaryotic chromosomes, whose large size and accompanying sensitivity to shear usually leads to fragmentation of the structures during isolation and handling.

Drug resistance plasmids (R plasmids) have several characteristics which make them particularly interesting subjects for studying the control and mechanism of DNA replication in bacteria. Many R plasmids are composite structures consisting of resistance transfer factor (RTF) and resistance determinants (*r*-determinants) components (*1,*

61, 103, 104), each of which is capable of autonomous replication under certain growth conditions (*15–18, 68, 76, 88, 89, 91, 93, 95*). Thus a composite R plasmid has at least two origins at which replication can be initiated (*77, 91, 92, 94*). Under certain conditions the *r*-determinants component can undergo extensive gene amplification and recombination to form R plasmids consisting of one RTF component and many tandem copies of the *r* determinants component. This phenomenon is interesting both as an example of gene amplification (*87–89, 91–93*) and as a model system for chromosomes containing multiple origins of replication, which may be analogous in structure to eucaryotic chromosomes (*41, 67*). In this chapter we will discuss various aspects of the control of R plasmid replication and the structure of both resting and replicating R plasmids.

1. Molecular Nature and Characteristics of R Plasmid DNA

The majority of the initial genetic and molecular studies on R plasmids were carried out using R plasmids which were isolated from *Shigella* and *Salmonella* species (*1, 15, 22, 24, 35, 61, 103*). Most of these R plasmids are transmissible among members of the Enterobacteriaceae. These R plasmids typically confer multiple drug resistance to tetracycline (TC), chloramphenicol (CM), streptomycin/spectinomycin (SM/SP), and sulfanilamide (SA) and also sometimes to kanamycin (KM) and/or ampicillin (AP) or to heavy metals. Genetic and molecular characterization revealed that these R plasmids consist of two distinguishable components: an RTF which mediates the transfer of the plasmids during bacterial mating and an *r*-determinants component which harbors the majority of the drug resistance genes (*1, 15–18, 61, 68, 76, 88, 89, 91, 93, 95, 103, 104*). In *Escherichia coli*, *Serratia marcescens*, and *Salmonella typhimurium* the RTF and *r*-determinants components are united to form a composite structure (*15, 16, 18, 27, 88*). In *E. coli*, occasional segregant cells can be isolated either spontaneously or in transduction experiments which have resistance to only TC and have lost resistance to all of the other drugs (*33, 62, 103–106, 108*). These segregant cells harbor only the RTF component on which the TC resistance genes reside (*78, 91, 98*) and have deleted the *r*-determinants component which carries the remainder of the drug resistance genes. In *S. typhimurium* spontaneous segregation of the r-determinants component occurs at such a high frequency that it is possible to do clonal analysis on the loss of drug resistance (*62, 106–108*). The formation of segregants which have simultaneously lost resistance to all of the drugs whose resistance genes reside on r-determinants is one method of identifying composite R plasmids which consist of the RTF and r-determinants components.

The DNA of most of the composite R plasmids which have been extensively characterized has a molecular weight of about 60×10^6 and a buoyant density of 1.710 to 1.712 g/ml (*15, 16, 18, 27, 64, 68, 69, 76, 88, 93, 95, 98*) which is similar to the density of the chromosomal DNA of *E. coli*, *S. typhimurium* and *Shigella* species (1.710 g/ml) (*97*). Consequently, the R plasmid DNA in these genera is not distinguishable as a satellite band to the host chromosomal DNA in a CsCl gradient. However, as will be discussed subsequently, the R plasmid DNA can be separated from the chromosomal DNA of these hosts by taking advantage of the unique properties of covalently closed circular DNA. In *S. marcescens* and *Proteus mirabilis*, whose chromosomal DNA has a density of 1.718 and 1.700 g/ml, respectively, composite R plasmid DNA forms a distinguishable satellite band in a CsCl gradient (*25, 85, 90*). The molecular and genetic characteristics of the composite R plasmids R_{NR1} (also called R_{222} and R_{100}) (*64, 76, 88, 93, 95, 98*), R_6 (*16, 18, 98*), and R_1 (*16, 18, 27, 98*) are included in Table I. RTF segregants which have lost the r-determinants component have a smaller molecular weight than the composite R plasmid, as would be expected (*17, 32, 76*). The density of the RTF DNA is approximately 0.002 g/ml less than that of the composite R plasmid DNA (Table I).

A number of other transmissible R plasmids have been isolated from other genera of the Enterobacteriaceae and from *Pseudomonas aeruginosa* which belong to a variety of compatibility groups (*21, 24*). These transmissible R plasmids have molecular weights which range from 25×10^6 to values as high as 120×10^6 and buoyant densities in a CsCl gradient which have ranged from 1.705 to 1.722 g/ml (Table I). Most of these transmissible R plasmids confer resistance to only one or two drugs whereas the majority of the composite R plasmids discussed previously usually confer resistance to four or five drugs. It is presently not known whether these other transmissible R plasmids consist of separable RTF and r-determinants components, as indicated by the formation of genetic segregants which have simul-

TABLE I. Molecular and Genetic Characteristics of Representative R Plasmids

R plasmid	Drug resistance pattern[a]	Compatibility group[b]
Transmissible R plasmids		
R_{NR1}	TC. CM. SM/SP. SA	FII
RTF (R_{NR1})	TC	FII
R_6	TC. CM. SM/SP. SA. KM/NM	FII
RTF (R_6)	TC	FII
R_1	AP. CM. SM/SP. SA. KM	FII
RTF (R_1)	—	FII
R_{64}	TC. SM	Iα
N-3	TC. SM. SA	N
R_{15}	SA. SM	N
RP4	TC. KM. AP	P
S-a	SA. SM. CM. KM	W
R_{6K}	AP. SM	X
R_{7K}	AP. SM. SA	W
Rts1	KM	T
Nontransmissible R plasmids		
R_{SF1010}	SM. SA	—
R_{SF1030}	AP	—
A (NTP1)	AP	—
NTP4	AP. SM. SA	—
ASu	AP. SA	—
SSu	SA. SM	—
SSu	SA. SM	—
pSC101	TC	—
Transfer factor and recombinant		
Δ^e	—	I
ΔT^f	TC	I

[a] Abbreviations used: TC, tetracycline; CM, chloramphenicol; SM/SP, strepto-neomycin; AP, ampicillin. Some R plasmids confer resistance to both SM and is denoted SM/SP. Other R plasmids confer resistance to only SM. In these cases
[b] See Chapters 10, 11.
[c] Small variations in these values have been reported by different laboratories and
[d] Estimated by comparing the ratio of plasmid DNA to host chromosome DNA chromosome ratio are observed in different experiments, particularly when the fraction of the plasmid DNA. If there is more than one chromosomal DNA equiv-portionately larger number of plasmid copies per cell than of plasmid copies per
[e] Transmissible plasmid (transfer factor) which does not carry drug resistance genes. resistance gene.

Base composition (% G+C)[c]	Buoyant density (g/ml)[c]	Molecular weight ($\times 10^6$)[c]	Number of copies per chromosome[d]
52	1.712	60	1–2
50	1.710	47	1–2
51	1.711	65	1–2
49	1.709	47	1–2
51	1.711	60	1–2
49	1.709	43	1–2
50	1.710	72	1–3
49	1.709	32	1–3
49	1.709	46	1–3
60	1.720	40	1–3
62	1.722	25	3–5
45	1.705	25	15–20
62	1.722	24	3–5
45	1.705	120	2–3
55	1.715	5.6	10–50
48	1.708	5.6	20–40
46	1.706	5.6	18
—	—	8.8	5–8
56	1.716	8.1	6–9
61	1.721	5.7	6–8
56	1.716	5.0	30–50
50	1.710	5.8	1–2
50	1.710	60	1.0
50	1.710	67	—

mycin/spectinomycin; SA, sulfonamide; KM, kanamycin; KM/NM, kanamycin/
SP using the same enzyme, SM adenylate synthetase. In these cases, the resistance
(or when resistance to SP has not been examined), the resistance is denoted SM.

the values listed are only approximate.
with the ratio of their respective molecular weights. Variations in the plasmid:
amount of plasmid DNA is estimated from the covalently closed circular (CCC)
alent per cell under the growth conditions of an experiment, there will be a pro-
chromosome.
[f] Recombinant between the transfer factor Δ and a nontransmissible TC drug

taneously lost a number of drug resistances or, as will be discussed subsequently, by molecular studies on the dissociation and reassociation of the RTF and *r*-determinants components of R plasmids.

In addition to transmissible R plasmids, a large number of R plasmids have been isolated in the Enterobacteriaceae (*1, 61, 63*) and in *Staphylococcus aureus* (*71–73*) which cannot mediate their own transfer from cell to cell. These nontransmissible R plasmids usually confer resistance to only one or two drugs, are present in multiple copies per cell, and have molecular weights of only $5–10 \times 10^6$ (Table I) (*24, 31, 60, 99*). Many bacterial genera also harbor transfer factors or sex factors which do not carry drug resistance genes. Nontransmissible R plasmids can be mobilized (transferred to a recipient cell) by a transfer factor or by a transmissible R plasmid when both are present in the same host cell (*1, 2, 61, 63*). The mechanism of transfer does not involve covalent linkage between the nontransmissible plasmid and the transfer factor. Transfer factors and small nontransmissible R plasmids can co-exist within the same host and do not recombine, as is true for any two compatible plasmids. Transfer factors which do not carry drug resistance genes would of course not be classified as R plasmids *per se*. Cells harboring both a transfer factor and a nontransmissible R plasmid would be able to transfer drug resistance whereas neither plasmid could do so in the absence of the other.

Anderson and his associates have extensively characterized a multiply drug resistant *Salmonella* strain which carries a transfer factor and two different small nontransmissible R plasmids (*1, 2*). The transfer factor (referred to as *Δ*) and the small nontransmissible R plasmids which conferred resistance to AP, SP, and SA remained as separate molecular entities upon successive intergeneric transfer of drug resistance and the transfer factor between *S. typhimurium* and *E. coli*. They also showed that the transfer factor could pick up a gene for TC resistance from the host bacterial chromosome (*1, 2*) which resulted in an increase in the size of the transfer factor-TC (*Δ*TC) complex (Table I) (*60*).

2. Dissociation and Reassociation of Composite R Plasmids

Many of the initial experiments on composite R plasmids were somewhat controversial (*15, 87, 91*), but it now appears that the molecular structure and physiological behavior of all of the composite R plasmids are quite similar (*87*; R. H. Rownd and N. Goto, unpublished data). In the following discussion we will summarize the characteristics of the composite R plasmid R_{NR1} (also called R_{222} and R_{100}) which has been characterized in several genera of Enterobacteriaceae.

In *E. coli*, *S. marcescens*, and *S. typhimurium*, the molecular weight (63×10^6), density (1.712 g/ml), and percentage of R plasmid R_{NR1} DNA relative to the host chromosome DNA (2–3%) are the same irrespective of whether the cells are cultured in a drug-free medium or medium containing drugs to which the R plasmid confers resistance. These findings have shown that R_{NR1} DNA exists as a composite structure consisting of the RTF and *r*-determinants components irrespective of the conditions of cell culture (*88, 93*; D. P. Taylor, D. Womble, and R. H. Rownd, unpublished data). From the very outset of studies on composite R plasmids in *P. mirabilis*, however, multiple R plasmid DNA bands have been observed in a CsCl density gradient (*25, 26, 85, 88, 90, 95*). In these experiments, the host cells were cultured in medium containing drugs to which the R plasmid confers resistance. The molecular weight, density, and percentage of the R plasmid DNA relative to the *P. mirabilis* chromosomal DNA were subsequently shown to depend characteristically upon the conditions under which the host cells are cultured (*22, 85, 88, 89, 95*). When R⁺ *P. mirabilis* is cultured in drug-free medium, R_{NR1} DNA forms a single satellite band of density 1.712 g/ml whose percentage is about 8% of the *P. mirabilis* chromosomal DNA in stationary phase cultures (Fig. 1A). After prolonged growth of the cells in medium containing any of the drugs to which R_{NR1} confers resistance (except TC), a much higher percentage DNA band of density 1.718 g/ml is observed; this band is usually markedly skewed toward the less dense side (Fig. 1C). As illustrated in Fig. 1, these two types of density profiles are interconvertible, depending on the conditions of cell culture. A diffuse intermediate density R_{NR1} DNA band (Fig. 1B) consisting of a collection of molecules having a broad spectrum of density between 1.712 and 1.718 g/ml is observed during the transition between these two states.

These systematic changes in the density profile of composite R plasmid DNA in *P. mirabilis* are due to the dissociation and the reassociation of the RTF and *r*-determinants components under different growth conditions (*22, 66, 87–89, 91–93, 95*). These events make pos-

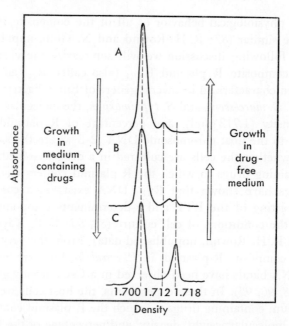

Fig. 1. Systematic changes in DNA density profiles of the R plasmid
R_{NR1} in *P. mirabilis*, depending on whether the host cells are cultured
in drug-free medium or medium containing appropriate drugs. The
band of density 1.700 g/ml is *P. mirabilis* chromosomal DNA. More
detailed analyses of the changes in the R_{NR1} DNA density profiles
during the transition and the back transition are described elsewhere
(*88, 89, 95*).

sible a novel mechanism of gene amplification which has been referred
to as a "transition." According to the transition model (Fig. 2), both
the RTF and *r*-determinants components are capable of autonomous
replication in *P. mirabilis*. The TC resistance genes of R_{NR1} reside on
the RTF component (referred to as RTF-TC), which has a molecular
weight of 49×10^6 and a density of 1.710 g/ml (*76, 78, 98*). The remainder of the drug resistance genes (CM, SM/SP, and SA) are located on the *r*-determinants component which has a molecular weight
of 14×10^6 and a density of 1.718 g/ml (*76*). Essentially all of the R
plasmids in *P. mirabilis* cells cultured in drug-free medium exist in a
composite form (63×10^6) consisting of a single copy of the RTF-TC
and *r*-determinants components (*76, 91, 93*). The composite R_{NR1} DNA
appears as a single satellite band of density 1.712 g/ml (Fig. 1A).

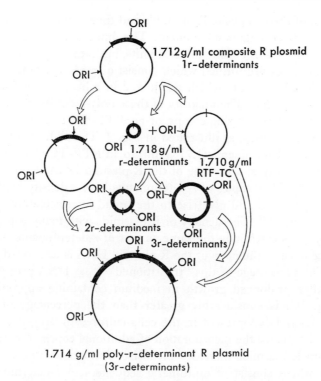

1.714 g/ml poly-r-determinant R plasmid
(3r-determinants)

Fig. 2. Schematic diagram illustrating the dissociation and the reassociation of the RTF-TC and *r*-determinants components of composite R plasmids in *P. mirabilis* and the density increase that accompanies the incorporation of multiple copies of the *r*-determinants component into individual R plasmids to form poly-*r*-determinant R plasmids. After the association of a large number of copies of the *r*-determinants component with a single copy of the RTF-TC component, the poly-*r*-determinant R plasmid DNA would have essentially the same density as *r*-determinants DNA (1.718 g/ml), since most of the mass of the DNA is due to the *r*-determinants component. The origins of replication in the RTF-TC component and the *r*-determinants component are designated ORI.

In medium containing drugs to which the *r*-determinants component confers resistance, there is selection for cells having a larger number of copies of *r*-determinants because these cells have a higher level of drug resistance and grow more rapidly (*34*). The amplification of *r*-determinants in these cells appears to be achieved by the dissociation of some of the composite R plasmids and the autonomous replication of the r-determinants component. The amplified r-determinants do not exist in the form of monomeric units, but rather "poly-r-determinant" molecules are formed which consist of repeated, tandem sequences of r-determinants which are joined in a head-to-tail fashion (*76, 78, 88, 89, 93, 95*). The majority of these poly-r-determinant molecules recombine with a single copy of an RTF-TC to form poly-r-determinant R plasmids, as illustrated in Fig. 2. The addition of multiple copies of r-determinants (1.718 g/ml) to an RTF-TC (1.710 g/ml) increases the density and the size of the R plasmid DNA. R plasmids containing only a few copies of r-determinants have a density between 1.712 and 1.718 g/ml and give rise to the broad intermediate density band seen in Fig. 1B. The density of R plasmids with many copies of r-determinants is essentially the same as that of r-determinants themselves, since most of the mass of the R plasmid DNA is due to r-determinants. The percentage of this "transitioned" R_{NR1} DNA present in the cells after prolonged growth in medium containing appropriate drugs (Fig. 1C) is considerably greater than the percentage of the 1.712 g/ml R_{NR1} DNA present in the cells cultured in drug-free medium (Fig. 1A), since the incorporation of additional copies of r-determinants into R plasmids increases their size. Autonomous poly-r-determinants which consist of multimeric sequences of r-determinants themselves are also present in transitioned cultures (*76, 78*).

The transition is a reversible phenomenon (*34, 88, 89, 93, 95*). During growth of transitioned cells of R+ *P. mirabilis* in drug-free medium, r-determinants dissociate from R plasmids that have tandem sequences of this component and smaller and less dense R plasmids are formed. As illustrated in Fig. 1, this results in a decrease in the percentage of the 1.718 g/ml R_{NR1} DNA and the reappearance of heterogeneous intermediate density R plasmid DNA. After several hundred generations of growth of the cells in drug-free medium, essentially all of the R plasmid DNA exists in the 1.712 g/ml form which consists of a single copy of the RTF and a single copy of the r-determinants component. These observations suggest that poly-r-determinant molecules are unstable, perhaps owing to the extensive homology of the repeated r-determinants sequences (*93*). Since there is no difference in the growth rates of transitioned and nontransitioned cells (*34*), it appears that r-determinants undergo only a limited amount of replication after dissociation from poly-*r*-determinant R plasmids and that the extra copies of *r*-determinants are diluted passively by cell division after dissociation.

The reversible amplification of the *r*-determinants component of composite R plasmids indicates a remarkable plasticity in the control of the replication of this genetic element (*34, 92, 94*). During growth in medium containing appropriate drugs, *r*-determinants apparently must be able to replicate, at least transiently, more frequently than the RTF-TC component in order to obtain amplification of the drug resistance genes. During subsequent growth of transitioned cells in drug-free medium, *r*-determinants are diluted from the cells and thus must replicate less frequently than the RTF-TC. Thus, some mechanism must exist for "turning on" and "turning off" the *r*-determinants replication system. On the other hand, there appears to be essentially no difference in the number of copies of the RTF-TC component per cell when the cells are cultured in either drug-free or drug-containing medium. The stability of the RTF-TC replication system may explain why *r*-determinants are incorporated into poly-*r*-determinant R plasmids during a transition rather than be allowed to remain autonomous. As a part of an R plasmid, *r*-determinants replication may be stabilized because they are duplicated under the control of the RTF replication system. Instability of *r*-determinants replication may also explain the relatively high frequency of loss of this component in *S. typhimurium* (*62, 106–108*). At present, the factors involved in the regulation of *r*-determinants replication are not understood. In any event, the behavior of composite R plasmids in *P. mirabilis* makes possible a novel mechanism by which the number of copies of specific gene segments can be regulated.

In *P. mirabilis*, the entire *r*-determinants component of R_{NR1} is amplified during a transition (*34, 76, 78*). As mentioned previously, many genetic segregants of composite R plasmids have been isolated which have deleted the entire *r*-determinants component. Taken together, these observations indicate that composite R plasmids have unique dissociation or excision sites which may be involved in the dissociation and reassociation of the *r*-determinants component. Recently, several of the insertion sequences which were previously shown to cause strong polar mutations in the galactose operon of *E. coli* (*28, 38, 96*) have been identified on a number of F, F-prime, and R plasmids (*40, 80*). These insertion sequences may be involved in site-specific recombination events. A copy of the insertion sequence IS1 is located at both interfaces between the RTF-TC and *r* determinants of several composite R plasmids (*40, 80*). These insertion sequences may play a role in the dissociation of the R plasmid structure and the formation of poly-*r*-determinant structures during a transition.

Recent studies with the F-like R plasmid R_{NR84}, which confers resistance to AP in addition to CM, SM/SP, SA, and TC, have shown that the nature of the density change of the R_{NR84} DNA in *P. mirabilis* and the patterns of the increased drug resistance of the cells depends upon the drug which is added to the growth medium (*87, 92, 93*; E. R. Appelbaum, N. Goto, and R. H. Rownd, unpublished data). Characterization of transitioned R_{NR84} DNA has shown that poly-*r*-determinant structures are formed. However, only a segment of the *r*-determinants component of R_{NR84} may be amplified during a transition and the region of the *r*-determinants component which is amplified in different experiments is not always the same. Selective amplification of specific drug resistance genes, either alone or in various combinations with other drug resistance genes, have been observed during the transition of R_{NR84}. This indicates that there may be multiple dissociation or excision sites on the composite R plasmid which makes possible the excision, amplification, and formation of multiple tandem sequences of different regions of the composite R plasmid genome (*87, 92*; E. R. Appelbaum, N. Goto, and R. H. Rownd, unpublished data).

Several groups have suggested that R plasmids exist in the composite form during exponential growth phase in *P. mirabilis* and dissociate spontaneously into the RTF and *r*-determinants components upon entry into stationary phase (*16, 18, 24, 26, 27, 52, 81*). The experiments which have been carried out in our laboratory, however, are not consistent with this suggestion (*66, 76, 87, 88, 93*). A detailed study of this question using the same strains and R plasmids used in these other investigations (*87, 91*; R. H. Rownd and N. Goto, unpublished data) has shown that R plasmids exist in the composite form in both exponential and stationary growth phases when the host cells are cultured in drug-free medium. This is also true in medium containing drugs if the cells are cultured for too short a period of time to obtain a transition. If the cells are cultured for longer periods in medium containing drugs, the R plasmid DNA is found to be in the transitioned form (high molecular weight poly-r-determinant R plasmids and autonomous poly-r-determinants) in both exponential and stationary phases. In the original experiments of Falkow *et al.* (*26, 27*) which led to the questionable conclusion that R plasmid dissociation occurs spontaneously in stationary phase, the R plasmid DNA density profiles of separate cultures which contained different kinds and concentrations of drugs were compared. It is likely that the differences observed between exponential and stationary phase R plasmid DNA density profiles in their experiments were due to different extents of transition of the cells in the separate cultures.

The transition has not been observed in *E. coli* harboring R_{NR1}. *E. coli* mutants which are resistant to very high concentrations of drugs have an increased number of copies of monomeric composite R_{NR1} (*64*) (or R_1 (*70*)) per cell. Poly-r-determinant R plasmid structures have been observed in a mutant of *E. coli* harboring the R plasmid R_{M201} (*74*). R_{M201} confers resistance to AP, CM, SM, SA, and TC. Although the R plasmid DNA in the mutant had an increased size, the mutant strain had an increased level of resistance to only AP, indicating that only the AP gene had been amplified in the formation of the poly-r-determinant structures. In other experiments, an *E. coli* mutant resistant to high levels of AP was found to contain a small circular DNA of contour length 3 μm in addition to the composite R plasmid (*74*). The AP resistance genes appear to reside on this minicircle which was stably maintained in the same host with the composite R plasmid. Using transformation, it was possible to separate the minicircle from the composite R plasmid. The "mini-R plasmid" was stably replicated when present alone in the host cells.

It has recently been shown that growth of a strain of *Streptococcus faecalis* harboring a nontransmissible R plasmid which confers resistance to TC in medium containing TC results in an increase in the molecular weight of the R plasmid DNA and an increase in the level of resistance of the host cells to TC (*14*). The data indicate that only a segment of the R plasmid DNA was amplified in the formation of the heterogeneous, higher molecular weight R plasmid molecules. This apparent gene amplification was reversible when the cells were subsequently cultured in drug-free medium. Thus, an R plasmid transition also appears to occur in the genus *Streptococcus*.

3. *Isolation and Characterization of Replicating R Plasmid DNA*

Whereas the small size of plasmid DNA is advantageous because it reduces the problem of breakage of the DNA during isolation and handling, it introduces the problem that only a small fraction of the plasmids in a random cell culture is replicating at any instant (5, 86). It is possible, however, to increase substantially the fraction of replicating R plasmid DNA in *P. mirabilis* as a consequence of decreasing the rate of DNA chain elongation by limiting the concentration of DNA precursors (75, 91, 94). Substrate limitation can be achieved by growth of a thymine auxotroph in medium containing limiting concentrations thymine (4, 75, 79) or by addition of hydroxyurea (an inhibitor of ribonucleoside diphosphate reductase) to the growth medium (75). Under these conditions, there is an increase in the time required for a DNA replication fork to traverse the plasmid DNA from the origin to the terminus of replication. Bacterial mass synthesis is not significantly affected during the first few hours of substrate limitation (4, 75). In *P. mirabilis* it appears that the rate of initiation of R plasmid replication continues at near the normal rate under these conditions (75). Since it requires a larger fraction of the bacterial division cycle to replicate the plasmid DNA, an increased fraction of the plasmids are in the process of replication throughout the period of substrate limitation. The substrate limitation technique does not appear to be effective in *E. coli* since an increase in the fraction of replicating R plasmid R_{NR1} DNA was not observed after thymine limitation or hydroxyurea treatment (D. D. Womble and R. H. Rownd, unpublished data). An undetermined degree of enhancement of R plasmid R_{6K} replication has been observed in *E. coli* after subjecting a thymine auxotroph to a period of thymine starvation and then adding thymine back to the growth medium (20, 57).

The density of the majority of the replicating molecules of composite R_{NR1} in *P. mirabilis* have a buoyant density intermediate between the covalently closed circular (CCC) and the nicked form of the plasmid DNA in an ethidium bromide-cesium chloride density gradient (D. D. Womble, R. L. Warren, S. Scallon, and R. H. Rownd, unpublished data). These observations indicate that R_{NR1} replicates as a CCC or supercoiled structure, as previously observed for replicating mitochondrial and SV40 and polyoma DNA (*6, 43, 45, 82*). An analysis of the positions of the two branch points in replicating R_{NR1} molecules using denaturation mapping has revealed that there are two different origins at which the replication of composite R plasmid DNA can be initiated. One is located in the RTF-TC component and the other is located in the *r*-determinants component (*77, 91, 92, 94*). The replicating R_{NR1} DNA molecules observed in an electron microscope were double-branched (*θ*-type) circular structures when either the RTF-TC origin or the *r*-determinants origin was used for the initiation of replication. Replicating molecules isolated from the same culture of cells were found to have initiated replication at either of the two origins of replication. In the case of either origin, replication could be either bidirectional or unidirectional in either sense. The replication branch points were usually not symmetrically arranged about either origin of replication. This asymmetry in the distribution of the replication branch points about either of the two origins may be due to the fact that the location of the terminus is not directly opposite either of the two origins on the circular plasmid molecule (*77, 92*). As a result, the arrival of one of the replication forks at the terminus before the other would interrupt replication in only one direction.

Poly-*r*-determinant R plasmids consisting of an RTF-TC plus multiple, tandem copies of *r*-determinants and autonomous poly-*r*-determinants must contain multiple origins of replication, the number depending on the number of copies of the *r*-determinants component as illustrated in Fig. 2.

Replicating molecules of the R plasmid R_{6K} (*57*) and a smaller deletion mutant of R_{6K} (designated R_{SF1040}) (*20*) have been isolated in the CCC form from *E. coli* cells. R_{6K} DNA replicates bidirectionally from a unique origin. There appears to be a terminus which is located approximately 20% of the genome size from this origin. In the majority of replicating molecules, replication proceeded sequentially from the origin to the terminus in only one direction and then from the origin to the terminus in the other direction to complete the replication of the R_{6K} molecule (*57*). In the case of the deletion mutant R_{SF1040}, replication is also bidirectional; however two different origins of replication were observed. In about 5% of the replicating molecules both origins were used simultaneously (*20*). It is presently not known whether either of the two origins of R_{SF1040} correspond to the single origin of R_{6K}. The reason that the deletion mutant R_{SF1040} utilizes a second origin of replication is also not understood.

A hybrid plasmid containing two origins of replication has been constructed *in vitro* by ligation of the EcoRI endonuclease-cleaved plasmid pSC101 and the colicin plasmid Col E1 (*101*). This hybrid plasmid (pSC134) was introduced into several strains of *E. coli* K12 by bacterial transformation in order to compare its replication characteristics with those of pSC101 and Col E1 as independent plasmids in the same host strains (*101*). When protein synthesis is inhibited by CM, Col E1 replication continues for more than 10 hr, whereas pSC101 replication is inhibited almost immediately. The hybrid plasmid pSC134 continues to replicate in the presence of CM. When pSC101 and Col E1 are both harbored by the same cell as independent plasmids, only Col E1 continues to replicate in the presence of CM. These results suggest that the hybrid plasmid can replicate under the control of the Col E1 replication functions in the presence of CM, but that these functions cannot be provided in *trans* to allow pSC101 to replicate when the cells harbor both plasmids as independent replicons. In a host carrying a temperature-sensitive mutation for DNA polymerase I (*ts polA* mutant) Col E1 is not maintained in the host cells at the nonpermissive temperature (*46*) which indicates that it is unable to replicate, whereas pSC101 and the hybrid plasmid pSC134 are maintained normally. In a host carrying both plasmids as independent replicons, pSC101 could not provide the functions in *trans* which would allow Col E1 to replicate at the nonpermissive temperature. These results suggest that the hybrid plasmid pSC134 can replicate at the nonpermissive temperature under the control of the pSC101 replication functions and that the replication of the Col E1 plasmid DNA requires physical attachment to the pSC101 plasmid to form a hybrid plasmid in order to allow its replication at the nonpermissive temperature. Electron microscopic studies of replicating molecules of pSC134 DNA have shown that the Col E1 origin of replication is exclusively used to initiate the replication of the hybrid plasmid in a wild-type host during exponential growth, whereas in the *polA*$^-$ mutant strain, the pSC101 origin of replication was used (*7*). Further experiments of this type involving hybrid plasmids formed from different replicons should provide valuable information about the mechanisms which control DNA replication in bacteria and the interaction between the replication systems of various bacterial plasmids.

4. Replication of R Plasmids and Synthesis of R Plasmid Gene Products

Most of the experiments on the replication of R plasmids and the synthesis of R plasmid gene products have been carried out in *P. mirabilis*, primarily because the total R plasmid DNA can be easily distinguished from the chromosomal DNA of this host in a CsCl gradient. The study of the synthesis of R plasmid gene products in this host strain is of particular interest because of the large variation in the number of copies of drug resistance genes per cell. *P. mirabilis* cells with R_{NR1} DNA in the transitioned (1.718 g/ml) form have much higher levels of drug resistance to those drugs whose resistance genes are on the *r*-determinants component than do cells with R_{NR1} DNA in the 1.712 g/ml form (*34, 88, 95*). This is as expected from gene dosage effects. If the average number of copies of *r*-determinants in transitioned cells is estimated from the percentage of the 1.718 g/ml R_{NR1} DNA, there is a linear dose-response relation between the number of copies of drug resistance genes per cell and the specific activity of CM acetyltransferase (*88, 95*).

The relation between the replication of R plasmids and the synthesis of CM acetyltransferase has been examined in considerable detail in *P. mirabilis*. In the majority of the *P. mirabilis* experiments, the R plasmid DNA was in the transitioned (1.718 g/ml) form so that the percentage of R plasmid DNA could be more accurately monitored in a CsCl gradient. Similar results have also been obtained with experiments with R_{NR1} in the nontransitioned (1.712 g/ml) form in *P. mirabilis* and also with R_{NR1} (H. Kasamatsu and R. H. Rownd, unpublished data) and other R plasmids (*51*) in *E. coli*. In Fig. 3 are shown the results of an experiment in which the percentage of R plasmid DNA and the specific activity of CM acetyltransferase were monitored at frequent intervals during exponential and stationary growth phases and after restoration of a stationary phase culture to exponential growth (*88, 95*). The percentage of R plasmid DNA is constant throughout exponential phase. This implies that there is a doubling of the multicopy pool of R plasmids during each bacterial division cycle, that is for each duplication of the host chromosome. Thus, even though there is more than one round of R plasmid replication in each division

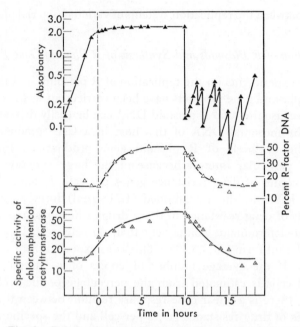

Fig. 3.   Relation between R plasmid R_{NR1} replication and synthesis of CM acetyltransferase in *P. mirabilis* harboring transitioned (1.718 g/ml form) R_{NR1} during exponential and stationary growth phases and after restoration of a stationary phase culture to exponential growth. The time of entry of the culture into stationary phase is denoted as zero time on the growth curve. After 10 hr in the stationary phase, the culture was diluted 20-fold into the same medium and maintained in exponential growth by periodic dilution (*22, 88, 95*).

cycle, there is a determined number of rounds (*44, 88*). After the culture enters stationary phase, the percentage of R plasmid DNA increases about 2.5-fold and the amount of *P. mirabilis* chromosomal DNA increases about 2-fold. Since the percentage of R plasmid DNA is measured relative to the amount of chromosomal DNA, it follows that the multicopy R plasmid pool must increase about 5-fold owing to continued R plasmid replication in stationary phase (*44, 88*). The specific activity of CM acetyltransferase also increases about 5-fold in stationary phase (*88, 95*). Thus, although the synthesis of host chromosomal gene products is arrested in stationary phase, R plasmid gene products continue to be synthesized.

After restoration of the culture to exponential growth, the percentage of R plasmid DNA decreases with time to the original exponential phase value. The kinetics of this process are consistent with a model in which the number of rounds of R plasmid replication per division cycle is equivalent to that characteristic of exponential growth. The remainder of the R plasmid DNA which accumulated during stationary phase is diluted passively with each cell doubling (*44, 88*). The specific activity of CM acetyltransferase decreases with the same kinetics, indicating that the rate of enzyme synthesis after restoration to exponential growth is proportional to the number of replicating R plasmids rather than to the total number of R plasmids per cell (*88, 95*). Taken together, these findings suggest that R plasmid replication and transcription are coupled in *P. mirabilis*.

The number of copies of R plasmid gene segments in *P. mirabilis* can apparently be regulated in two different ways: (1) the dissociation and reassociation of the RTF-TC and *r*-determinants components under different growth conditions, and (2) the continued replication of R plasmids in stationary phase. As a result of these two mechanisms of gene amplification, the specific activity of CM acetyltransferase may be varied over a 100-fold range in *P. mirabilis* (*88*).

In *E. coli* and *S. marcescens* composite R plasmids do not dissociate and reassociate as they do in *P. mirabilis* (*88, 93*). However, in these two genera some R plasmids continue to replicate in stationary phase, and this is accompanied by a corresponding increase in the specific activity of R plasmid gene products (*51*; H. Kasamatsu and R. H. Rownd, unpublished data).

DNA density labeling experiments have shown that R plasmids are selected at random for replication in all phases of a growth cycle such as the one shown in Fig. 3: *i.e.*, during balanced exponential growth (*64, 86, 100*), when the R plasmid pool size is increased due to continued replication in stationary phase (*44*), and when the pool size is decreased after a stationary culture is restored to exponential growth (*44*). In the latter situation, R plasmids are selected at random from the entire stationary phase pool of plasmids. These findings have shown that the initiation of the replication of the entire multicopy pool of R plasmids in bacterial cells does not occur simultaneously and the initiation of the replication of R plasmids is not simultaneous with the initiation of the replication of the host chromosome. They also show that the time required for the replication of an R plasmid (S period) is only a small part of the division cycle (*86*). Since one or more proteins appear to be required for the initiation of R plasmid replication (see below), it appears that these initiator proteins interact with individual copies of R plasmids in a random way. Since R plasmid replication continues in stationary phase, it also appears that the synthesis of R plasmid initiator proteins also continues in stationary phase.

5. Covalently Closed Circular (CCC) R Plasmid DNA

All of the plasmids which have been examined can be isolated in the form of CCC or supercoiled molecules, that is, molecules in which there are no breaks in either of the two strands of the circular duplex DNA (*36*). In the majority of instances, however, it is not known whether 100% of the plasmid DNA actually exists in the CCC form within the cells. Many of the plasmid DNA isolation procedures which have been used yield only the CCC form in the purified plasmid DNA preparation; plasmid DNA molecules containing one or more single-strand nicks would have been lost during isolation and handling of the DNA.

The CCC nature of plasmids gives them a number of properties which are useful for the isolation and the study of the structure of these molecules (*15*). Since the two strands of CCC DNA cannot unwind and separate completely, the plasmid DNA can be reversibly denatured. After exposure of the DNA to denaturing conditions, it is possible to separate the plasmid DNA molecules which have restored the native duplex structure from the irreversibly denatured host chromosome (or plasmid) DNA, which is in the single-stranded form, by using a number of common techniques. It is also possible to separate CCC DNA from nicked circular or linear DNA in a CsCl density gradient containing a dye such as ethidium bromide due to the restricted binding of the intercalating dye to the CCC form of the DNA (*83*). This results in a smaller decrease in buoyant density of the CCC plasmid molecules compared to linear or nicked circular DNA. CCC DNA also has a higher buoyant density than nicked circular or linear DNA in an alkaline CsCl density gradient (pH 12.5), thus allowing separation of the plasmid DNA by this technique (*102*). Owing to their compact structure, and thus smaller frictional coefficient, CCC or supercoiled molecules also sediment more rapidly in an ultracentrifuge than either nicked circular or linear forms (*84, 102*).

Some plasmids have been ioslated from *E. coli* by a process of gentle lysis which is followed by a short period of low-speed centrifugation (*10*). Under these conditions, most of the host chromosomal DNA sediments to the bottom of the centrifuge tube, while the plasmid DNA remains in the supernatant (referred to as a "cleared lysate") which is relatively free of chromosomal DNA contamination. The fraction of the total plasmid DNA which is present in the supernatant depends on the nature of the plasmid. For example most of the Col E1 plasmid DNA or R plasmid DNA is present in the supernatant of a cleared lysate, whereas most of F plasmid DNA sediments to the bottom of the centrifuge tube with the chromosomal DNA under these conditions unless the lysate is subjected to several successive cycles of freezing and thawing (*49, 50*). Most of the plasmid DNA isolated by the cleared lysate procedure has a sedimentation rate in a neutral pH sucrose gradient which is similar to the value of CCC plasmid molecules.

Many colicin plasmids, F plasmids, and R plasmids which have been isolated using the cleared lysate procedure have the interesting property of being susceptible to conversion to the nicked circular form by agents which disrupt protein structure, such as certain detergents or proteolytic enzymes (*10–12, 42, 49, 59*). As a result of such treatment, there is a reduction in the sedimentation rate of the plasmid DNA from that characteristic of the CCC form to the sedimentation rate of nicked circular molecules. These findings have been interpreted as an indication that the plasmid molecules exist in the form of DNA-protein "relaxation complexes." The percentage of the CCC plasmid DNA which can be converted to the nicked circular form varies with the culture conditions of the cells and the agent used to induce relaxation (*13, 53*). Treatments which cause relaxation of some plasmids have been shown to convert other plasmids to authentically CCC molecules which are no longer susceptible to relaxation (*53, 59*). Thus not all plasmid relaxation complexes have identical properties.

It has also been found that the percentage of R plasmid R_{NR1} DNA and R_{ROR12} DNA in the CCC form when isolated from *P. mirabilis* depends upon the conditions used for isolation of the DNA

(*65*). R_{ROR12} is a round of replication mutant derived from R_{NR1} in which there is an increased number of R plasmid copies per cell. By varying the pH of the buffer used to resuspend the cells for lysis, it has been shown that the percentage of the R plasmid DNA in the CCC form ranges from 0 to 100%. When isolated in the nicked circular form, the R plasmid DNA contains a single nick in a unique strand of the duplex. Not all R plasmids isolated from *P. mirabilis* have identical properties with respect to closed circularity. Under conditions which yield 100% of the DNA of R_{ROR12} as CCC molecules, only 35% of R_{NR1} DNA is CCC (C. F. Morris and R. H. Rownd, unpublished data). This is particularly interesting since R_{ROR12} was derived from R_{NR1}. Only a small fraction of transitioned R_{NR1} DNA which contains multiple tandem copies of the *r*-determinants component can be isolated in the CCC form, but this may be due to the much larger molecular weight (up to 200×10^6 daltons) of transitioned DNA, and thus greater susceptibility to breakage during isolation and handling.

Studies in this laboratory on the nature of the relaxation complex of the R plasmid R_{NR1} in cleared lysates prepared from *E. coli* have also shown that the state of the plasmid DNA after isolation depends upon the method used to prepare the DNA (D. D. Womble and R. H. Rownd, unpublished data). If a cleared lysate containing R_{NR1} DNA which has been prepared according to the methods described by Clewell and Helinski is examined directly, the sedimentation rate of the DNA is not changed by treatment with either sodium dodecylsulfate (SDS) or pronase; that is, the R_{NR1} DNA continues to sediment at the rate characteristic of CCC DNA. Under these same conditions, approximately 60% of Col Ib-P9 DNA can be converted to the nicked circular form in agreement with the previous results of Clewell and Helinski (*11*). However, if an R_{NR1} cleared lysate prepared according to the method of Clewell and Helinski is first sedimented in a preparative sucrose gradient and the fractions containing the CCC R_{NR1} DNA then treated with SDS, most of the R_{NR1} DNA is converted to the nicked circular form. These findings raise the interesting question of what fraction of the plasmid DNA actually exists in the form of a DNA-protein relaxation complex within the cells. The percentage could be as high as 100% and the lower values which have been observed in many experiments employing cleared lysates could be due to a conversion of an undetermined part of the plasmid DNA to the CCC form. In any case, these studies in *E. coli* and *P. mirabilis* indicate that the form of purified plasmid DNA can be highly dependent on the methods used for its isolation.

It has been suggested that DNA-protein relaxation complexes may play an important role in the replication and maintenance of plasmids (*35*). The relaxation complex proteins could serve as a point of attachment of the plasmid DNA to the cell membrane or they could function in the initiation of plasmid replication. It is also possible that these proteins could be involved in the mechanism of plasmid transfer during bacterial mating. The possibility of the involvement of the relaxation complex proteins in plasmid replication is particularly attractive since it is necessary for a closed circular molecule to have a nick or a swivel mechanism in order to relieve the strain introduced by unwinding of the duplex DNA during replication. Studies with Col E1 and R_{6K} have shown that the site of the nick induced by the relaxation event is in a unique strand of the DNA duplex and is located at or near the origin used for the initiation of the replication of these two plasmids (*37, 55–57*).

6. Number of Plasmids per Chromosome

The number of copies of a plasmid per chromosome is usually estimated by comparing the ratio of plasmid DNA to chromosome DNA with the ratio of their respective sizes (molecular weights). For example, the ratio of nontransitioned (1.712 g/ml) R plasmid R_{NR1} DNA to *P. mirabilis* chromosomal DNA is 0.025 during exponential growth at rapid growth rates (*76*; D. P. Taylor, C. F. Morris, D. D. Womble, and R. H. Rownd, unpublished data). Since the ratio of the molecular weight of R_{NR1} DNA (63×10^6) to the estimated size of the *P. mirabilis* chromosome (2.8×10^9) is also about 0.025, there must be about one copy of nontransitioned R_{NR1} per chromosomal equivalent of DNA in *P. mirabilis* during exponential growth at rapid growth rates. In this example, the plasmid:chromosome ratio could be determined directly since R_{NR1} DNA and *P. mirabilis* chromosomal DNA have different buoyant densities in a CsCl gradient. In cases where the plasmid and chromosomal DNA densities are so similar that they are not resolved, such as R_{NR1} in *E. coli*, one must rely on the separation of the CCC plasmid DNA from the chromosomal DNA for an estimate of the plasmid: chromosome ratio. This estimate may be a minimum value if not all of the plasmid DNA is isolated in the CCC form under the conditions used for DNA preparation. The molecular weight of plasmid DNA can be determined by a number of methods, the most useful of which are sedimentation velocity in a sucrose gradient and contour length measurements by electron microscopy (*15, 76*). Sedimentation analysis has the advantage that the whole population of plasmid molecules can be examined, while electron microscopy has the advantage that features of individual molecules can be seen. A combination of both of these methods usually gives the most satisfactory analysis.

There is usually a constant ratio of plasmid DNA to chromosomal DNA throughout the exponential phase of growth which indicates that there is a fixed number of rounds of plasmid replication each division cycle (*44, 100*). The number of rounds of plasmid replication is a characteristic of each type of plasmid and is one of the features of the control of its replication. In order for a plasmid to be maintained stably in a population of cells, there must be at least one round of plasmid replication during each division cycle. Many plasmids, particularly the larger plasmids such as F plasmids and the transmissible R plasmids, are present as approximately one or two copies per chromosome (*15*). In those cases where the same plasmid has been examined in several hosts, the same ratio of plasmid to chromosomal DNA has been observed within the accuracy of the measurements. This indicates that the same number of plasmid copies per chromosome are present in different hosts. For example, there is approximately one copy of R_{NR1} per chromosome in *E. coli*, *P. mirabilis*, *S. typhimurium*, and *S. marcescens* (D. D. Womble, D. P. Taylor, H. Hashimoto, and R. H. Rownd, unpublished data). Many of the smaller plasmids, such as Col E1 and the nontransmissible R plasmids, have a much larger number of copies per chromosome (*15, 24, 31, 60, 72, 99*). Plasmids with as many as 40 copies per host chromosome have been studied.

By selecting for increased levels of drug resistance, it has been possible to isolate R plasmid mutants which have an increased number of copies per cell (*64, 70*). These mutants have an increased level of drug resistance owing to gene-dosage effects. These mutants have been referred to as round of replication (ROR) mutants since they undergo an increased number of rounds of replication during the bacterial division cycle *(64)* or as copy mutants since they have an increased number of copies per cell *(70)*. ROR mutants of the R plasmids R_1 and R_{NR1} have been isolated in *E. coli*. These ROR mutants have the same size as the wild-type R plasmids, showing that the number of copies of the drug resistance genes has not been increased by the formation of multimeric structures, as in a transition in *P. mirabilis*. It is expected that the characterization of these mutants will reveal important features of the control of plasmid replication. In the case of R_{ROR12}, which was derived from R_{NR1}, there are 3–4 copies of the plasmid per chromosome *(64)*. Cells harboring R_{ROR12} have a 3–4 times higher specific activity of CM acetyltransferase, the enzyme which inactivates CM. The mutation which results in the increased number of rounds of replication of R_{ROR12} has been shown to reside on the RTF-TC component of the composite R plasmid. An RTF-TC segregant of R_{ROR12} has the same increased number of copies that are characteristic of the *ror* mutant.

7.   Requirement of Macromolecular Synthesis for Plasmid Replication

Studies on bacterial chromosome replication have shown that protein synthesis is required for the initiation of replication, but not for the completion of rounds of replication once the initiation event has occurred *(54, 58)*. These observations suggest that one or more proteins are required for the initiation of chromosome replication. At the present time, very little is known about the function of these "initiator proteins."

When protein synthesis is inhibited in *E. coli* or *P. mirabilis* harboring the R plasmid R_{NR1} (either in the nontransitioned or transitioned state) by starving an auxotrophic strain for a required amino acid or treatment of cells harboring a CM-sensitive mutant of R_{NR1} with CM, there is approximately a 25% increase in the amount of plasmid DNA whereas the amount of residual chromosomal DNA synthesis is about 40–50% *(88, 94)*. Although the residual chromosomal replication during inhibition of protein synthesis requires 60–90 min for completion, the 25% increase in R_{NR1} DNA is usually completed within 10–15 min (M. H. Barnes, T. M. Twose, D. D. Womble, and R. H. Rownd, unpublished data). Since only a small fraction of the R plasmids in the cells will be in the process of replication at the time protein synthesis is arrested, the 25% increase in the amount of R plasmid DNA indicates that new rounds of R plasmid replication are initiated in the absence of protein synthesis. The observation that R plasmid replication continues for only 10–15 min after protein synthesis is arrested suggests that protein synthesis is also required for replication of the R plasmid DNA. Taken together, these findings suggest that one or more proteins are required for the initiation of R plasmid replication and that a small pool of "initiator protein" is present in the cells during exponential growth. The utilization of this initiator protein would account for the residual R plasmid replication which takes place when protein synthesis is arrested.

Similar experiments have shown that the nontransmissible R plasmids R_{SF1010} and R_{SF1020} undergo only a limited amount of replication in the absence of protein synthesis (*24*). The R plasmids R_{SF1030} and R_{6K} (*24*) and the colicin plasmid Col E1 (*8*), on the other hand, continue to replicate for more than 10 hr in the absence of protein synthesis. Col E1, the F plasmid, R_{6K}, and R_{SF1030} also appear to require RNA synthesis for replication (*9, 24, 48*) since rifampicin, an inhibitor of RNA polymerase, inhibits the replication of these plasmids in the absence of protein synthesis. Inhibition of RNA synthesis by rifampicin, however, has no effect on the replication of R_{NR1} in *P. mirabilis* or *E. coli* during amino acid starvation or treatment of the cells with CM, which indicates that rifampicin-sensitive RNA synthesis is not required for R_{NR1} replication (*94*). Thus, either R_{NR1} does not require RNA synthesis for replication, or uses a rifampicin-insensitive RNA polymerase for its replication.

8. Genetic Requirements for Plasmid Replication

Mutations which affect R plasmid replication have been found both on the plasmids themselves and on the host chromosome. Examples of plasmid-located mutations include the round of replication mutants discussed previously. Host-specified mutations include those which affect chromosome replication as well as plasmid replication. Two types of temperature-sensitive host mutants have been isolated and characterized (*39*). One type seems to affect only the initiation of chromosome replication; at the restrictive temperature, rounds of chromosome replication which are in progress are completed but the initiation of new rounds of replication does not take place. The second type of host mutant, elongation mutants, arrests DNA chain elongation immediately when the cells are cultured at the restrictive growth temperature. Of the initiation mutants in *E. coli*, *dna*A is not required for replication of most R plasmids (*3, 24, 30*), while *dna*C does appear to be required for plasmid replication (*30*). The elongation mutations, such as *dna*B, are also required for R plasmid replication (*24*). Among the plasmids which have been examined, only Col E1 appears not to require the *dna*B gene products at the restrictive temperature (*24*).

Like the host bacterial chromosome, most plasmids also require DNA polymerase III (which is temperature-sensitive in *dna*E or *pol*C mutants) for their replication (*24*), but are able to replicate normally in host mutants lacking an active DNA polymerase I (*pol*A mutants) (*24*). However, Col E1 (*46*) and R_{SF1030} (*24*) both require polymerase I for replication and R_{SF1010} is slightly unstable in DNA polymerase I mutants (*24*). These last three plasmids have no requirement for DNA polymerase III (*24, 29*). Taken together, these results suggest that much of the replication machinery of a bacterial cell is shared by the host chromosome and various plasmids, including R plasmids.

Host mutations which affect the replication of specific plasmids or groups of plasmids have been isolated (*47*). These mutants appear to undergo normal chromosome replication. For example, three groups of mutants were identified by their inability to replicate all of the plasmids which were examined (group I), their inability to replicate Col E1 and F-like plasmids (group II), or their inability to replicate Col E1 (group III). It is hoped that further studies of these various mutants will eventually help to elucidate the role of each of these gene products in the replication process.

9. Time of Plasmid Replication during the Cell Division Cycle

Density transfer experiments in *P. mirabilis* and in *E. coli* have shown that individual copies of several different plasmids are selected at random for replication during the duplication of the multicopy plasmid pool during the cell division cycle (*86*). These experiments have revealed that not all copies of the plasmids are replicated simultaneously and that some copies of the plasmids are replicated more than once during the cell division cycle to the exclusion of an equivalent number of copies which are not replicated at all. The random selection of plasmids for replication during the duplication of a multicopy pool does not necessarily mean that plasmid replication takes place randomly throughout the bacterial division cycle. Experiments in which *E. coli* and *P. mirabilis* cells were fractionated in a sucrose gradient on the basis of cell age indicate that R plasmids are replicated preferentially in the latter part of the cell cycle, although the resolution of these experiments is limited by technical problems with the fractionation procedure (*94*; W. E. Hill, R. A. Stickgold, and R. H. Rownd, unpublished data). Yabe and Mitsuhashi have also presented evidence that the replication of an R plasmid does not take place uniformly throughout the division cycle of *E. coli* (*109*). In their experiments with cultures of *E. coli* whose chromosome replication cycles had been aligned by treatment with phenethyl alcohol, R plasmid replication occurred after the replication of the galactose genes on the host chromosome. Unfortunately, the resolution obtained in all of these experiments is not sufficient to determine whether R plasmid replication takes place at only a particular stage in the cell division cycle or whether replication takes place throughout the cell division cycle even though replication occurs preferentially in older cells. Experiments with synchronous cultures of *E. coli* have also indicated that the F-*lac* plasmid does not replicate randomly throughout the cell division cycle (*19*, *23*). In these experiments the time of F-*lac* replication was found to vary with the growth rate of the cells, although at the present time, the relationship (if any) between the replication of F-*lac* and the initiation of chromosome replication is a controversial subject.

When a better resolution of the time in the cell cycle at which plasmids are replicated can be obtained, a number of interesting questions concerning the control of plasmid replication and gene expression can be examined. For example, are initiator proteins synthesized at a specific time during the cell division cycle and are they immediately used for the initiation of replication? Are plasmid DNA-protein relaxation complexes present throughout the cell cycle, *i.e.* in cells of all ages, or are there only specific periods of the cell cycle when the plasmid molecules exist in the complexed form? These and many other questions are basic to our understanding of the control of plasmid replication during the cell division cycle.

REFERENCES

1 Anderson, E. S. 1968. *Annu. Rev. Microbiol.*, **22**, 131–180.
2 Anderson, E. S. and Lewis, M. J. 1965. *Nature*, **208**, 843–849.
3 Arai, T. and Clowes, R. 1975. *In* Microbiology—1974, ed. by D. Schlessinger, pp. 141–155, American Society for Microbiology, Washington, D.C.
4 Barnes, M. H. and Rownd, R. 1972. *J. Bacteriol.*, **111**, 750–757.
5 Bazaral, M. and Helinski, D. R. 1970. *Biochemistry*, **9**, 399–406.
6 Bourgaux, P. and Bourgaux-Ramoisy, D. 1972. *J. Mol. Biol.*, **70**, 399–413.
7 Cabello, F., Timmis, K., and Cohen, S. N. 1976. *Nature*, **259**, 285–290.
8 Clewell, D. B. 1972. *J. Bacteriol.*, **110**, 667–676.
9 Clewell, D. B., Evenchik, B., and Cranston, J. W. 1972. *Nature New Biol.*, **237**, 29–31.
10 Clewell, D. B. and Helinski, D. R. 1969. *Proc. Natl. Acad. Sci. U.S.*, **62**, 1159–1166.
11 Clewell, D. and Helinski, D. 1970. *Biochem. Biophys. Res. Commun.*, **41**, 150–156.
12 Clewell, D. and Helinski, D. 1970. *Biochemistry*, **9**, 4428–4440.
13 Clewell, D. B. and Helinski, D. R. 1972. *J. Bacteriol.*, **110**, 1135–1146.
14 Clewell, D. B., Yagi, Y., and Bauer, B. 1975. *Proc. Natl. Acad. Sci. U.S.*, **72**, 1720–1724.
15 Clowes, R. 1972. *Bacteriol. Rev.*, **36**, 361–405.
16 Cohen, S. and Miller, C. 1970. *J. Mol. Biol.*, **50**, 671–687.
17 Cohen, S. N. and Miller, C. A. 1970. *Proc. Natl. Acad. Sci. U.S.*, **67**, 510–516.
18 Cohen, S. N., Silver, R. P., Sharp, P. A., and McCoubrey, A. E. 1971. *Ann. N.Y. Acad. Sci.*, **182**, 172–187.
19 Collins, J. and Pritchard, R. H. 1973. *J. Mol. Biol.*, **78**, 143–155.
20 Crosa, J. H., Luttropp, L. K., Heffron, F., and Falkow, S. 1975. *Mol. Gen. Genet.*, **140**, 39–50.
21 Datta, N. 1975. *In* Microbiology—1974, ed. by D. Schlessinger, American Society for Microbiology, Washington, D.C.
22 Davies, J. E. and Rownd, R. H. 1972. *Science*, **176**, 758–768.
23 Davis, D. B. and Helmstetter, C. E. 1973. *J. Bacteriol.*, **114**, 294–299.
24 Falkow, S. 1975. Infectious Multiple Drug Resistance, Pion, Ltd., London.
25 Falkow, S., Citarella, R. V., Wohlheiter, J. A., and Watanabe, T. 1966. *J. Mol. Biol.*, **17**, 102–116.

26 Falkow, S., Haapala, D., and Silver, R. 1969. *In* Ciba Foundation Symposium on Bacterial Episomes and Plasmids, ed. by G. Wolstenholme and M. O'Connor, pp. 136–158, Little Brown, Boston.

27 Falkow, S., Tompkins, L. S., Silver, R. P., Guerry, P., and LeBlanc, D. J. 1971. *Ann. N.Y. Acad. Sci.*, **182**, 153–171.

28 Fiandt, M., Szybalski, W., and Malamy, M. H. 1972. *Mol. Gen. Genet.*, **119**, 223–231.

29 Goebel, W. 1970. *Eur. J. Biochem.*, **15**, 311–320.

30 Goebel, W. 1973. *Biochem. Biophys. Res. Commun.*, **51**, 1000–1007.

31 Guerry, P., van Embden, J., and Falkow, S. 1974. *J. Bacteriol.*, **117**, 619–630.

32 Haapala, D. K. and Falkow, S. 1971. *J. Bacteriol.*, **106**, 294–295.

33 Hashimoto, H. and Mitsuhashi, S. 1970. *In* Progress in Antimicrobial and Anticancer Chemotherapy (Proc. 6th Int. Congr. Chemother.), pp. 545–551, University of Tokyo Press, Tokyo.

34 Hashimoto, H. and Rownd, R. 1975. *J. Bacteriol.*, **123**, 56–68.

35 Helinski, D. R. 1973. *Annu. Rev. Microbiol.*, **27**, 437–470.

36 Helinski, D. R. and Clewell, D. B. 1971. *Annu. Rev. Biochem.*, **40**, 899–942.

37 Helinski, D. R., Lovett, M. A., Williams, P. H., Katz, L., Kupersztock-Portnoy, Y. M., Guiney, D. G., and Blair, D. G. 1975. *In* Microbiology —1974, ed. by D. Schlessinger, pp. 104–114, American Society for Microbiology, Washington, D.C.

38 Hirsch, H. J., Starlinger, P., and Brachet, P. 1972. *Mol. Gen. Genet.*, **119**, 191–206.

39 Hirota, Y., Mordoh, J., Scheffler, I., and Jacob, F. 1972. *Fed. Proc.*, **31**, 1422–1427.

40 Hu, S., Ohtsubo, E., Davidson, N., and Saedler, H. 1975. *J. Bacteriol.*, **122**, 764–775.

41 Huberman, J. A. and Riggs, A. D. 1968. *J. Mol. Biol.*, **32**, 327–341.

42 Humphreys, G. O., Grindley, N. D. F., and Anderson, E. S. 1972. *Biochim. Biophys. Acta*, **287**, 355–360.

43 Jaenisch, R., Mayer, A., and Levine, A. 1971. *Nature New Biol.*, **233**, 72–75.

44 Kasamatsu, H. and Rownd, R. 1970. *J. Mol. Biol.*, **51**, 473–489.

45 Kasamatsu, H. and Vinograd, J. 1974. *Annu. Rev. Biochem.*, **43**, 695–719.

46 Kingsbury, D. T. and Helinski, D. R. 1971. *Biochem. Biophys. Res. Commun.*, **41**, 1538–1544.

47 Kingsbury, D. T. and Helinski, D. R. 1973. *J. Bacteriol.*, **114**, 1116–1124.

48 Kline, B. C. 1974. *Biochemistry*, **13**, 139–145.

49 Kline, B. C. and Helinski, D. R. 1971. *Biochemistry*, **10**, 4975–4980.

50 Kline, B. C. and Miller, J. R. 1975. *J. Bacteriol.*, **121**, 165–172.

51 Kontomichalou, P., Mitani, M., and Clowes, R. 1970. *J. Bacteriol.*, **104**, 34–44.

52 Kopecko, D. and Punch, J. 1971. *Ann. N.Y. Acad. Sci.*, **182**, 207–216.

53 Kupersztoch-Portnoy, Y. M., Miklos, G. L. G., and Helinski, D. R. 1974. *J. Bacteriol.*, **120**, 545–548.

54 Lark, K. G. 1969. *Annu. Rev. Biochem.*, **38**, 569–604.

55 Lovett, M. A., Guiney, D. G., and Helinski, D. R. 1974. *Proc. Natl. Acad. Sci. U.S.*, **71**, 3854–3857.

56 Lovett, M. A., Katz, L., and Helinski, D. R. 1974. *Nature*, **251**, 337–340.

57 Lovett, M. A., Sparks, R. B., and Helinski, D. R. 1975. *Proc. Natl. Acad. Sci. U.S.*, **72**, 2905–2909.

58 Maaløe, O. 1963. *J. Cell Comp. Physiol.*, **62** (Suppl. I), 31–44.

59 Messing, J., Staudenbauer, W. L., and Hofschneider, P. H. 1972. *Biochim. Biophys. Acta*, **281**, 465–471.

60 Milliken, C. E. and Clowes, R. C. 1973. *J. Bacteriol.*, **113**, 1026–1033.

61 Mitsuhashi, S. 1969. *J. Infect. Dis.*, **119**, 89–100.

62 Mitsuhashi, S., Harada, K., and Kameda, M. 1961. *Japan. J. Exp. Med.*, **31**, 119–123.

63 Mitsuhashi, S., Harada, K., and Kameda, M. 1969. *Japan. J. Genet.*, **44**, 367–375.

64 Morris, C., Hashimoto, H., Mickel, S., and Rownd, R. 1974. *J. Bacteriol.*, **118**, 855–866.

65 Morris, C., Hershberger, C., and Rownd, R. 1973. *J. Bacteriol.*, **114**, 300–308.

66 Morris, C. and Rownd, R. 1974. *J. Bacteriol.*, **118**, 867–879.

67 Newlon, C. S., Petes, T. D., Hereford, L. M., and Fangman, W. L. 1974. *Nature*, **247**, 32–35.

68 Nisioka, T., Mitani, M., and Clowes, R. C. 1969. *J. Bacteriol.*, **97**, 376–385.

69 Nisioka, T., Mitani, M., and Clowes, R. C. 1970. *J. Bacteriol.*, **103**, 166–177.

70 Nordström, K., Ingram, L., and Landbäck, A. 1972. *J. Bacteriol.*, **110**, 562–569.

71 Novick, R. 1969. *Bacteriol. Rev.*, **33**, 210–264.

72 Novick, R. and Bouanchaud, D. 1971. *Ann. N.Y. Acad. Sci.*, **182**, 279–294.

73 Novick, R., Wyman, L., Bouanchaud, D., and Murphy, E. 1975. *In*

Microbiology—1974, ed. by D. Schlessinger, pp. 115–129, American Society for Microbiology, Washington, D.C.

74 Odakura, Y., Hashimoto, H., and Mitsuhashi, S. 1974. *J. Bacteriol.*, **120**, 1260–1267.

75 Perlman, D. and Rownd, R. H. 1975. *Mol. Gen. Genet.*, **138**, 281–291.

76 Perlman, D. and Rownd, R. 1975. *J. Bacteriol.*, **123**, 1013–1034.

77 Perlman, D. and Rownd, R. H. 1976. *Nature*, **259**, 281–284.

78 Perlman, D., Twose, T. M., Holland, M. J., and Rownd, R. 1975. *J. Bacteriol.*, **123**, 1035–1042.

79 Pritchard, R. H. and Zaritsky, A. 1970. *Nature.* **226**, 126–131.

80 Ptashne, K. and Cohen, S. N. 1975. *J. Bacteriol.*, **122**, 776–781.

81 Punch, J. D. and Kopecko, D. J. 1972. *J. Bacteriol.*, **109**, 336–349.

82 Robberson, D. L. and Clayton, D. A. 1972. *Proc. Natl. Acad. Sci. U.S.*, **69**, 3810–3814.

83 Radloff, R., Bauer, W., and Vinograd, J. 1967. *Proc. Natl. Acad. Sci. U.S.*, **57**, 1514–1522.

84 Rhoades, M., MacHattie, L. A., and Thomas, C. A., Jr. 1968. *J. Mol. Biol.*, **37**, 21–40.

85 Rownd, R. 1967. *In* Symposium on Infectious Multiple Drug Resistance, ed. by S. Falkow, pp. 17–33, U.S. Government Printing Office, Washington, D.C.

86 Rownd, R. 1969. *J. Mol. Biol.*, **44**, 387–402.

87 Rownd, R. H., Goto, N., Appelbaum, E. R., and Perlman, D. 1975. *In* Microbial Drug Resistance, ed. by S. Mitsuhashi and H. Hashimoto, pp. 3–25, University of Tokyo Press, Tokyo / University Park Press, Baltimore and London.

88 Rownd, R., Kasamatsu, H., and Mickel, S. 1971. *Ann. N.Y. Acad. Sci.*, **182**, 188–206.

89 Rownd, R. and Mickel, S. 1971. *Nature New Biol.*, **234**, 40–43.

90 Rownd, R., Nakaya, R., and Nakamura, A. 1966. *J. Mol. Biol.*, **17**, 376–393.

91 Rownd, R. H., Perlman, D., and Goto, N. 1975. *In* Microbiology—1974, ed. by D. Schlessinger, pp. 76–94, American Society for Microbiology, Washington, D.C.

92 Rownd, R. H., Perlman, D., Goto, N., and Appelbaum, E. R. 1975. *In* DNA Synthesis and Its Regulation, ed. by M. Goulian and P. Hanawalt, pp. 537–559, W.A. Benjamin, Inc., Menlo Park, California.

93 Rownd, R., Perlman, D., Hashimoto, H., Mickel, S., Appelbaum, E., and Taylor, D. 1973. *In* Cellular Modification and Genetic Transformation by Exogenous Nucleic Acids (Proc. 6th Miles Int. Symp. on Molec-

ular Biology), ed. by R. F. Beers, Jr. and R. C. Tilgham, pp. 115–128, The Johns Hopkins University Press, Baltimore.

94 Rownd, R. H., Perlman, D., Womble, D. D., Taylor, D. P., Morris, C. F., and Hill, W. E. 1975. *In* Microbial Drug Resistance, ed. by S. Mitsuhashi and H. Hashimoto, pp. 27–50, University of Tokyo Press, Tokyo / University Park Press, Baltimore and London.

95 Rownd, R., Watanabe, H., Mickel, S., Nakaya, R., and Gargan, R. 1970. *In* Progress in Antimicrobial and Anticancer Chemotherapy (Proc. Int. Congr. Chemother.), pp. 536–544, University of Tokyo Press, Tokyo.

96 Saedler, H. and Heiss, B. 1973. *Mol. Gen. Genet.*, **122**, 267–277.

97 Schildkraut, C., Marmur, J., and Doty, P. 1962. *J. Mol. Biol.*, **4**, 430–443.

98 Sharp, P. A., Cohen, S. N., and Davidson, N. 1973. *J. Mol. Biol.*, **75**, 235–255.

99 Smith, H. R., Humphreys, G. O., and Anderson, E. S. 1974. *Mol. Gen. Genet.*, **129**, 229–242.

100 Terawaki, Y. and Rownd, R. 1972. *J. Bacteriol.*, **109**, 492–498.

101 Timmis, K., Cabello, F., and Cohen, S. N. 1974. *Proc. Natl. Acad. Sci. U.S.*, **71**, 4556–4560.

102 Vinograd, J. and Lebowitz, J. 1966. *J. Gen. Physiol.*, *Part 2*, **49**, 103–125.

103 Watanabe, T. 1973. *Bacteriol. Rev.*, **27**, 87–115.

104 Watanabe, T. 1967. *In* Symposium on Infectious Multiple Drug Resistance, ed. by S. Falkow, pp. 5–16, U.S. Government Printing Office, Washington, D.C.

105 Watanabe, T., Furuse, C., and Sakaizumi, S. 1968. *J. Bacteriol.*, **96**, 1791–1795.

106 Watanabe, T. and Lyang, K. W. 1962. *J. Bacteriol.*, **84**, 422–430.

107 Watanabe, T. and Ogata, Y. 1970. *J. Bacteriol.*, **102**, 363–368.

108 Watanabe, T., Ogata, C., and Sato, S. 1964. *J. Bacteriol.*, **88**, 922–928.

109 Yabe, Y. and Mitsuhashi, S. 1971. *Japan. J. Microbiol.*, **15**, 21–28.

9 BIOCHEMICAL MECHANISMS OF PLASMID-MEDIATED RESISTANCE

Susumu Mitsuhashi,* Saburo Yamagishi,** Tetsuo Sawai,** and Haruhide Kawabe***

Department of Microbiology, School of Medicine, Gunma University, Maebashi, Japan, Faculty of Pharmaceutical Sciences, Chiba University, Chiba, Japan,** and Episome Institute, Fujimi, Gunma, Japan****

The demonstration of the drug-resistance plasmid and its wide distribution in gram-negative and gram-positive bacteria has proven to be of great importance in both medicine and genetics. Since the demonstration of drug-resistant strains of bacteria, many investigators in the medical and pharmaceutical sciences have sought to determine biochemical mechanisms of such resistance.

The fact that many research workers did not notice the differences between *in vitro*-developed resistance and naturally occurring resistance in bacteria has hindered progress in the investigation of mechanisms of bacterial resistance that are of clinical importance. Therefore, studies on the biochemical mechanisms of the drug resistance in naturally occurring resistant strains made little advancement for a long time, while biochemical studies on the mode of action of antibacterial agents made the rapid progress.

The establishment of *in vitro* systems of protein, nucleic acids, and peptidoglycan syntheses, the use of radioisotopes, and advances in techniques for separation and purification of protein and nucleic acids, all contributed to the analysis of the antimicrobial actions of drugs.

In conjunction with this progress, the biochemical mechanisms of R-plasmid resistance were also investigated, and the results therefrom have opened the way for research into the origin of genes determining drug resistance of R plasmids.

In 1961, Miyamura (*113*) reported that resistant dysentery bacilli isolated from patients inactivated chloramphenicol (CM). Okamoto and Suzuki (*123*) observed that *E. coli* carrying R factor could inactivate dihydrostreptomycin (DH-SM), kanamycin (KM) and CM in the presence of ATP or acetyl CoA as a cofactor. Owing to these findings, rapid progress has been made in studies of biochemical mechanisms of plasmid-mediated resistance. We soon noticed that the mechanisms of *in vitro*-developed resistance are different from those of naturally occurring resistances in bacteria, and that the biochemical mechanisms of plasmid-mediated resistance are the same in bacteria isolated in every country. With these facts we were able to develop a method of tailoring known chemotherapeutic agents to be effective again against bacteria carrying plasmids. Thus, we obtained many drugs that became effective again against drug-resistant bacteria by modifying known chemotherapeutic agents, such as β-lactam antibiotics, aminoglycoside antibotics, nalidixic acid, *etc*. Unfortunately, bacteria were able to develop drug resistance against the new tailored drugs, mainly by the development of drug-resistance plasmids.

Studies on biochemical mechanisms of plasmid-mediated resistance have also provided a method for studying the origins of the drug-resistance determinants on plasmids and their evolutional processes in microorgainsms.

1. Mechanism of Resistance to Aminoglycoside Antibiotics

The mechanisms of resistance to aminoglycoside antibiotics have been extensively characterized by many research workers. One type of resistance in Enterobacteriaceae is the result of the mutation of certain chromosomal genes that causes insensitivity of the 30 S ribosome component which is the site of action of aminoglycoside antibiotics. Hence, this ribosome component no longer binds to antibiotics. However, this type of resistance is rare among clinical isolates resistant to aminoglycoside antibiotics.

In 1961, Miyamura (*113*) reported that resistant dysentery bacilli isolated from patients inactivated CM. Furthermore, Okamoto and Suzuki *(123)* observed that *Escherichia coli* carrying an R factor could inactivate DH-SM, KM, and CM using ATP or acetyl CoA as a co-factor. It was later found that the acetylated product of KM by *E. coli* carrying an R factor was 6'-N-acetyl KM-A *(170)*. Umezawa *et al.* *(169)* described another type of KM inactivation by *E. coli* carrying an R factor, *i.e.*, phosphorylation of the 3'-hydroxyl group of KMs. Thus, studies on the biochemical mechanisms of aminoglycoside resistance were initiated, and many types of drug inactivation were reported. The resistances described were found to be due to enzymatic inactivation of aminoglycoside antibiotics by phosphorylation, adenylylation, or acetylation of the hydroxyl or amino group of the drugs using ATP or acetyl CoA as coenzyme *(12, 30, 31, 110)*.

1) Aminoglycoside antibiotic phosphotransferase
The enzyme which catalyzes the phosphorylation of the 3'-hydroxyl group of aminoglycoside antibiotics was found in *E. coli* carrying an R factor *(19, 86, 87, 126, 128, 172, 177, 180, 189, 199)*, *Pseudomonas aeruginosa (34, 35, 78, 81, 87, 98)*, *Staphylococcus aureus (33, 73, 82)*, and *Providencia stuartii (99)*.

Recently, three types of the KM phosphotransferase, *i.e.*, APH (3'), were confirmed in R-bearing *E. coli* strains resistant to KM. APH

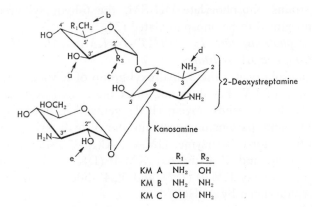

Fig. 1. Chemical structure of KMs. Arrows indicate the site of inactivation: phosphorylation(a), acetylation(b, c, d) and adenylylations(e).

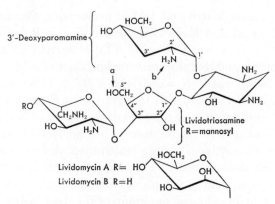

Fig. 2. Chemical structure of lividomycins. Arrows indicate the site of inactivation: phosphorylation(a) and acetylation(b).

(3')-I phosphorylates the 5"-hydroxyl group of KM, neomycin (NM), and lividomycin (LV), but has no effect on butirosins (BTs). APH (3')-II phosphorylates the 3'-hydroxyl group of BTs, but is ineffective with LV. APH(3')-III phosphorylates the 3'-hydroxyl group of both BTs and the 5"-hydroxyl group of LV in addition to KM and NM.

Ozanne *et al.* (*128*) reported that *E. coli* R+ strains resistant to streptomycin (SM) were capable of phosphorylating the 3"-hydroxyl group of the drug. It was further found that crude extracts from *P. aeruginosa* strains phosphorylate DH-SM, the 6-hydroxyl group of SM being presumed to be phosphorylated (*75*).

i) *KM phosphotransferase I; APH(3')-I—KM, NM, RM, paromomycin (PM), and LV resistance*
APH(3')-I phosphorylates the 3'-hydroxyl group of KMs and the 5"-hydroxyl group of LV, but does not affect the 3'-hydroxyl group of BTs. KM-A, -B, -C, ribostamycin (RM), gentamicin (GM)-A, NM, PM, neamine, and paromamine contain the 3'-hydroxyl group and are the substrates for this enzyme. GM-C_1, -C_{1a}, -C_2, sisomicin (SS), tobramycin (TM), and 3', 4'-dideoxy KM-B (DKB) (*174*), 3'-deoxy KM-A (*173*), 3'-deoxy KM-B (*161*), and 3', 4'-dideoxyneamine (*175*) are not phosphorylated by APH(3')-I.

The LV-phosphorylating enzyme was demonstrated in LV-resistant *P. aeruginosa* strains (*81*) and in LV-resistant *E. coli* strains carrying the R factor (*198*), and the inactivated product of LV was a

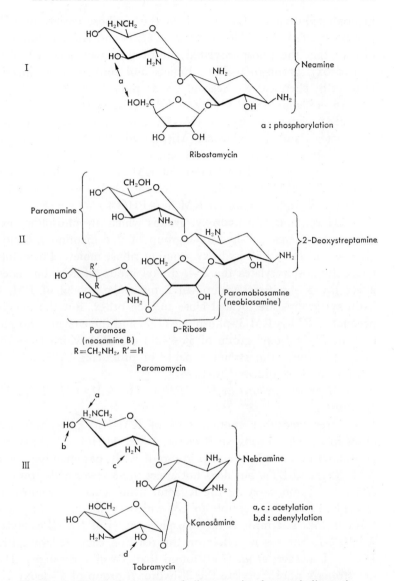

Fig. 3. I. Chemical structure of ribostamycin. Arrows indicate the site of inactivation: phosphorylation(a). II. Chemical structure of paromomycin. III. Chemical structure of tobramycin. Arrows indicate the site of inactivation: acetylation(a, c) and adenylylation(b, d).

monophosphorylated LV, in which the D-ribose moiety of LV was phosphorylated *(199)*. Umezawa *et al.* *(177)* and Kondo *et al.* *(87)* indicated that the phosphorylated site of the inactivated LV was the 5″-hydroxyl group of D-ribose moiety and confirmed the inactivated product by chemical synthesis of LV 5″-phosphate *(201)*.

An epidemiological survey of KM-resistant strains isolated from clinical specimens shows the KM-LV cross resistance in gram-negative bacteria and staphylococci (Mitsuhashi *et al.*, unpublished observations). It was proved that this type of resistance is due to phosphorylation of the 3′-hydroxyl group of KM and the 5″-hydroxyl group of LV *(177)*. KM-A inhibits the phosphorylation of LV and LV inhibits the phosphorylation of KM by APH(3′)-I.

RM contains two hydroxyl groups which are phosphorylated by phosphotransferase, 3′-hydroxyl group of 2, 6-diamino-2, 6-dioxy-D-glucose moiety and 5″-hydroxy group of ribose moiety. Phosphotransferase I phosphorylates the 3′-hydroxyl group of RM but does not affect the 5″-hydroxyl group. In a molecular model of RM, these hydroxyl groups are located close to each other. But the inactivated product of RM is RM 3′-phosphate *(177)* and the enzyme phosphorylates the 5″-hydroxyl group of 3′, 4′-dideoxy RM which lacks the 3′-hydroxyl group, the strains capable of producing APH(3′)-I being resistant to 3′, 4′-dideoxy RM *(181)*.

ii) KM phosphotransferase II; APH(3′)-II—KM, NM, RM, PM, and BT resistance

It was reported that another type of KM-NM phosphotransferase exists in *E. coli* carrying an R factor, called APH(3′)-II. This enzyme phosphorylates the 3′-hydroxyl group of KMs, paromamine, neamine, NM, RM, and BTs, but does not affect the 5″-hydroxyl group of LV *(19, 189)*. *E. coli* carrying the R factor which encodes the production of APH(3′)-II is susceptible to LV which is not phosphorylated by this enzyme. TM inhibits the phosphorylation of NM-B catalyzed by APH(3′)-I, but has no effect on the reaction catalyzed by APH(3′)-II *(19)*. Umezawa *et al.* *(180)* found that phosphotransferase II does not strongly phosphorylate the 3′-hydroxyl group of 4′-deoxy KM-A compared with that of KM-A, suggesting that the 4′-hydroxyl group is involved in binding this enzyme to the drug. But APH(3′)-I phosphorylates the 3′-hydroxyl group of 4′-dideoxy KM-A as well as KM-A to the same degree. Recently, Umezawa *et al.* *(179)* found that, if the enzymes are immobilized, the inactivated products are easily purified.

iii) KM phosphotransferase III; APH(3′)-III—KM, RM, BT, and LV resistance

Marengo *et al.* (*99*) reported that crude enzyme extracts of *P. stuartii*, resistant to KM, LV, and BT-B, phosphorylate KM, LM, BT-B using ATP as a coenzyme. It is not certain whether the phosphorylation of these drugs is due to a single enzyme or the presence of two enzymes. APH(3′)-III phosphorylates the 3′-hydroxyl group of KM-A, RM and BT-A, and 5″-hydroxyl group of LV. This enzyme was strongly inhibited by KM-A and RM at concentrations of 6 μM or more. The enzyme was labile and its molecular weight was estimated to be 25,500 by gel-filtration (*182*).

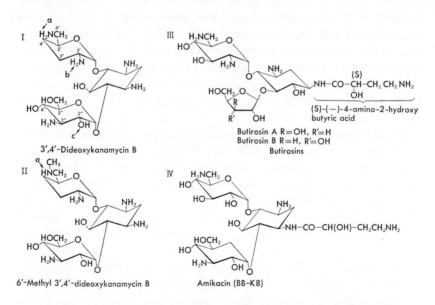

Fig. 4. I. Chemical structure of 3′,4′-dideoxykanamycin B. Arrows indicate the site of inactivation: acetylation(a, b) and adenylylation(c). II. Chemical structure of 6′-methyl 3′,4′-dideoxykanamycin B. Arrow indicates the site of inactivation: acetylation(a). III. Chemical structure of butirosins. IV. Chemical structure of amikacin (BB-K8).

iv)   RM 5″-phosphotransferase; APH(5″)

RM was found to be converted to two kinds of inactivated RM (*74, 76*). RM 5″-phosphate accounted for approximately 99% of the inactivated RMs, and the remaining portion corresponded to RM 3″-phosphate. The hydroxyl group at the C-5 position of the ribose moiety was preferentially phosphorylated by the inactivating enzyme in *P. aeruginosa* even though the hydroxyl group at the C-3 position of the 2, 6-diaminoglucose moiety was available.

v)   KM phosphotransferase from various organisms

P. aeruginosa strains are mostly resistant to aminoglycoside antibiotics, such as KMs, NM, PM, and RM, and have enzymes that inactivate these antibiotics by phosphorylation of the 3′-hydroxyl group of the drugs. KM phosphotransferase was also found in *P. aeruginosa* (*34, 35, 78, 81, 172*), *S. aureus* (*33, 82*) and *Providencia* (*99*). Kida *et al.* (*74*) reported that a crude extract from *P. aeruginosa* preferentially phosphorylates the 5″-hyroxyl group rather than the 3″-hydroxyl group of RM. KM phosphotransferase has been found in KM-resistant staphylococci and cross resistance between KMs and LV is frequently observed, suggesting the presence of APH(3′)-I. Kobayashi *et al.* (*82*) reported that the inactivated product of LV by an enzyme prepared from a KM-resistant *S. aureus* strain was identical with that produced by *E. coli* carrying an R factor, *i.e.*, 5″-phosphoryl LV.

vi)   SM phosphotransferase

SM is also inactivated by phosphorylation of the drug by SM-resistant strains in the presence of ATP, *i.e.*, SM 3″-phosphotransferase and SM 6-phosphotransferase. SM-phosphorylating enzymes have been reported in SM-resistant strains of *E. coli* (*126, 128, 169, 179*) and of *P. aeruginosa* (*15, 34, 63, 77, 80*).

a)   SM 3″-phosphotransferase; APH(3″)—SM resistance. Ozanne *et al.* (*128*) reported that *E. coli* strains carrying an R factor which are SM-resistant and spectinomycin(SP)-sensitive, have been found to phosphorylate the 3″-hydroxyl group of SM. Although the phosphorylating enzyme as well as the adenylylating enzyme reacts with the same hydroxyl group on the N-methyl-L-glucosamine, the chemical structure of the inactivated product of SP has not been fully investigated. SM-resistant but SP-sensitive strains produce the SM-phosphorylating enzyme, and the strains resistant to both SM and SP produce the adenylylating enzyme (*13*). It was reported that DH-SM

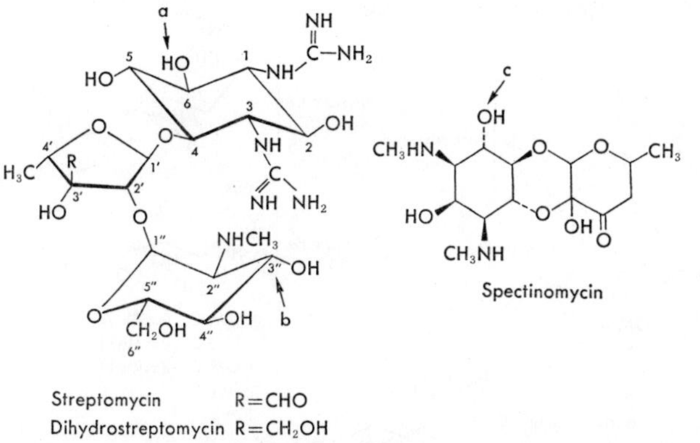

Streptomycin   R=CHO
Dihydrostreptomycin R=CH₂OH

Fig. 5. Chemical structure of streptomycins and spectinomycin. Arrows indicate the site of inactivation: adenylylation(a, b, c) and phosphorylation(a, b).

was phosphorylated by *P. aeruginosa* (*77*), and the phosphorylated product was determined to be the 3″-hydroxyl group of DH-SM (*63, 116*).

b) SM 6-phosphotransferase; APH(6)—SM resistance. Kida *et al.* (*75*) reported that crude extracts from *P. aeruginosa* phosphorylated DH-SM and the phosphorylated product showed the same *Rf* value as that of DH-SM 6-phosphate, which was formed by an extract prepared from a SM-producing strain of *Streptomyces*, as reported by Walker and Skorvaga (*183*).

SM 6-kinase is known to be present in extracts from SM-producing strains of *Streptomyces* (*104*) but SM 3″-kinase activity occurs in a nonstreptomycin-producing strain of *Streptomyces* (*183*). 3″-Kinase from *Streptomyces* will be studied in the future to ascertain whether or not there is an evolutionary relationship between these enzymes, *i.e.*, APH(6) from SM-resistant *P. aeruginosa* and APH(3″) from SM-resistant *Pseudomonas* and enteric bacteria carrying R plasmids (*11*).

2) Aminoglycoside antibiotic acetyltransferase
Okamoto and Suzuki (*123*) reported that a cell-free extract from *E. coli* strain carrying an R factor inactivated KM-A in the presence of acetyl coenzyme A. Umezawa *et al.* (*170*) purified the inactivated product of KM-A and determined that it was 6′-N-acetyl KM-A.

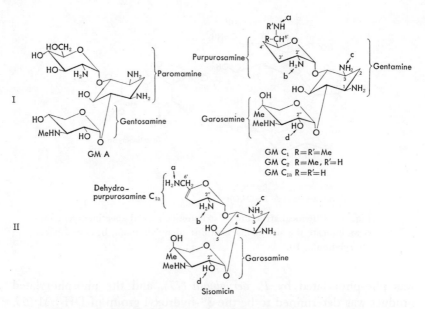

Fig. 6. I. Chemical strucure of gentamicins. Arrows indicate the site of inactivation: acetylation(a, b, c) and adenylylation(d). II. Chemical structure of sisomicin. Arrows indicate the site of inactivation: acetylation(a, b, c) and adenylylation(d).

Mitsuhashi (*107, 111*) classified the aminoglycoside-aminocyclitol 6′-N-acetyltransferase into four groups, *i.e.*, AAC(6′)-I, -II, -III, and -IV, owing to its substrate profiles and susceptibility to the drugs. The strains capable of producing AAC(6′)-I, -II, -III and -IV are resistant, respectively, to (KMs-NM), (KMs, NM, GM-C_{1a}, -C_2), (KMs, NM, GM-C_{1a}, -C_2, DKB), and in addition to amikacin (AK) (*71*), resulting from the acetylation of these drugs using acetyl CoA as a coenzyme.

GM 3-acetyltransferase in *P. aeruginosa* was reported by Mitsuhashi *et al.* (*106*), and the same enzyme was also demonstrated from R-bearing *Klebsiella* strains resistant to GM (*76*). GM was also inactivated by acetylation of the 2′-hydroxyl group of GM (*22, 115, 200*).

i) *Aminoglycoside 6′-N-acetyltransferase; AAC(6′)—KM, GM, SS, DKB, and AK resistance*

KM was found to be inactivated by *E. coli* carrying an R factor (*123*,

125) and the inactivated product of KM-A was determined to be 6'-N-acetyl KM-A (*170*). Similarly, Benveniste and Davies (*9*) purified the products acetylated by *E. coli* carrying an R factor, *i.e.*, N-acetyl KM-A, N-acetyl KM-B, N-acetyl NM-B, and N-acetyl GM-C_{1a}. Moreover, KM 6'-N-acetyltransferase inactivates SS (*120, 121*), KM-A (*170*), RM (*202*), DKB (*66, 188*), and AK (*69*). Based on these findings, Mitsuhashi (*111*) classified 6'-N-acetyltransferases encoded by R plasmids into four groups, *i.e.*, AAC(6')-I, -II, -III, and -IV, owing to its substrate profiles and susceptibility of R^+ strains to drugs. The enzyme AAC(6')-I acetylates KM-A, -B, and NM, but does not affect other aminoglycoside antibiotics, such as GMs, DKB, and AK. The enzyme AAC(6')-II from *Moraxella* strains (*96*) inactivates KM-A, -B, NM, GM-C_{1a}, but does not affect DKB and AK. We were able to further demonstrate from our stock cultures two types of *P. aeruginosa* strains resistant to DKB, *i.e.*, (DKB^r. AK^r. 6'-methyl DKB^s) and (DKB^r. AK^s. 6'-methyl DKB^r) (r, resistant; s, sensitive) (*67–69, 112, 176*), which can inactivate the drugs by acetylation. Two acetylating enzymes were extracted and purified by affinity chromatography. Enzymological studies on the inactivation reaction and chemical studies on the inactivated products indicated that these drugs were inactivated by acetylation of the 6'-amino group. One enzyme, aminoglycoside 6'-N-acetyltransferase III (*67*), acetylates KM-A, -B, GM-C_{1a}, -C_2, DKB, 6'-N-methyl KM-B, but does not affect AK. Another enzyme, aminoglycoside 6'-N-acetyltransferase IV (*69*), acetylates KM-A, -B, GM-C_{1a}, -C_2, DKB, and AK.

Based on epidemiological studies of aminoglycoside antibiotic resistance in *P. aeruginosa*, we were able to demonstrate (DKB^r. AK^s) or (DKB^r. AK^r) strains, whose resistance was encoded by R plasmids. AK was produced by acylation of the 1-amino group of KM-A with γ-amino-α-hydroxybutyric acid, but still has the hydroxyl groups at the C-3' and C-2'' positions. The 3'-hydroxyl and 2''-hydroxyl groups of KM-A are known to be phosphorylated or adenylylated by enzymes from R-bearing strains, but strains capable of inactivating KM-A by 3'-phosphotransferase or 2''-adenylyltransferase were found to be susceptible to AK and could not inactivate the drug (*130*). Furthermore, AK has an amino group at the C-6' and C-3 positions, but the strains possessing R plasmid encoding the formation of 6-N-acetyltransferases of AAC(6')-I, -II, and III, are susceptible to AK. But the strains carrying R plasmid encoding the formation of AAC(6′)-IV is resistant to AK and inactivates the drug. These results indicate that the acylation of 1-amino group of KM-A can protect the acetylation of the 6-amino group from some 6′-N-acetyltransferases, such as AAC(6′)-I,-II, and -III.

ii) *Aminoglycoside 3-acetyltransferase*

a) *GM 3-acetyltransferase I; AAC(3)-I—GM and SS resistance.* This enzyme inactivates GMs and SS by acetylation of the amino group at the C-3 position of 2-deoxystreptamine moiety. Mitsuhashi *et al.* (*106, 107*) reported that the crude extracts from *P. aeruginosa* strains inactivate GM-C_1, -C_{1a}, and -C_2 in the presence of acetyl CoA. The acetylated position of the inactivated product of GM-C_1 was concluded to be the amino group at the C-3 position of 2-deoxystreptamine moiety of the drug (*79*). A similar acetylating enzyme AAC(3)-I was also demonstrated in *E. coli* (*178*). Brzezinska *et al.* (*18*) partially purified this enzyme and reported that the enzyme inactivates GMs and SS as excellent substrates, whereas closely related antibiotics, such as TM, KM-A, -B, and -C, are either poor substrates or are not acetylated. Witchitsz (*186*) isolated *Enterobacter, Serratia, Klebsiella,* and *E. coli* strains possessing R-mediated resistance to GMs. They are resistant to GMs by acetylation of the amino group at the C-3 position of the drugs (*178*). The enzyme AAC(3)-I acetylates the 3-amino group of GM-C_1, -C_{1a}, -C_2, and SS, but does not affect KMs, TM, DKB, NM, and LV.

b) *Aminoglycoside 3-acetyltransferase II; AAC(3)-II—GM, SS, TM, and KM resistance.* Le Goffic *et al.* (*95*) described a GM acetyltransferase prepared from *Klebsiella* strain possessing R-mediated resistance to GM, TM, and KM. This enzyme, AAC(3)-II, acetylates the amino group at the C-3 position of GM, SS, TM, and KM. It is different from AAC(3)-I in substrate profiles, the resulting resistance patterns and isoelectric point, the isoelectric points of AAC(3)-I and -II being 7.4 and 6.4, respectively.

iii) *Aminoglycoside 2′-acetyltransferase; AAC(2′)—LV, RM, BT, GM, KM-B, -C, DKB, and NM resistance*

Providencia strains resistant to many aminoglycoside antibiotics, except KM-A and AK, were isolated and their resistance was due to the acetylation of the 2′-amino group (*22, 115, 200*). This enzyme AAC(2′) catalyzes the acetylation of the 2′-amino group of GMs, KM-B, -C,

TM, DKB, NM, BT, RM, and SS, but can not inactivate KM-A and AK, which lack the 2'-amino group.

3) Aminoglycoside antibiotic adenylyltransferase

i) SM adenylyltransferase; AAD(3")—SM, SP resistance

Umezawa *et al.* (*171*) reported on an *E. coli* strain with R-mediated SM resistance resulting from adenylylation of the drug. The inactivated product of the drug was determined to be 3"-adenylyl SM (*194, 162*). A similar enzyme was reported by Harwood and Smith (*49*), which adenylylates SP, DH-SM, actinamine, SM, and bluensomycin (*151*). Benveniste and Davies (*13*) reported the enzymatic adenylylation of SM and SP by *E. coli* R+ strain. They isolated a mutant sensitive to both SM and SP from an *E. coli* strain resistant to both drugs and showed that this mutant can not produce an enzyme adenylylating both drugs. But the revertant mutants resistant to SM and SP regained the activity of adenylylation of both drugs.

ii) SM 6-adenylyltransferase; AAD(6)—SM resistance

Kawabe and Mitsuhashi (*64*) describe intermediate SM-resistance in *S. aureus* strains, which inactivates the drug by adenylylation. They further disclosed, by epidemiological surverys, that there are three types of resistance to SM and SP in staphylococci: (SM[s]. SP[r]), (SM[r]. SP[s]), and (SM[s]. SP[r]). The (SM[s]. SP[r]) and (SM[r]. SP[s]) mutants of *S. aureus* could be obtained from a strain (SM[r]. SP[r]) by transduction or by elimination of resistance. *S. aureus* (SM[r]. SP[r]) was found to inactivate both SM and SP by adenylylation. Genetic analysis disclosed that the genes governing resistance to SM and SP are located separately on different nonconjugative(r) plasmids. They purified an inactivated product of SM by *S. aureus* (SM[r]. SP[r]) and were shown to be different from 3"-adenylyl SM using electrophoresis (*65*). Adenylylstreptidine was obtained from the methanolysis product of adenylyl SM and was determined to be 6-adenylylstreptidine by elemental analysis and periodate consumption. The adenylylated product of SM was, therefore, determined to be 6-adenylyl SM (*158*). These facts indicate that there is a type of SM resistance in staphylococci resulting from the production of 6-adenyl SM which is different from R-mediated (SM. SP)-resistance resulting from adenylylation of the 3"-hydroxyl group of SM.

iii)   GM-KM 2''-adenylyltransferase; AAD(2'')—GMs, KMs, TM, and DKB resistance

It was reported that *Klebsiella pneumoniae* carrying R plasmid inactivated KM, GM-C_1, -C_{1a}, -C_2, SS (*10, 76*), and DKB (*117, 187*) by adenylylation of the drugs. The adenylylated DKB was concluded to be a monoadenylylated DKB by UV adsorption at 260 nm, chemical analyses, and by the formation of both DKB and adenylic acid by

TABLE I.   Proposal for a Rational Nomenclature for Aminoglycoside-Aminocyclitol

Enzyme activity	Enzyme trivial name
1. Phosphorylation	
1-(1) Phosphorylation of 3''-OH of SM	A-A 3''-PHase
1-(2) Phosphorylation of 3'-OH of KM, RM (not BT), and 5''-OH of LV	A-A 3'-PHase I
1-(3) Phosphorylation of 3'-OH of KM, RM (not LV), and BT	A-A 3'-PHase II
1-(4) Phosphorylation of 3'-OH of KM, RM, BT, and 5''-OH of LV	A-A 3'-PHase III
1-(5) Phosphorylation of 6-OH of SM	A-A 6-PHase
1-(6) Phosphorylation of 5''-OH of RM	A-A 5''-PHase
2. Acetylation	
2-(1) Acetylation of 6'-NH_2 of KM-A, -B, and NM	A-A 6'-ACase I
Acetylation of 6'-NH_2 of KM-A, -B, NM, and GM[a]	A-A 6'-ACase II
Acetylation of 6'-NH_2 of KM-A, -B, NM, GM[a], and DKB	A-A 6'-ACase III
Acetylation of 6'-NH_2 of KM-A, -B, NM, GM[a], DKB, and AK	A-A 6'-ACase IV
2-(2) Acetylation of 3-NH_2 of GMs, and SS	A-A 3-ACase I
2-(3) Acetylation of 3-NH_2 of GMs, SS, KM-B, and TM	A-A 3-ACase II
2-(4) Acetylation of 2'-NH_2 of A-A antibiotics except KM-A and AK	A-A 2'-ACase
3. Adenylylation	
3-(1) Adenylylation of 3''-OH of SM and adenylylation of SP	A-A 3''-ADase
3-(2) Adenylylation of 2''-OH of GMs, KMs, and DKB	A-A 2''-ADase
3-(3) Adenylylation of 6-OH of SM	A-A 6-ADase
3-(4) Adenylylation of 4'-OH of TM, KM, NM, PM, BT, and AK	A-A 4'-ADase

A-A, aminoglycoside-aminocyclitol; PHase, phosphotransferase; ACase, acetyltrans-

hydrolyzation of the inactivated product by snake venom phosphodiesterase. Thus, the adenylyl DKB was found by NMR analysis to be DKB-2″-adenylate, that is, the 2″-hydroxyl group of the 3-amino-3-deoxy-D-glucose moiety is adenylylated (117). A synthesized 2″-deoxy GM-C$_2$ was not inactivated by K. pneumoniae carrying R plasmid encoding the production of AAD(2″) and inhibited the adenylylation of GMs by this enzyme (27), indicating that the 2″-hydroxyl group is

Modifying Enzymes

Enzyme systematic name	Abbreviation of enzyme name	Gene symbol
ATP: A-A 3″-PHase	APH(3″)	aph(3″)
ATP: A-A 3′-PHase	APH(3′)-I	aph(3′)
ATP: A-A 3′-PHase	APH(3′)-II	aph(3′)
ATP: A-A 3′-PHase	APH(3′)-III	aph(3′)
ATP: A-A 6-PHase	APH (6)	aph(6)
ATP: A-A 5″-PHase	APH(5″)	aph(5″)
Acetyl CoA: A-A 6′-ACase	AAC(6′)-I	aac(6′)
Acetyl CoA: A-A 6′-ACase	AAC(6′)-II	aac(6′)
Acetyl CoA: A-A 6′-ACase	AAC(6′)-III	aac(6′)
Acetyl CoA: A-A 6′-ACase	AAC(6′)-IV	aac(6′)
Acetyl CoA: A-A 3-ACase	AAC(3)-I	aac(3)
Acetyl CoA: A-A 3-ACase	AAC(3)-II	aac(3)
Acetyl CoA: A-A 2′-ACase	AAC(2′)	aac(2′)
ATP: A-A 3″-ADase	AAD(3″)	aad(3″)
ATP: A-A 2″-ADase	AAD(2″)	aad(2″)
ATP: A-A 4′-ADase	AAD(4′)	aad(4′)
ATP: A-A 6-ADase	AAD(6)	aad(6)

ferase; ADase, adenylyltransferase. ^{a} Gentamicin C$_{1a}$ and C$_2$.

adenylylated. A similar adenylylating enzyme was also demonstrated in *P. aeruginosa* (*16, 62*).

iv) *TM 4'-adenylyltransferase; AAD(4')—TM, KM, NM, BTs, PM, and AK resistance*

Kayser and Santanam (*72*) reported that *Staphylococcus epidermidis* strains resistant to aminoglycoside antibiotics have been shown to contain an enzyme, which inactivates KMs, NM, BTs, PM, GM-A, AK, and TM by adenylylation. The chemical structure of the adenylylated products was not studied but it is most probable that the 4'-hydroxyl group of the antibiotics mentioned above is adenylylated.

4) Resistance mechanisms without inactivation of aminoglycoside antibiotics

Tanaka (*164*) described GM resistance in *P. aeruginosa* strain that did not inactivate the drug. Biochemical studies of this resistance disclosed that *in vitro* protein synthesis, using the ribosome of this strain, was not inhibited by GM, while the ribosomes prepared from other *Pseudomonas* strains were sensitive to the drug, the resistance mechanism of this strain being due to decrease in the ribosome sensitivity to the drug.

The levels of SM resistance in *P. aeruginosa* were classified into three groups, *i.e.*, susceptible, intermediate- and high-resistant (*17, 57, 168*). There are two types of high SM resistance: (1) R-mediated resistance due to phosphorylation of the drug and (2) decrease in the ribosome sensitivity to SM. Intermediate SM resistance cannot be accounted for by either inactivation of the drug or decrease in the SM sensitivity of ribosome. R plasmids encoding intermediate SM resistance were not demonstrated from these strains whose SM resistance was explainable by their reduced permeability to SM and hence by the diminished uptake of SM (*168*).

Kawabe *et al.* (*70*) reported that plasmid-mediated SM resistance in gram-negative enteric bacteria is mostly due to inactivation of the drug, *i.e.*, by phosphorylation or adenylylation. In *P. aeruginosa* strains, 20% of the R-mediated SM resistance is not due to inactivation of the drug. Biochemical studies of this type of SM resistance have disclosed the following facts: (1) decrease in the accumulation of SM into the strains possessing this type of R plasmid, (2) enhancement of antibacterial activity of SM toward these strains by EDTA treatment, (3) increase in the whole cell accumulation of SM into these strains after treatment with EDTA, and (4) no differences of ^{3}H-dihydro SM binding to ribosomes prepared from R$^+$ and R$^-$ cells. We can conclude therefore that the mechanism of SM resistance mediated by this type of R plasmid is due to decrease in the penetration of SM into bacterial cells (*70, 89*).

2.   Mechanism of Penicillin (PC)/Cephalosporin (CS) Resistance

1)   β-Lactamase (PC/CS β-lactam amidohydrolase, EC 3. 5. 2. 6)

Synthetic PCs which are effective against gram-negative bacteria, *i.e.*, APC, permitted the wide use of such drugs for bacterial infections caused by both gram-positive and gram-negative bacteria. Soon after APC introduction for clinical use, APC-resistant strains of *E. coli*, *Salmonella*, and *Shigella* were isolated in Europe (*5, 6, 21*) and later in Japan (*36, 163*), and the R factors capable of conferring APC resistance were demonstrated from such strains, and penicillinase (PC β-lactamase, PCase) was found to be the main factor for the APC resistance (*28, 37*). PCase is an enzyme which hydrolyzes the C-N bond in the β-lactam ring of PCs causing irreversible inactivation (Fig. 7). The plasmid-mediated PCases are cell-associated and their synthesis is constitutive.

This laboratory also isolated R plasmids capable of conferring APC resistance on their host organisms from *E. coli* and *Shigella* strains (*36, 163*). APC resistance was due to synthesis of PCase in the host bacterium. The PCase produced by the most of them was similar

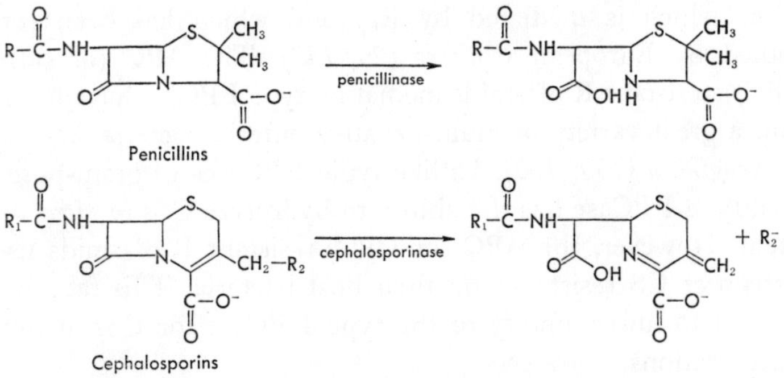

Fig. 7.   Inactivation of penicillins and cephalosporins by β-lactamases.

to the PCase of R_{6K} in substrate profile. However, the PCases mediated by two other R plasmids were greatly different from those reported thus far and were capable of efficiently hydrolyzing both APC and cloxacillin. According to the extensive investigations of many PCases produced by R-bearing bacteria, it was found that these plasmid-mediated PCases were not homogeneous in their enzymological, physicochemical, and immunological properties. Datta and Konto-michalou (28) demonstrated that R plasmids originally isolated from E. coli, Salmonella typhimurium, and Salmonella paratyphi are capable of producing PCases. They studied the enzymological properties of the PCases produced by E. coli strains harboring R plasmids which were transferred conjugally from naturally isolated strains, and found that three R plasmids, R_{6K} (original name: R_{TEM}), R_{46} (original name: R_{1818}) and R_{7268}, were capable of conferring APC resistance on their host bacterium and the PCases produced by the three R plasmids were different from each other in both substrate specificity and specific activity per dry weight of bacterial cell. Succeeding investigations revealed that these two types of PCases differ in physicochemical, enzymological, and immunological properties (137, 195). We designated the former enzyme, which is represented by the enzyme of R_{GN14} (renamed R_{ms212}), type I PCase, and the latter enzyme, which is also represented by the enzyme of R_{GN238} (renamed R_{ms213}), type II PCase. The properties of the two PCases are summarized in Tables II and III.

The APC-resistant R plasmids which have been isolated from clinical sources in Japan during the past decade mostly mediated the synthesis of type I PCase. Type I PCase may be identical to TEM-PCase which is mediated by R_{6K} and which has been extensively studied by European workers (29, 132). The APC (or carbenicillin (CPC))-resistant R plasmids mediating type I PCase have been isolated from a great variety of gram-negative enteric bacteria, and also from P. aeruginosa (159, 160). Unlike typical PCases of gram-positive bacteria, type I PCase has the ability to hydrolyze CSs in vitro to a good extent. However, the APC (or CPC)-resistant R plasmids usually do not confer CS resistance on their host bacteria. This fact may be attributed to lower affinity of the type I PCase for CSs at lower drug concentrations.

Ooka et al. (127) isolated an APC-resistant R plasmid, designated

TABLE II. Summary of Comparison between Types I and II Penicillinases Mediated by R Plasmids

Properties	Penicillinase		
	Type Ia penicillinase (R_{GN114}, renamed R_{ms212})	Type Ib penicillinase (R_{GN823})	Type II penicillinase (R_{GN238}, renamed R_{ms213})
Penicillinase activity[a] per mg of dry weight of bacteria	0.6	16.7	0.025
Specific penicillinase activity per mg of enzyme protein	1,330	1,670	20
pH optimum	6.5–7.0	6.5–7.0	7.6
Temperature optimum (°C)	45	40–45	30
Inhibition of activity by chloride ion	No	No	Yes
Inhibition of activity by anti-(type Ia penicillinase) serum	Yes	Yes	No
Molecular weight[b]	20,600	24,000	25,400
Isoelectric point[c]	5.1 (5.4)	6.9 (5.6)	8.3 (7·4)
$s_{20,W}$	—	2.45	2.66
Secondary structure[d]	α25%	α25%	$\alpha+\beta$
Substrate specificity[e] and *Km* Substrate			
Benzylpenicillin	100 (27 μM)	100 (24 μM)	100 (5 μM)
Phenethicillin	33 (32 μM)	27 (14 μM)	155 (6 μM)
Ampicillin	115 (30 μM)	112 (32 μM)	450 (16 μM)
Cloxacillin	2	1	292 (13 μM)
6-Aminopenicillanic acid	87 (222 μM)	89 (200 μM)	263 (26 μM)
Cephaloridine	130 (400 μM)	111 (500 μM)	36 (111 μM)

[a] Penicillinase activity is expressed in units; one unit of the enzyme activity is defined as the activity which hydrolyzes 1 μmole of benzylpenicillin in min at 30°C.
[b] The molecular weight was estimated by the gel filtration method.
[c] Isoelectric points were determined by the use of agar-gel electrophoresis. The values in parenthesis were taken from the data of Matthew *et al.* (*102, 103*), which were determined by the use of analytical isoelectric focusing.
[d] α-Helix content was determined by ORD spectrum.
[e] Substrate specificity is expressed as the percentage of hydrolysis of benzylpenicillin.

TABLE III.   Amino Acid Composition of Types I and II Penicillinases (196)

Amino acid	Type I penicillinase		Type II penicillinase
	R_{GN14} (R_{ms212})	R_{GN823}	R_{GN238} (R_{ms213})
Lys	52.0	47.4	105.9
His	22.0	25.2	15.2
Arg	60.7	90.1	21.4
Asp	94.4	100.4	130.4
Thr	80.0	84.4	61.5
Ser	58.0	62.0	53.5
Glu	117.6	123.8	100.6
Pro	56.2	58.4	32.7
Gly	82.0	90.2	71.4
Ala	100.0	100.0	100.0
Val	61.9	50.6	71.3
Met	33.7	37.7	18.6
Ile	57.3	57.3	56.0
Leu	106.7	125.9	87.8
Tyr	15.5	13.0	18.5
Phe	24.0	22.9	38.4
Trp[a]	10.3	7.8	13.1
$CysO_3$[b]	5.0	9.3	3.3

[a] Estimated spectrophotometrically and given as a ratio relative to tyrosine.

[b] Given by performic acid oxidation and indicated as a ratio relative to alanine.

as R_{GN823}, from a clinical isolate of *K. pneumoniae*, and found that it mediated highly active PCase production in the host bacteria; PCase activity is about 28 times higher than the activity of the bacteria harboring R_{GN14}.

Plasmid R_{GN823} confers moderate CS resistance together with high APC resistance on its host bacteria. PCase mediated by R_{GN823} was purified by Sawai *et al.* (139), and its properties were investigated in detial (see Tables II and III). The enzyme of R_{GN823} showed very similar characteristics to type I PCase, and its enzymological and immunological properties could not be distinguished from this type of enzyme (196). However, the two PCases were not identical in physicochemical properties, such as molecular weight and isoelectropoint (139). Recently, Matthew and Hedges (103) found that R_{PI} PCase, originally isolated from a *P. aeruginosa* strain, is identical with R_{GN823} PCase. These facts suggest that the origin of type I PCase is hetero-geneous.

As mentioned above, the highly active production of type I PCase results in moderate cephalosporin resistance of the host bacteria al-though the enzyme is of the PCase type. With increasing amounts of CS antibiotics being used in practical medicine, more clinical isolates harboring the R_{GN823}-type R plasmid will appear in the future. Type II PCase mediated by R plasmid is a unique β-lactamase which is able to hydrolyze methicillin, oxacillin, and its derivatives. These PCs are known to be the semisynthetic PCs resistant to hydrolysis by many β-lactamases. APC-resistant R plasmids mediating this type PCase have been isolated from various gram-negative species (*25, 37*). As seen in Tables II and III, the R_{GN238} enzyme, a representative of type II PCase, is very different from type I PCase in enzymological, im-munological, and physicochemical properties.

Type II PCase has been given the general name "oxacillin-hydro-lyzing β-lactamase" based on its unique substrate profile. Oxacillin-hydrolyzing PCases are more heterogeneous than type I PCase. Dale and Smith (*25*) arranged the unique enzymes mediated by R plasmid into seven subgroups. Comparison among the representative enzymes from the seven subgroups are presented in Table IV. This type of PCase has a common characteristic in that their activities are affected by the presence of monovalent anions such as halides (*195*). Five of seven PCases listed in Table IV have a molecular weight of 41,000 to 45,200. These values are unusually high compared with β-lactamases from many gram-negative species. However, Dale and Smith (*26*) have produced evidence suggesting that the high molecular weight of the enzymes is due to the dimerisation of the monomeric PCases.

All known β-lactamases of R plasmid, except the enzyme mediated by R_{22K}, can be classified as PC β-lactamase according to their substrate specificity although their properties are not homogeneous. The R plas-mid, R_{22K}, was originally isolated from *Proteus mirabilis*, and mediates the constitutive production of a β-lactamase that hydrolyzes CSs more rapidly than PCs (*90*). The β-lactamase is the first CS β-lactamase mediated by plasmid. Recently, Bobrowski *et al.* (*14*) reported an interesting fact showing that the cephalosporinase (CSase) could not

TABLE IV.   Classification of Oxacillin-hydrolyzing Penicillinases

R plasmid	β-Lactamase activity (milli-units/10^9 bacterial cells)	Concn. of NaCl to cause 50% inhibition of enzyme activity (mM)	Substrate	
			Methicillin	Oxacillin
1. R_{455}	9.1	5	281	184
2. R_{GN238} (R_{ms213})	5.8	8	332	197
3. R_{55}	7.2	49	32.8	376
4. R_7	1.7	38	36.1	513
5. R_{Ox176}	5.3	30	26.9	595
6. R_{46} (R_{1818})	25.2	15	23.3	646
7. R_{Ox179}	261	11	40.2	870

^{a} Substrate specificity is expressed as a percentage of the activity against benzyl-

TABLE V.   Properties of Cephalosporinase of R_{22K} and Its Comparison with a Chromosomal β-Lactamase of *E. coli*

Properties	β-Lactamase	
	E. coli K-12 strain D3	R_{22K}
β-Lactamase activity (nmole of benzylpenicillin hydrolyzed per min/10^9 bacteria)	13.2	15.9
Activity relative to benzylpenicillin:		
Benzylpenicillin	100	100
Cephaloridine	324	325
Ampicillin	5	5
Oxacillin	0	0
Sensitivity to 100 mM of NaCl	Nonsensitive	Nonsensitive
Sensitivity to 100 mM of p-chloromercuri-benzoate	Nonsensitive	Nonsensitive
Molecular weight	31,800	31,800
Starch gel electrophoretic mobility (mm/hr towards cathode)	+10.0	+10.0
Km values (μM)		
Benzylpenicillin	5.5	3.5
Penicillin V	8.6	8.1
Cephalosporin C	50	51
Cephaloridine	134	202

specificity[a]		Molecular weight	Binding to blue dextran	Electrophoretic mobility (cm/hr towards cathode)
Ampicillin	Cephaloridine			
161	32.6	24,300	−	−0.12
382	30.0	23,300	−	−0.08
173	44.7	41,200	+	−0.13
133	61.9	45,200	+	+0.49
178	64.6	44,800	+	+0.48
179	36.6	44,600	+	+0.51
247	67.2	45,200	+	+0.51

penicillin.

be distinguished from the chromosomally mediated (species-specific) β-lactamase of *E. coli* in enzymological, physical, and immunological properties. The properties of the R_{22K} CSase and the comparison of the enzyme with the species-specific β-lactamase of *E. coli* are presented in Table V.

The *P. mirabilis* strain originally harboring R_{22K} was found in 1963 from a patient in Greece. However, with the exception of R_{22K}, no such R plasmid mediating the production of CSase has been reported thus far. This fact can be regarded as exceptional on the basis of our experiences that the newly emerged R plasmid can be found in many places several years after its first appearance.

When the enzymological properties of the CSase of R_{22K} are compared with those of chromosomal CSase of various gram-negative bacteria, the R_{22K} enzyme is not a typical CSase. Fortunately, as far as we know, the plasmid that mediates a typical CSase has not been isolated. The bacteria producing typical CSase are usually highly resistant to both PCs and CSs, but the bacteria producing PCase are usually susceptible to CSs.

Yaginuma *et al.* (*193*) reported that the PCase specified by an R_{te16} plasmid in *Bordetella bronchiseptica*. The enzyme, designated type III PCase, has a molecular weight of $46,000 \pm 3,000$ and is found to be different from R-mediated PCases, *i.e.*, type I and type II, in various enzymological properties. It has an isoelectric point of 8.3, is highly active against phenethicillin, oxacillin, and PC, and is inhibited by sodium chloride but not by ferrous ion.

Sawada *et al.* (*136*) investigated the *Pseudomonas* R plasmid-mediated β-lactamases in the same host *P. aeruginosa* ML4259. They demonstrated two types of β-lactamase mediated by R plasmids in *P. aeruginosa*. One group of β-lactamase was found to be quite similar to the type I PCase. Another type of PCase was extracted from *P. aeruginosa* R_{ms139}^+ and purified by means of column chromatography. Based on enzymological studies, *i.e.*, isoelectric point, optimal pH for the hydrolysis of PCs, optimal temperature, molecular weight, effects of inhibitors and ions, and substrate profiles, it was concluded that this enzyme is a new type of PC β-lactamase different from the type I, type II, or type III PCases, and was designated type IV PCase.

2) Relationship between R plasmid-mediated β-lactamases and species-specific β-lactamases in gram-negative bacteria

A transmissible R plasmid consists of two or more initially independent genetic elements, namely a transfer factor (7) and drug-resistant determinant(s). Although R plasmids which mediated PCase were isolated for the first time from *E. coli*, *Salmonella*, and *Shigella*, these three bacterial species do not have the genetic ability to produce PCase as their species-specific β-lactamases. It is apparent that the PCase determinants on plasmid might originate from outside these

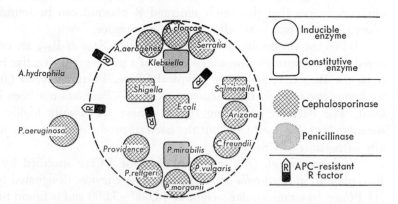

Fig. 8. Distribution map of β-lactamases of enteric bacteria and related gram-negative bacteria.

three bacterial species. The origin of the PCase determinant is a subject of great interest because it may offer the key to an understanding of the evolution of R plasmid in nature.

Figure 8 is a distribution map of β-lactamase among enteric bacteria and related gram-negative rod bacteria. The map was made up mainly from data from our laboratory (*37, 100, 101, 139, 140, 152, 191, 192*). Sawal *et al.* (*100, 137, 140*) attempted to estimate the phylogenetical relationship between the species-specific β-lactamases and the R plasmid PCases on the basis of enzymological, physical, and immunological properties. The chromosomal PCases of *Klebsiella* group were found to be similar to type I R plasmid PCase with respect to substrate profile, pH optimum, temperature optimum, heat stability, behavior to inhibitors and molecular weight. The antiserum against type Ia PCase reacted with the enzymes of *Klebsiella* group. Although the PCases of the *Klebsiella* strains examined were not identical with any of the type I PCases, many common properties observed suggested a close relationship between the chromosome-mediated and the plasmid-mediated PCases.

As shown in Table III, type II PCase is different from type I PCase even in overall amino acid compositon (*196*). A similar observation was found by Richmond and Sykes (*131*) between the amino acid compositions of the TEM-PCase (the type Ia PCase) and an oxacillin-hydrolyzing PCase (R_{46} enzyme). They also suggested that β-lactamases of gram-negative enteric bacteria, including TEM-PCase, are very similar to each other in overall amino-acid composition, but the oxacillin-hydrolyzing R_{46} PCase is distinct from TEM-PCase and species-specific β-lactamases of enteric bacteria. Sawai *et al.* extensively sought a species-specific PCase with a unique substrate specificity capable of hydrolyzing oxacillin, but they could not find such a PCase among chromosomal β-lactamases of various enteric bacteria.

It is possible to imagine that type I PCase is derived from enteric bacteria, presumably from *Klebsiella* group. On the other hand, type II PCase may have its origin outside the Enterobacteriaceae. Recently, *Aeromonas hydrophila* was found to produce an oxacillin-hydrolyzing PCase as a chromosomally mediated β-lactamase (*138*). Although the PCase is an inducible enzyme, other enzymological characteristics are very similar to the type II PCase mediated by R plasmids. The PCase of *A. hydrophila* can hydrolyze oxacillin about twice as rapidly as benzyl PC, and the enzyme activity is inhibited by sodium chloride. It showed the unusual property of binding to blue dextran, and had a molecular weight of 23,000. These characteristics are common to many oxacillin-hydrolyzing PCases mediated by R plasmids. It is a very interesting fact that such a unique PCase is produced as a species-specific enzyme by *A. hydrophila*, while R plasmids can be transferred from the species to the Enterobacteriaceae (7).

3) PC resistance which is not attributed to β-lactamase production
Curtis *et al.* (*24*) suggested the possibility that an R plasmid, R_{P1} originally isolated from *P. aeruginosa* carries a locus which specifies resistance of the host bacteria to PCs by a mechanism other than β-lactamase production. However, the mechanism for the resistance has not yet been analyzed.

3. Mechanisms of Chloramphenicol (CM) Resistance

1) CM acetyltransferase (CATase, EC 2. 3. 1. 28)
There are two schools of thought regarding the explanation of the mechanism of CM resistance conferred by R factors; the first is CM inactivation by an R factor-resistant strain (*113, 114*), and the second is the decrease in the membrane permeability for CM in the resistant strains (*122, 204*). The latter theory is based on results showing the incorporation of amino acids into polypeptide fractions in the cell-free polypeptides synthesizing system containing $MgSO_4$ was inhibited by a low concentration of CM to the same extent in both *E. coli* R^+ and *E. coli* R^-. However, in 1965, Okamoto and Suzuki (*123*) reported that the strain of *E. coli* harboring an R factor capable of conferring resistance to four antibiotics, namely, TC, CM, SM, and KM, was able to produce enzymes which inactivated CM, SM, and KM. They found that an acetyl CoA forming system containing CoA, ATP, and $Mg(OAs)_2$ is essential for the inactivation of both CM and KM in the cell-free system, and that for the inactivation of CM the enzyme is functional only in the presence of acetyl CoA. Further studies revealed that the enzyme capable of inactivating CM by acetylation was different from that responsible for the inactivation of KM-A. Chemical studies on the inactivated CM showed that it was modified by an enzyme in the presence of acetyl CoA resulting in the formation of 3-O-

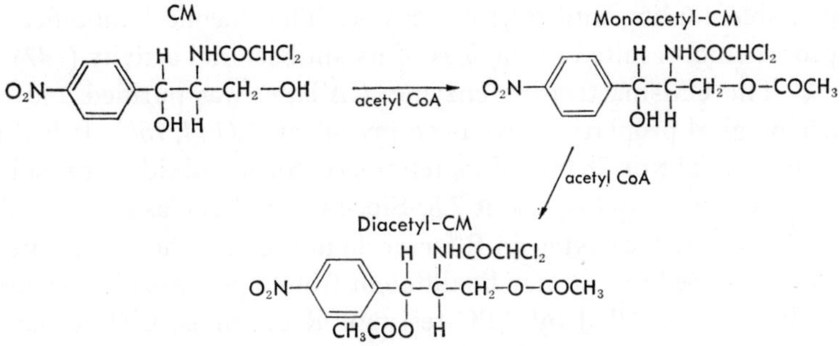

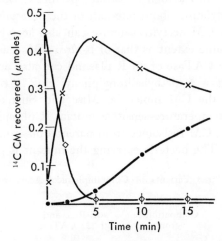

Fig. 9.   Inactivation of chloramphenicol by CM acetyltransferase.

Fig. 10.   Time course of the disappearance of chloramphenicol and the appearance of metabolites in crude extracts of *E. coli* R⁺ (*143*). × 3-O-monoacetyl-CM ; ● 1,3-O-diacetyl-CM ; ◇ CM.

acetyl CM and 1, 3-O-diacetyl CM (*142, 143, 156*). The enzyme responsible for monoacetylation of CM was also capable of reacetylating monoacetyl CM to diacetyl CM. Neither monoacetyl CM nor diacetyl CM retained any antibacterial activity. Chemical structures of the acetylated CMs and the time course of the CM acetylation are shown in Figs. 9 and 10. Many reports on the relation between the chemical structure of CM and its antibacterial activity have been presented with the conclusion that the propanediol moiety of the molecule is indispensable for its antibacterial activity. The chemical modification of propanediol resulted in the loss of its antibacterial activity (147).

The CM-inactivating enzyme, CATase, was purified and its enzymological properties have been investigated (144, 156). It had a molecular weight of 78,000 in its tetrameric form with identical sub-units and an optimal pH of about 7.8. Since the spheroplasts prepared from an E. coli strain carrying an R factor do not release the enzyme into surrounding medium, it may be different from a periplasmic enzyme such as PCase controlled by APC-resistant R plasmids. CM (D-threo) has three stereoisomers: L-threo, D-erythro, and L-erythro. CATase cannot inactivate the L-threo or D-erythro isomer, but only D-threo isomer, indicating that the enzyme has a high substrate specificity. Since the enzyme is capable of acetylating about one-half of the DL-erythro isomer, it was thought that CM acetyltransferase can also acetylate the L-erythro isomer to the same extent as that of D-threo-CM. Casacci et al. (20) reported that the CATase of an R plasmid can also acetylate thiamphenicol possessing a p-methylsulfonylphenyl ring in place of p-nitrophenyl moiety of the CM molecule. Mise and Suzuki (105) isolated E. coli carrying temperature-sensitive mutant R plasmids derived from R_{NR1} encoding CM resistance from parental plasmid at the frequency of about 10^{-4}. The bacteria carrying the mutant R grew at

TABLE VI. Properties of Three Variants of Chloramphenicol Acetyltransferase

R plasmid	fi type	Compatibility group	Cross reaction anti-R_{6-S} and anti-222 CATase[a] serum	MIC[b] of CM (μg/ml)
R_1	+	FII	+	175
222	+	FII	+	175
R_{6-S}	+	FII	+	175
R_{390}	−	N	+	175
R_{57b}	−	N	+	175
S-a	−	W	−	75
R_{A3}	−	W	−	75
R_{A4}	−	W	−	75
R_{387}	−	−	−	100

[a] CATase: chloramphenicol acetyltransferase.   [b] MIC (minimum inhibitory concen- 5, 5′-dithiobis-2-nitrobenzoate.

34°C but not at 43°C in the presence of CM. CATase obtained from bacteria carrying the mutant R plasmids was heat-labile in contrast with that from a strain harboring the wild-type R factor, and both enzymic activities producing the monoacetyl CM and the diacetyl CM were heat-labile to the same extent. These facts strongly suggest that the CM resistance gene on the R plasmids is the structure gene of CATase itself, and just one active site of the enzyme molecule plays a role in two steps of CM acetylation. The suggestion is supported by the genetical study of Foster and Howe (*38*). The result of their recombination experiments between single-site and multisite CM-sensitive mutants of R_1 and R_{100-1} indicated that the CM reistance region is a single cistron for the 20,000-molecular weight sub-unit of CATase.

Foster and Shaw (*39*) proposed the classification of CATases controlled by R plasmids. As indicated in Table VI, they grouped these enzymes into three classes, I, II, and III, and suggested a correlation between the *fi* type of CM-resistant plasmid and the class of CATase. Recently, the three variants of the CATases were purified to homogeniety by affinity chromatography. The variants behaved differently in binding response of the buffer, the length of spacer arms, and the extent of substitution by the ligand in the affinity column containing CM or *p*-amino CM attached to the free carboxyl group of a substituted Sepharose (*207*). Although the variants of the enzymes were

Specified by R Plasmids (*39*)

Km for CM (μM)	Electrophoretic mobility	Inhibition by DTNB[c]	Class of CATase[a]
8–10.5	Slow	−	I
8–10.5	Slow	−	I
8–10.5	Slow	−	I
10.6	Slow	−	I
8–10.5	Slow	−	I
19.6	Intermediate	+	II
17.2	Intermediate	+	II
17.5	Intermediate	+	II
17.8	Fast	−	III

tration) was measured with *E. coli* J5-3 *pro⁻*, *met⁻* as the host organism.   [c] DTNB:

classified into the three groups according to certain enzymological properties, a class III CATase has a native molecular weight of 80,000 composed of four identical subunits which give a hybrid form with a class I enzyme. Furthermore, it is suggested that class II and class III CATases are highly homologous with class I enzymes in their protein-chemical nature. Thus it may be considered that three variants of these enzymes differ with each other in a few amino acid residues.

CATase was detected in CM-resistant strains of *S. aureus* and inactivated CM in the presence of acetyl CoA. It was quite similar to that from the R plasmid-resistant strains in its enzymological properties (*88, 146, 157*). However, CATase in staphylococci is an inducible enzyme and staphylococcal CM-resistance is elevated by pretreatment of the CM-resistant staphylococci with subinhibitory concentrations of CM. On the other hand, CATase mediated by R plasmids is a constitutive enzyme. Nevertheless, Harwood and Smith (*50*) found catabolite repression of CATase synthesis in *E. coli* harboring a CM-resistant R plasmid which was caused by glucose or glucose 6-phosphate. Such a decrease in the enzymic activity was completely restored by the presence of cyclic 3′, 5′-AMP at 5 mM but not by 5′-AMP. This finding suggests the possibility that the CATase gene may be closely linked to a cAMP-sensitive promotor region.

Iyobe *et al.* (*56, 58*) isolated various mutants of an *E. coli* K12 strain, in which a CM-resistance gene (*cml*) derived from an R_{100-1}, was integrated into the chromosome. The CATase activity of these strains and the strain carrying R_{100-1} were determined during exponential growth with the following results: (1) CATase activity varied, depending upon the site of integration of the *cml* gene on the chromosome. Activity was found to be higher when the *cml* gene was integrated nearer the replication origin of the chromosome. (2) When two or three *cml* genes were integrated on the same chromosome, the total enzyme activity was the sum of activities coded by each gene separately. (3) When the *cml* gene was in a cytoplasmic state on R factor R_{100-1}, the expressed enzyme activity was four to eightfold higher than that in the chromosomal state, suggesting the existence of about four to eight copies of R factor per chromosome. The CATase activity returned to the level expressed by R_{100-1} when the chromosomal *cml* gene was detached and picked up by an R factor. Davis and Vapnek (*32*) reported recently that the level of R plasmid transcription was increased by twofold in a strain carrying the derepressed plasmid in comparison to an isogenic strain carrying the parental repressed plasmid, and the level of CATase activity was also notably increased, especially in a mutant strain of *E. coli* carrying the derepressed R, and was resistant to high levels of antibiotics.

2) Species-specific CATase

Surveys have disclosed that CATases are widely distributed among the CM-resistant strains of gram-negative bacteria including *E. coli*, *Klebsiella-Aerobacter* group, *Proteus*, and *Pseudomonas* which do not carry R plasmid (*124, 142*). The CM-acetylating activity is demonstrated in CM-sensitive strains of bacteria even though the activity is very weak. These facts strongly suggest that the enzymes capable of acetylating CM are widely distributed in gram-negative bacteria and play possible physiological roles in such bacterial strains, the enzyme being different from the CATase. This enzyme may be capable of acetylating CM more efficiently following mutation, and when strains capable of producing this enzyme become resistant to CM. These facts furthermore suggest the origin of genes determining CM resistance on the R plasmid and the evolutional changes in bacterial drug resistance. In fact, Shaw (*145*) has isolated single-step CM-resistant mutants of a *P. mirabilis* strain which appeared to be devoid of R plasmids. These mutants were highly resistant to CM and produced a large amount of CATase. This enzyme consists of four subunits with a molecular weight of 20,000 and is quite similar to that specified by fi^+ R plasmids (see Table VI) in enzymological, physicochemical, and serological properties. For example, the fingerprints of tryptic peptides from the *P. mirabilis* enzyme were compared with those from the fi^+ R specified monomer, indicating that there are several peptides which appeared to be common to both enzymes, although the two enzyme molecules are not perfectly equal.

3) Decrease in the permeability of CM

Nagai and Mitsuhashi (*118*) isolated four fi^+ R plasmids conferring CM resistance on *E. coli* of clinical origin. Bacterial strains harboring these plasmids were found to be incapable of acetylating CM in the presence of acetyl CoA. They found that one of these plasmids, R_{ms70}, confers the impermeability of CM on its host strain. CM resistance specified by R_{ms70} was considered to be inducible, since the preincubation with subinhibitory concentrations of CM remarkably elevated the growth rate of the R^+ bacterial cells in the presence of CM at 25 μg/ml and the preincubation effect was lost after overnight growth in the CM-free medium. This is the first finding that some R plasmids confer change in permeability of CM on the host organism, but the biochemical mechanism of the apparent decrease in permeability of the antibiotic remains unsolved. Another paper supports the universal validity that this type of mechanism for CM resistance is generally observed in bacteria.

Mitsuhashi et al. (48, 109) reported that among 11 Pseudomonas R plasmids, four plasmids could not inactivate CM in the presence of ATP, CoA, and magnesium acetate or in the presence of acetyl CoA. The mechanism of CM resistance encoded by these R plasmids was accounted for by a decrease in the permeability of the drug. This finding was also confirmed by Kono and O'hara (89) that an R plasmid, R_{kr102}, originated from P. aeruginosa K-Ps 102 confers the decreased membrane permeability of CM on its host strain. They failed to detect either inactivation of CM by CATase activity or some alteration of ribosomes causing the decrease in affinity for CM, and suggested that the CM-resistance barrier specified by R_{kr102} is in the surface layer of cells harboring the R plasmid because of the elevated sensitivity to CM in glycine-spheroplasts prepared from the R^+ cells. From these findings, it might be postulated that some proteins, if compared to the "TET" protein exhibiting tetracycline (TC) resistance in R^+ bacterial cells, could be inducibly formed in the cells.

4. Mechanism of Tetracycline (TC) Resistance

It is well known that TC and its derivatives inhibit protein synthesis in cell-free systems prepared from TC-sensitive, in vitro-developed TC-resistant, and R plasmid-resistant strains of E. coli to the same extent (94, 122, 204). Moreover, the in vitro-developed TC-resistant or R-mediated TC-resistant strains are incapable of inactivating antibiotic (123). These facts indicate that the mechanism of TC resistance controlled by R plasmids is different from the inactivating mechansisms of APC, CM, and aminoglycoside antibotics resistance in R plasmid-resistant strains. Izaki et al. (59, 60) and Franklin et al. (40, 42, 43) reported that TC-sensitive *E. coli* strains accumulate a large amount of TCs in cells from the surrounding medium through some energy-requiring system, and the accumulation is inhibited by the presence of inhibitors such as dinitrophenol or sodium azide. The apparent rate of the accumulation of TC should be defined as the difference between the rates of its influx and its efflux, but the mechanism of the energy-requiring accumulation of the drug still remains unsolved.

Izaki and Arima (*59*) showed that *E. coli* harboring an R plasmid become highly resistant even to 400 μg/ml of TC after the cells have been preincubated in a subinhibitory dose of 20 μg/ml. Franklin and Godfrey (*42*) also indicated that an *in vitro*-developed TC-resistant *E. coli* strain is only inhibited for about 1 hr when treated with 20 or 200 μM TC and thereafter the cells resumed the exponential growth in the presence of a high concentration of TC. Such an inducible resistance to TC was further demonstrated by several workers with various species of gram-negative and gram-positive bacteria.

It was also found that the gene encoding TC resistance in staphylococci is located on the nonconjugative resistance(r) plasmid (*54, 108*; see Chapter 3). Genetic and biochemical studies disclosed that prior treatment of *S. aureus* carrying r(TC) plasmid with low concentrations of the drug induced TC resistance. Rapid loss of TC resistance in induced populations took place after they were inoculated in a medium without TC. The aquisition of TC resistance after induction was found to be parallel with a decrease in accumulation of TC in microorganisms (*52–55*).

The induction of strains carrying R plasmids encoding TC resistance as well as *in vitro*-developed TC-resistant strains to one TC leads to the corresponding resistance to other TCs. Not only TCs but also TC derivatives, which could not inhibit the growth of bacteria such as β-apo-oxy TC or 4-epi TC, can induce TC resistance. However, cross resistance was not observed with other antibiotics, such as aminoglycoside antibiotics, macrolide antibiotics, CM, or β-lactam antibiotics. Connamacher (*23*) suggested that minute quantities of TC, as little as 2nM of the drug, could induce the resistance and thus the receptors for induction differed from those for inhibition of protein synthesis. Nevertheless, Franklin (*40*) and Inoue *et al.* (*53*) observed that the induction of TC resistance in *E. coli* R+ and TC-resistant *S. aureus*, respectively, was blocked by actinomycin D at 1.5 μg/ml or CM, and these facts suggest that some RNA synthesis or protein synthesis is required for the induction of TC resistance in these organisms. It may be postulated that, in the presence of TC at concentrations too high to cause induction of the resistance, a part of protein synthesis in cultures occurs and consequently, induction is possible. Franklin and Cook (*41*), and Robertson and Reeve (*133*) isolated the R plasmid mutants which conferred the constitutive TC resistance on host organisms. These findings indicate the participation of a regulatory gene apparently coding for a repressor of the resistance gene(s) in the induction of TC resistance.

Inoue *et al.* (*54*) investigated the antibacterial and inducer activities of TC resistance in *S. aureus* using 13 TC derivatives and analogues. Four compounds of the TC derivatives used were not able to induce TC resistance in *S. aureus* carrying a nonconjugative plasmid r-ms7 (TC) harboring an inducible TC-resistance determinant. The 12a-hydroxy position seems to be essential for inducer activity of TC resistance.

Levy and McMurry (*97*) reported the presence of a new protein occurring in membrane of minicells of *E. coli* containing R(TC) plasmids when they were incubated in the presence of the antibiotic. The "TET protein" was not demonstrated in minicells carrying R plasmids which lack TC resistance but was uniquely detectable in minicells harboring TC-resistant plasmids such as R_{222}. When placed on a sodium dodecylsulfate (SDS) polyacrylamide gel, the protein was electrophoretically detected as a single band when either a whole minicell containing a TC-resistant R plasmid, supernatants of sonically disrupted lysates that had been centrifuged at 55,000 rpm, or purified membrane preparations of the cells was used. Thus, TET protein was easily solubilized and its molecular weight was estimated to be about 50,000 on gel using a phosphate buffer system. It was suggested that the protein behaves at the level of the cell membrane by antagonizing the active accumulation of the antibiotic either by reducing its influx or accelerating its efflux. In addition, a similar mobility on gel electrophoresis of the TET protein specified by R plasmids of at least five different compatibility groups was demonstrated, and hence the TC-resistance gene on R plasmids might have evolved from one common origin. Yang *et al.* (*203*) investigated the gene expression concerning the

TET synthesis. They compared the synthesis of proteins encoded by R_{222} plasmid in a DNA-directed cell-free system containing the S-30 fraction with that in *E. coli* minicells containing the R plasmid, through observations of fluorograms on SDS polyacrylamide gels. A greater number of proteins specified by the plasmid was detected in the cell-free system (30 distinct proteins) than in the minicells (about 10 proteins). This result indicates the presence of control factors for the negatively regulated gene expression of the plasmid in the minicells. Synthesis of the TET protein specified by R_{222} was observed in the minicells only after induction by TC, whereas the TET protein was synthesized *in vitro* in a cell-free system in the absence of the drug though the amounts of the protein were much less than in the minicells after the induction. However, the TET protein synthesis in the cell-free system was specifically repressed by adding fractionated extracts from cells containing R_{222} plasmid to the system, and the inhibition was reversed by the addition of TC or a TC analog, 5α, 11α-dehydro-7-chloro TC, which is not a protein synthesis inhibitor. Such a cytoplasmically diffusible inhibitor of TET protein synthesis could be a negative control protein presumably specified by the R plasmid working at the level of either transcription or translation. Young and Hubball (*206*) investigated the function of the TET protein mediated by an *fi+* F-like R plasmid, FR1 in *E. coli* K12. They used a mutant plasmid, FR1*tet-ts*1, which is a temperature-sensitive mutant plasmid encoding TC resistance (sensitive at 42°C and resistant at 30°C). This R plasmid mutant is not temperature-sensitive as its plasmid replication and the mutation has occurred on the TC-resistance gene. While *E. coli* R⁻ cells accumulate TC at a rate dependent on temperature in a range of 30–42°C, the cells carrying FR1*tet-ts*1 do not take up detectable amounts of the antibiotic at 30 or 33°C but accumulate it at rates comparable to those of R⁻ cells above 36°C. However, the apparent rate of TC efflux from *E. coli* FR1*tet-ts*1 is very similar to that from the R⁻ cells at both 42 and 30°C. These results are consistent with the speculation that the TET protein plays a role in decreasing the influx rate of TC rather than accelerating the efflux rate of the drug.

The alternative mechanism to explain TC resistance on the basis of gene-dosage effect has been reported by several investigators.

Yagi and Clewell (*190*) reported that a gradual increase in the size of pAMα1 plasmid in *Streptococcus faecalis* was observed during growth of the cells in the presence of TC. The analyses of the enlarged plasmids using sucrose density-gradients sedimentation, electron microscopy, and the EcoR1 enzyme indicated that the plasmid contained repeated units of a 2.65 megadalton segment, including the TC-resistant gene. Apparent gene amplification such as that which occurs with pAMα1 may also explain the mechanism of the TC induction.

5. Resistance to Macrolide Antibiotics

It is well-known that plasmids which confer macrolide antibiotics-resistance on host cells are widely distributed among staphylococci and other gram-positive bacteria, and the macrolide-resistance in most of these bacteria can be induced by pretreating the bacterial cells with a subinhibitory dose of a proper inducer such as erythromycin. No inactivating mechanism of erythromycin or other macrolides could be detected in cultures of macrolide-resistant *S. aureus* (*134, 135, 197*).

Yamagishi *et al.* (*197*) noted that sensitive and uninduced cells had an uptake of erythromycin into *S. aureus* of between 5 and 7.5×10^{-2} μg/mg dry weight of cells whereas macrolide-resistant cells of the induced or constitutively resistant *S. aureus* contained only 1.2×10^{-2} μg/mg dry weight of cells or less. They suggested that level of the intracellular accumulation of the antibiotic could be reflected by the binding affinity of the ribosomes of the bacterial strains for it. This mechanism of macrolide resistance in *S. aureus* was confirmed by the investigation of Saito *et al.* (*134, 135*). They found that the inhibition of cell growth by erythromycin was proportional to the intracellular concentration for macrolide-sensitive strains which was 44–90 times that of the medium. Since the inhibitors of oxidative phosphorylation or respiration, such as 2, 4-dinitrophenol, cyanide or sodium azide, did not affect the uptake of erythromycin in cells, the decrease in the active accumulation of the antibiotic is excluded from the mechanism of erythromycin resistance in *S. aureus*.

According to them, the amount of erythromycin-ribosome complex in induced cells, as well as constitutively resistant cells, was about one-eighth of that in uninduced cells, and such a decrease in the drug binding affinity of ribosomes can satisfactorily explain the decrease in intracellular accumulation of erythromycin in macrolide-resistant *S. aureus.*

Several investigators tried to make the biochemical mechanism of the inducible resistance in *S. aureus* manifest through studies to detect some altered proteins in 50S subunits of ribosomes from the induced cells after successfully finding an altered 50S subunit protein from an *in vitro*-developed erythromycin-resistant strain of *E. coli*, but none of them were able to do so. However, Lai and Weisblum (*91*) demonstrated, for the first time, that an altered methylated base is contained in 23S rRNA from the induced cells or the cells of constitutively resistant strains but not in that from uninduced or sensitive cells of *S. aureus*, and the methylated base was identified as 6-dimethyladenine. The methylation of the adenine residue(s) in a specific sequence of 23S rRNA may result in a weaker binding of the modified ribosomes for erythromycin or other macrolides as compared with the normal ribosomes, and this mechanism may explain the resistance to the antibiotics in *S. aureus.* Later, they found that dimethylation occurred at a heptamer sequence Pu_6Py (tentatively identified as GGAAAGC or GAAAGGC) in a single fragment obtained by treating (Me-^{14}C)-labelled 23S rRNA from the induced cells with T_1 ribonuclease and then pancreatic ribonuclease, while seven other methyl-labelled fragments were found to be common to rRNA from uninduced, induced and constitutively resistant cells. Lai *et al.* (*92*) succeeded in reconstituting functionally active 50S subunits from 23S rRNA of the induced or the uninduced *S. aureus* and ribosomal proteins together with 5S rRNA of *Bacillus stearothermophilus.* They tested poly(U)-directed poly(phe) synthesis activity with a combined system composed of heterologously reconstituted 50S subunits or native 50S subunits and 30S subunits of *E. coli.* The addition of spiramycin or lincomycin to the system inhibited phenylalanine incorporation into poly(phe) fractions when the 23S rRNA came from the uninduced cells of *S. aureus* whereas inhibition to a much lesser degree was observed in the presence of the antibiotics when the 23S rRNA came from the induced cells as well as the constitutive resistant cells. This result also indicates that methylation of one of the adenine residues in 23S rRNA is the principal mechanism for resistance to erythromycin and other macrolide antibiotics in *S. aureus.* However, details of the mechanism of methylation, the enzymologically phenotypic trait corresponding to gene(s) of erythromycin resistance and so on are still unknown.

6. Mechanisms of Sulfonamide (SA) Resistance

Since p-aminobenzenesulfonamide (sulfanylamide: SA) was established as the active antibacterial moiety of the prontosil molecule, a large number of effective derivatives have been synthesized by substitution on the amide group. However, all of the SA and its derivatives have the common mode of the inhibitory action being antagonized by p-aminobenzoate (PABA). SAs are antagonized not only by PABA, but also by a variety of other compounds including folic acid analogs, purines, and unknown constituents of peptone. Antibacterial acitivity of SAs can be reversed by a large amount of PABA, whether its source is intrinsic manufacture by the cell or it is provided by external milieu or media. In SA-resistant strains of staphylococci isolated from clinical sources, it was found that they produce a 20-fold greater amount of PABA and 5-fold greater amount of folate than SA-sensitive strains (184). Similarly, in vitro-developed SA-resistant strains of staphylococci produce a larger amount of both PABA and folate than the [parental SA-sensitive strains (93, 184). Thus, SAs inhibit the biosynthesis of tetrahydrofolate by competing at the site of PABA in dihydropteroate synthetase (dihydropteroate-synthase, EC 2. 5. 1. 15) and this inhibition causes the prevention of the formation of a number of raw materials of protein, DNA and RNA biosynthesis. The route of the synthesis of tetrahydropteroate and the inhibition sites of SAs as well as trimethoprim (TP) are illustrated in Fig. 11.

1) Altered dihydropteroate synthetase
Pato and Brown (129) reported that there are two types of mechanism in artificially developed SA-resistant E. coli strains: (1) SAs sensitivity of a dihydropteroate synthetase (Fig. 11), which decreases in accordance with an increase in SA resistance, and (2) decrease in permeability of SAs in SA-resistant strains of E. coli. In the latter case the folate synthesizing system in SA-resistant strains is still inhibited by SA as much as that in SA-sensitive strains. The former mechanism was found also in in vitro developed SA-resistant strains of pneumococci.

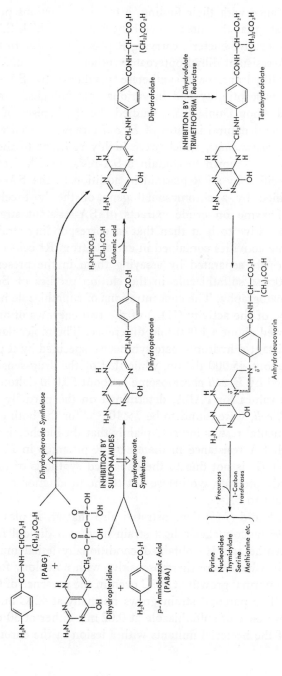

Fig. 11.   Pathways for enzymatic synthesis of tetrahydrofolate.

In accordance with their finding, a few investigations published recently indicate that the most general mechanism of high SA resistance in gram-negative bacteria carrying R plasmids is due to the production of SA-resistant dihydropteroate synthetase which differs from SA-sensitive dihydropteroate synthetase produced by SA-sensitive strains in SA susceptibility and in various enzymological properties.

Wise and Abou-Donia (*185*) studied the mechanism of SA resistance in several natural isolates of *E. coli* strains, as well as *Citrobacter* and *K. pneumoniae*, which were highly resistant to the drugs. These strains were shown to contain a SA-resistant dihydropteroate synthetase specified by an R plasmid in addition to the SA-sensitive enzyme specified by a chromosomal gene of the host cells. The SA-resistant enzyme on crude extracts of SA-resistant strains was much more sensitive to heat than that in corresponding strains, and the two enzyme activities contained in extracts from R+ cells of *E. coli* strains were easily separated by assaying them in the presence and absence of 10^{-4} M sulfathiazole in the elution profiles of Sephadex column chromatography. The concentrations of sulfathiazole necessary to inhibit 50% of the activity (ID_{50}) of the two enzymes of an *E. coli* R+ strain showed about a 1,000-fold difference. The molecular weight of the SA-resistant dihydropteroate synthetase specified by R plasmids in *E. coli* is about 45,000 dalton, while that of the drug-sensitive enzyme controlled by *E. coli* chromosome is about 50,000 daltons. However, the *Km* values for PABA, determined on the partially purified enzymes of *E. coli*, were found to be 7×10^{-7} M for the both enzymes. These experimental results indicate plainly that the biochemical mechanism of high SA resistance mediated by R plasmids in *E. coli* and its related bacteria is not due to the enhanced synthesis of the drug-sensitive dihydropteroate synthetase but to the production of the new enzyme resistant to SAs.

Recently, Sköld (*148*) demonstrated also that an R plasmid mediating SA resistance makes a host strain of *E. coli* diploid for dihydropteroate synthetase. He obtained conditionally lethal mutants of *E. coli* C strain which were thermosensitive with no colony formed at 42°C but with normal growth at 30°C even in the presence of 0.02 mM sulfathiazole. The parental strain grows normally at 42°C but cannot grow in the presence of sulfathiazole at 0.02 mM either at 30 or 42°C. The rescue of the bacterial mutants with a lesion in the chromosomal dihydropteroate synthetase from temperature sensitivity was achieved by a derepressed R plasmid, R_{1dr19}, encoding resistance to SAs, CM, ampicillin (APC), SM, and KM. Other evidence was obtained by direct measurements of the dihydropteroate synthesizing activity and the degrees of its inhibition by sulfathiazole in partly purified extracts from the parental strain with and without the plasmid. The result was that the dihydropteroate synthetase activity of the extracts from R+ cells was significantly less inhibited at a concentration of sulfathiazole where the extracts from R− cells is inhibited more than 95%. This interesting finding indicates that SA resistance mediated by some R plasmids can be explained by a drug-resistant target enzyme, dihydropteroate synthetase, specified by the R plasmids. Such a biochemical mechanism of drug resistance is analogous to that of TP resistance specified by R plasmids, as stated later.

Nagate and Mitsuhashi (*119*) investigated the biochemical mechanism of SA resistance mediated by conjugative (R) and nonconjugative (r) plasmids. The rate of incorporation of ^{14}C-PABA into the dihydropteroate fraction with extracts prepared from *E. coli* ML1410 carrying an R_{ms248} encoding SA resistance, was notably less sensitive to SA inhibition than that with extracts from its host strain of *E. coli* ML1410. They found out that many plasmids carrying SA resistance or (SA. SM) resistance specify the SA-resistant and thermosensitive dihydropteroate synthetase while the majority of R plasmids mediating resistance to more than three drugs, including SAs, may specify other mechanisms of SA resistance such as the decrease in permeability of the drug because of the sensitivity of the cell-free folate synthesizing system from these R+ cells to SAs. This finding supports their interesting postulation that the evolutionary routes of SA or some of the (SA. SM) plasmids specifying the SA-resistant dihydropteroate synthetase may differ from those of R plasmids which mediate resistance to more than three drugs, including SM and SA. It may be considered that a transposon (SA. SM) specifying the dihydropteroate synthetase as well as the SM resistance occurs widely in gram-negative bacteria (see Chapter 4).

2) Decrease in permeability

The mechanisms of SA resistance in *E. coli* carrying R plasmids have been extensively studied by Yokota *et al.* (*1, 2, 205*) who found that the cell-free system capable of synthesizing folate prepared from R+ cells is equally inhibited by SAs as is the SA-sensitive strain. From these results it may be concluded that the mechanism of SA resistance in the R+ strain is ascribed to the decrease in permeability of the drug through the cell membrane, and not by increase in the amounts of either the folate or its precursors and also not by the decrease in SA sensitivity of enzymes responsible for folate synthesis.

According to tracer experiments using ^{35}S-sulfathiazole, it was found that the amount of SA incorporated in R+ cells is decreased by about one-third from that in SA-sensitive R− cells of *E. coli*, and they suggested that the decrease in SA permeability may be the main factor responsible for SA resistance in strains harboring SA-resistant R plasmids. However, whether the 200- to 500-fold elevation of SA resistance in R+ strains is explainable by such a difference in the permeability of the drug is as yet unknown.

7. Mechanisms of TP Resistance

TP (2, 4-diamino-5-(3′, 4′, 5′-trimethoxybenzyl)pyrimidine) is the most active and selective antibacterial agent among various inhibitors of dihydrofolate reductase (5, 6, 7, 8-tetrahydrofolate: NADP oxidoreductase, EC 1. 5. 1. 3), and it has been used clinically in combination with a SA, sulfamethoxazole. The loci of TP as well as SAs inhibition are shown in Fig. 11. R plasmids encoding very high resistance to TP were isolated from clinical sources just 3 years after the introduction of the drug. Skold and Widh (149) found that an R plasmid, R_{483}, mediating high resistance to TP, specifies the production of a large amount of dihydrofolate reductase which differs from that of *E. coli* host in the enzymological properties. The R plasmid confers a 7- to 20-fold increase in dihydrofolate reductase activity on host cells of *E. coli* K12, B or C. They demonstrated that this increased enzymic activity could not be due simply to enhanced synthesis of the normal chromosomal enzyme but to the introduction into the resistant cells of a new enzyme encoded by the R plasmid: (1) dihydrofolate reductase of the R plasmid is far more heat-labile than that of the *E. coli* chromosome since the former was inactivated about 70 times faster than the chromosomal enzyme, and (2) the purified dihydrofolate reductase controlled by R_{483} is about 10,000 times less sensitive to TP inhibition than the enzyme from R⁻ cells, and this can be explained partly from the fact that a Ki value of 0.6×10^{-9} M was obtained for the enzyme from R⁻ cells while the enzyme of the R plasmid has Ki of 0.4×10^{-5} M, although both activities of the enzymes were inhibited competitively by TP.

The mechanism of TP resistance mediated by R plasmids has been confirmed by recent investigations by Amyes and Smith (*3, 4*). The TP-resistant dihydrofolate reductase mediated by an R plasmid, R_{388}, in *E. coli* could be separated from the TP-sensitive enzyme of the host chromosome by DEAE-cellulose ion-exchange chromatography and obtained in a homogeneous state. The pH optima of the R-mediated enzyme and the host enzyme were 6.0 and 6.5, respectively, but the pH activity curve of the R plasmid enzyme showed a much sharper peak. The purified R plasmid enzyme was about 20,000 times less sensitive to TP than the host chromosomal enzyme since the doses of the drug giving 50% inhibition (ID_{50}) of the chromosomal enzyme and the R-plasmid enzyme were 10×10^{-9} and 18×10^{-5} M, respectively, at pH 6.0. This difference in the susceptibility to TP between the two enzymes coincides with that in Ki values between those enzymes, as the previous investigators demonstrated, even though the Km for the chromosomal enzyme and the R-plasmid enzyme were 20 and 8.3 μM, respectively. Moreover, they found that the molecular weight of the R_{388}-mediated enzyme was 35,000 whereas that of the chromosomal enzyme was 21,000. They postulated that the origin of the gene coding dihydrofolate reductase in the R plasmid may have arisen from that of the T even phage since the dihydrofolate reductase of the T_6 phage has a molecular weight of 31,000 and the T_4-phage mutants were isolated which produced dihydrofolate reductases that were less sensitive to antifolate drugs than was the wild-type T_4 enzyme.

These investigations indicate that the biochemical mechanism of TP resistance mediated by R plasmids is analogous to that of SA resistance specified by R plasmids, and the formation of a drug-resistant target enzyme is very important in the consideration of biochemical mechanisms mediated by R plasmids as well as two other general types of mechanisms for R plasmid-mediated drug resistance which are modifications of the drugs and the induction of permeation change.

Barth *et al.* (*8*) investigated the transposition of a DNA sequence encoding TP and SM resistance from R_{483}, which was used in the study by Skold and Widh (*149*) as described above, to other replicons, *i.e.*, to *E. coli* chromosome or to related and unrelated plasmids. A segment of DNA of about 9×10^6 daltons containing both resistance genes could be transposed to other replicons but the colicin Ia or pilus genes of R_{483} were not transposed. It appeared that (TP^r. SM^r) transposition was very site-specific and the *recA* gene product is not necessary for this transposition. They speculated that the (TP^r. SM^r) segment of R_{483} is a transposon with a specific boundary sequence. It is interesting that the TP resistance gene in the T even phages may be picked up resulting in the formation of the (TP^r. SM^r) transposon.

8.   Mechanisms of Mercury Resistance

Since 1957 when Smith (*150*) reported the isolation of R plasmids conferring resistance either to mercuric ion Hg(II) or to mercuric, cobalt and nickel ions on an *E. coli* host, a large number of drug resistant plasmids containing a Hg(II)-resistance determinant have been reported by many investigators. While a variety of strains of *Pseudomonas* species exhibiting the resistance to both Hg(II) and organomercurials, such as phenylmercuric acetate (PMA), had been isolated and the biochemical mechanism of the Hg(II) resistance in one of these strains was clarified by Tonomura *et al.* (*166, 167*), no organomercurials-resistant R plasmids in gram-negative species had been described until 1974 when Schottel *et al.* (*141*) isolated 8 R plasmids encoding the resistance to both Hg(II) and PMA out of 30 mercury-resistant R plasmids. According to their paper, the majority of those Hg(II)- and PMA-resistant R plasmids, originally isolated from *Serratia marcescens*, carry an APC resistance gene simultaneously and L or S incompatibility determinants. Moreover, the PMA resistance of those plasmids is expressed as an inducible function for the expression of Hg(II) resistance.

1)   Resistance to mercuric ion and organomercurials in pseudomonad
Investigations of the biochemical mechanism of resistance to mercury specified by enteric R plasmids were preceded by the studies of Tonomura *et al.* (*44–47, 166, 167*) with a mercury-resistant strain of pseu-

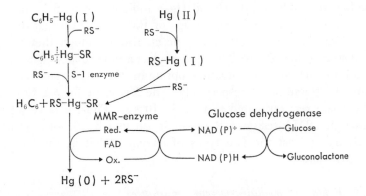

RS⁻ : SH compound
S-1 enzyme : C–Hg linkage splitting enzyme 1
MMR-enzyme : metallic mercury-releasing enzyme

Fig. 12. The postulated pathway for the reductive decomposition of organomercurials in mercury-resistant *Pseudomonas* K-62 strain.

domonad in which the mercury-resistance could be controlled by chromosomal determinants.

At first, they demonstrated that the mechanism of Hg(II) and organomercurials resistance in a strain K-62 is due to the enzymatic reduction of Hg(II) and organomercurials (R-Hg(I)) to metallic mercury (Hg(0)) which is volatile and lost from its culture medium. Later, one of the pathways by which Hg(II) is reduced to Hg(0) with metallic mercury-releasing enzyme (MMR) enzyme (see Fig. 12), as found by Furukawa and Tonomura, has been investigated more minutely with strains of *E. coli* carrying Hg(II)-resistant R plasmids as described in the following section. However, the analysis of the pathway for R-Hg(I) → Hg(0) remains unclear.

Tezuka and Tonomura (*165*) recently proposed a pathway for the reductive decomposition of PMA as well as Hg(II), as indicated in Fig. 12, because of their interesting finding of the organomercurials-decomposing enzyme in strain K-62. They succeeded in the purification of "a splitting enzyme" (or S-1 enzyme) from "the crude cytochrom C-1" fraction by repeated Sephadex, DEAE-Sephadex, and DEAE-cellulose column chromatographies. This enzyme catalyzes the cleavage of ≡C-Hg⁺ bond in the presence of an SH-compound like thioglycolate to produce $\equiv$C-H and Hg-S-moieties. The S-1 enzyme can cleave not only the C-Hg linkage of PMA, but also that in aliphatic methylmercuric and ethylmercuric chlorides, though they are poorer substrates than PMA. This enzyme has a molecular weight of 19,000, and its pH and temperature optimum for its enzyme activity are about 7.0 and 50°C, respectively. The Km value for p-chloromercuribenzoate was estimated to be 5.3×10^{-5} M. Thus, it is very probable that the PMA-resistant R plasmids isolated by Schottel et al. (141) specify at least the two types of enzymes, that is, the S-1 and the MMR-enzymes.

2)   R plasmid-mediated mercury resistance

After the discovery of the volatilization of Hg(II) from the culture broth of pseudomonad by Tonomura et al., Izaki and his co-workers (83–85) demonstrated that E. coli cells carrying a Hg(II)-resistant R plasmid (R_{100}) converted Hg(II) into volatile Hg(0) and crude cell-free extracts from the cells were also capable of catalyzing the vaporization of Hg(II) in the presence of NADPH, 2-mercaptoethanol and Mg^{2+} in the assay medium whereas no Hg(II) vaporizing activity could be detected with the extracts of R⁻ cells. NADPH is an essential cofactor for the vaporization process but NADH had only a slight effect on the reductive vaporization of Hg(II).

On the other hand, Furukawa and Tonomura (44–47) observed, as described above, that cell-free extracts of a K-62 strain of *Pseudomonas* sp. containing glucose dehydrogenase activity was active in the reductive vaporization of Hg(II) or PMA in the presence of SH compounds, such as thioglycolate, NAD(P) and glucose. Thereafter, they found that the glucose dehydrogenase, MMR (Fig. 12) and cytochrome c-1 fraction in the extracts participate in vaporizing Hg(II) from the assay medium. The MMR enzyme purified mainly by DEAE-Sephadex chromatography was found to be a flavoprotein containing FAD, and its molecular weight was about 67,000. Moreover, they demonstrated that the *Pseudomonas* strain produces the MMR enzyme in an inducible manner by the presence of a variety of mercury salts.

The Hg(II)-reducing enzyme specified by the R plasmid in E. coli was purified about 100-fold from the crude extracts by Izaki et al. (61). The purified enzyme had a characteristic absorption spectrum indicating the presence of a flavin compound in its molecule which was identified as FAD from the result of analysis using thin-layer chromatography and D-amino acid oxidase apoenzyme. Rapid reduction of Hg(II) was observed in the presence of both the purified enzyme and NADPH, but the reduction of organomercurials, such as PMA, did not occur under the same condition. A notable difference between this enzyme mediated by the R plasmid and the MMR enzyme of *Pseudomonas* was seen in the cofactor requirement that NADH acts as an electron donor for the enzymatic reduction of Hg(II) to a remarkably lesser extent than NADPH in the reaction with the R plasmid-mediated enzyme. The *Km* value of the enzyme for $HgCl_2$ was 20×10^{-5} M. The enzymatic activity was severely inhibited by Ag^+, Cu^{2+}, and Cd^{2+}, and the vaporization of Hg(0) from Hg(II) was intensively inhibited by the presence of an equimolecular amount of Ag^+. Therefore, the MMR enzyme and the R plasmid-mediated reductase appear to be very similar though they are not identical. Similarly, Summers *et al.* (*153, 154*) also reported that the inducible and heat-labile volatilization of Hg(II) was observed with *E. coli* cells carrying a mercury-resistant R plasmid and the strain converted 95% of 10^{-5} M Hg(II) to Hg(0) at a rate of 4 to 5 nmoles of Hg(II) per min per 10^8 cells at 37°C. According to them, the volatile form of mercury produced by Hg(II)-resistant *E. coli*, which is soluble in common solvents, are not volatile dimethylmercury but metallic mercury, Hg(0), from the result of analysis using gas chromatography-mass spectroscopy of the toluene or chloroform extracts of the induced cells. In accordance with the finding by Izaki *et al.* (*61*), it was found that Ag^+ and Au^{3+} are intensive inhibitors of mercury volatilization. Thereafter, Summers and Sugarman (*155*) also obtained the partly purified Hg(II)-reducing enzyme specified by an R plasmid and suggested that the enzyme is located in the cytoplasm rather than in the periplasmic space of the cell. However, it may be more reasonable to consider that the Hg(II)-reducing activity is loosely associated with the cytoplasmic membrane and works there. They investigated also the inhibitors of this enzyme in detail. Among those inhibitors, Ag^+ and Au^{3+} salts markedly inhibited the Hg(II)-reducing activity in whole cells and Ag^+ inhibited the cell-free activity. But both Au^{3+} and Ag^+ may serve as substrates for the enzyme because it was found that Au^{3+} was reduced to metallic colloidal Au(0) with the cell-free system.

Anyway, the R plasmid-mediated Hg(II)-reducing enzymes isolated by both groups of investigators *(83–85, 153–155)* were able to convert just Hg(II) to Hg(0), and its activity was rather inhibited by the presence of PMA. It was apparently observed that *E. coli* strains harboring R plasmids conferring only Hg(II) resistance could volatilize only Hg(II). However, strains carrying R plasmids which confer the resistance to both Hg(II) and PMA, isolated by Schottel *et al. (141)*, cause the volatilization of the both compounds. Thus, it is very probable that the latter group of the R plasmids contain the gene(s) specifying R-Hg(I) splitting activity besides in the genome that specifying the Hg(II)-reducing enzyme.

The mechanisms of resistance to other heavy metallic ions, such as nickel or cobalt mediated by R plasmids, remain unsolved.

REFERENCES

1 Akiba, T. and Yokota, T. 1961. *Med. Biol. (Tokyo)*, **58**, 161–165 (in Japanese).
2 Akiba, T. and Yokota, T. 1962. *Med. Biol. (Tokyo)*, **63**, 155–159 (in Japanese).
3 Amyes, S. G. B. and Smith, J. T. 1974. *Biochem. Biophys. Res. Commun.*, **58**, 412–418.
4 Amyes, S. G. B. and Smith, J. T. 1976. *Eur. J. Biochem.*, **61**, 597–603.
5 Anderson, E. S. and Datta, N. 1965. *Lancet*, **i**, 407–409.
6 Anderson, E. S. and Lewis, M. J. 1965. *Nature*, **206**, 579–583.
7 Aoki, T., Egusa, S., Ogata, Y., and Watanabe, T. 1971. *J. Gen. Microbiol.*, **65**, 343–349.
8 Barth, P. T., Datta, N., Hedges, R. W., and Grinter, N. J. 1976. *J. Bacteriol.*, **125**, 800–810.
9 Benveniste, R. and Davies, J. 1971. *Biochemistry*, **10**, 1787–1796.
10 Benveniste, R. and Davies, J. 1971. *FEBS Letters*, **14**, 293–296.
11 Benveniste, R. and Davies, J. 1973. *Proc. Natl. Acad. Sci. U.S.*, **70**, 2276–2280.
12 Benveniste, R. and Davies, J. 1973. *Annu. Rev. Biochem.*, **42**, 471–505.
13 Benveniste, R., Yamada, T., and Davies, J. 1970. *Infect. Immunol.*, **1**, 109–119.
14 Bobrowski, M. M., Matthew, M., Barth, P. T., Datta, N., Grinter, N. J., Jacob, A. E., Kontomichalou, P., Dale, J. W., and Smith, J. T. 1976. *J. Bacteriol.*, **125**, 149–157.

15 Bryan, L. E., Van Den Elsen, H. M., and Tseng, J. T. 1972. *Antimicrob. Agents Chemother.*, **1**, 22–29.

16 Bryan, L. E., Shahrabadi, M. S., and Van Den Elzen, H. M. 1974. *Antimicrob. Agents Chemother.*, **6**, 191–199.

17 Bryan, L. E., Van Den Elzen, H. M., and Shahrabadi, M. H. 1975. *In* Microbial Drug Resistance, ed. by S. Mitsuhashi and H. Hashimoto, pp. 475–490, University of Tokyo Press, Tokyo / University Park Press, Baltimore and London.

18 Brzezinska, M., Benveniste, R., Davies, J., Daniels, P. J. L., and Weinstein, J. 1972. *Biochemistry*, **11**, 761–765.

19 Brzezinska, M. and Davies, J. 1973. *Antimicrob. Agents Chemother.*, **3**, 266–269.

20 Casacci, F., Sassi, A., and Marca, G. 1974. *Boll. Chim. Farm.*, **113**, 488–494.

21 Chabbert, Y. A. and Bandens, J. G. 1966. *Antimicrob. Agents Chemother.*, *1965*, 380–383.

22 Chevereau, M., Daniels, P. J. L., Davies, J., and LeGoffic, F. 1974. *Biochemistry*, **13**, 598–603.

23 Connamacher, R. H. and Pratt, E. A. 1972. *Adv. Antimicrob. Antineopl. Chemother.*, **1-I**, 521–524.

24 Curtis, N. A. C., Richmond, M. H., and Stanisich, V. 1973. *J. Gen. Microbiol.*, **79**, 163–166.

25 Dale, J. W. and Smith, J. T. 1974. *J. Bacteriol.*, **119**, 351–356.

26 Dale, J. W. and Smith, J. T. 1976. *Biochem. Biophys. Res. Commun.*, **68**, 1000–1005.

27 Daniels, P. J. L., Weinstein, J., Tkach, R. W., and Morton, J. 1974. *J. Antibiot.*, **27**, 150–154.

28 Datta, N. and Kontomichalou, P. 1965. *Nature*, **208**, 239–241.

29 Datta, N. and Richmond, M. H. 1966. *Biochem. J.*, **98**, 204–209.

30 Davies, J. 1971. *J. Infect. Dis.*, **124** (Suppl.), 7–10.

31 Davies, J., Brzezinska, M., and Benveniste, R. 1971. *Ann. N.Y. Acad. Sci.*, **182**, 226–233.

32 Davis, R. and Vapnek, D. 1976. *J. Bacteriol.*, **125**, 1148–1155.

33 Doi, O., Miyamoto, M., Tanaka, N., and Umezawa, H. 1968. *Appl. Microbiol.*, **16**, 1282–1284.

34 Doi, O., Ogura, M., Tanaka, N., and Umezawa, H. 1968. *Appl. Microbiol.*, **16**, 1276–1281.

35 Doi, O., Kondo, S., Tanaka, N., and Umezawa, H. 1969. *J. Antibiot.*, **22**, 273–282.

36 Egawa, R., Hiraishi, H., Atsumi, K., and Mitsuhashi, S. 1966. *Japan. J. Bacteriol.*, **21**, 591–592 (in Japanese).

37 Egawa, R., Sawai, T., and Mitsuhashi, S. 1967. *Japan. J. Microbiol.*, **11**, 173–178.

38 Foster, T. J. and Howe, T. G. B. 1973. *J. Bacteriol.*, **116**, 1062–1063.

39 Foster, T. J. and Shaw, W. V. 1973. *Antimicrob. Agents Chemother.*, **3**, 99–104.

40 Franklin, T. J. 1967. *Biochem. J.*, **105**, 371–379.

41 Franklin, T. J. and Cook, J. M. 1971. *Nature*, **229**, 273–274.

42 Franklin, T. J. and Godfrey, A. 1965. *Biochem. J.*, **94**, 54–60.

43 Franklin, T. J. and Higginson, B. 1970. *Biochem. J.*, **116**, 287–297.

44 Furukawa, K., Suzuki, T., and Tonomura, K. 1969. *Agr. Biol. Chem.*, **33**, 128–130.

45 Furukawa, K. and Tonomura, K. 1971. *Agr. Biol. Chem.*, **35**, 604–610.

46 Furukawa, K. and Tonomura, K. 1972. *Agr. Biol. Chem.*, **36**, 217–226.

47 Furukawa, K. and Tonomura, K. 1972. *Agr. Biol. Chem.*, **36**, 2441–2448.

48 Fuse, A., Kawabe, H., Hasuda, K., Sagai, H., Iyobe, S., and Mitsuhashi, S. 1975. *Japan. J. Bacteriol.*, **30**, 354–355 (in Japanese).

49 Harwood, J. and Smith, D. H. 1969. *J. Bacteriol.*, **97**, 1262–1271.

50 Harwood, J. and Smith, D. H. 1971. *Biochem. Biophys. Res. Commun.*, **42**, 57–62.

51 Holmes, R. K., Minshew, B. H., Gould, K., and Sanford, J. P. 1974. *Antimicrob. Agents Chemother.*, **6**, 253–262.

52 Inoue, M., Hashimoto, H., and Mitsuhashi, S. 1969. *In* Progress in Antimicrobial and Anticancer Chemotherapy (Proc. 6th Int. Congr. Chemother., Tokyo), ed. by H. Umezawa, pp. 433–439, University of Tokyo Press, Tokyo.

53 Inoue, M., Hashimoto, H., and Mitsuhashi, S. 1970. *J. Antibiot.*, **23**, 68–74.

54 Inoue, M., Okubo, T., Oshima, H., and Mitsuhashi, S. 1975. *In* Microbial Drug Resistance, ed. by S. Mitsuhashi and H. Hashimoto, pp. 153–164, University of Tokyo Press, Tokyo / University Park Press, Baltimore and London.

55 Inoue, M., Kazawa, T., and Mitsuhashi, S. 1976. *Japan. J. Microbiol.*, in press.

56 Iyobe, S., Hashimoto, H., and Mitsuhashi, S. 1970. *Japan. J. Microbiol.*, **14**, 463–471.

57 Iyobe, S., Hasuda, K., Fuse, A., and Mitsuhashi, S. 1974. *Antimicrob. Agents Chemother.*, **5**, 547–552.

58 Iyobe, S., Kono, M., Ohara, K., Hashimoto, H., and Mitsuhashi, S. 1974. *Antimicrob. Agents Chemother.*, **5**, 68–74.

59 Izaki, K. and Arima, K. 1965. *J. Bacteriol.*, **89**, 1335–1339.

60 Izaki, K., Kiuchi, K., and Arima, K. 1966. *J. Bacteriol.*, **91**, 628–633.
61 Izaki, K., Tashiro, Y., and Funaba, T. 1974. *J. Biochem.*, **75**, 591–599.
62 Kabins, S., Nathan, C., and Cohen, S. 1974. *Antimicrob. Agents Chemother.*, **5**, 565–570.
63 Kawabe, H., Kobayashi, F., Yamaguchi, M., Utahara, R., and Mitsuhashi, S. 1971. *J. Antibiot.*, **24**, 651–652.
64 Kawabe, H. and Mitsuhashi, S. 1971. *Japan. J. Microbiol.*, **15**, 545–548.
65 Kawabe, H., Inoue, M., and Mitsuhashi, S. 1974. *Antimicrob. Agents Chemother.*, **5**, 553–557.
66 Kawabe, H. and Mitsuhashi, S. 1972. *Japan. J. Microbiol.*, **16**, 436–437.
67 Kawabe, H., Kondo, S., Umezawa, H., and Mitsuhashi, S. 1975. *Antimicrob. Agents Chemother.*, **7**, 494–499.
68 Kawabe, H. and Mitsuhashi, S. 1975. *In* Microbial Drug Resistance, ed. by S. Mitsuhashi and H. Hashimoto, pp. 449–461, University of Tokyo Press, Tokyo / University Park Press, Baltimore and London.
69 Kawabe, H., Naito, N., and Mitsuhashi, S. 1975. *Antimicrob. Agents Chemother.*, **7**, 50–54.
70 Kawabe, H., Umezawa, H., Iyobe, S., and Mitsuhashi, S. 1976. 3rd Int. Symp. on Antibiotic Resistance, Czechoslovakia, June.
71 Kawaguchi, H., Naito, T., Nakagawa, S., and Fujisawa, K. 1972. *J. Antibiot.*, **25**, 695–708.
72 Kayser, F. H. and Santanam, P. 1975. 9th Int. Congr. Chemother., London.
73 Kayser, F. H. 1976. 3rd Int. Symp. on Antibotic Resistance, Czechoslovakia, June.
74 Kida, M., Igarashi, S., Okutani, T., Asako, T., Hiraga, K., and Mitsuhashi, S. 1974. *Antimicrob. Agents Chemother.*, **5**, 92–94.
75 Kida, M., Asako, T., Yoneda, M., and Mitsuhashi, S. 1975. *In* Microbial Drug Resistance, ed. by S. Mitsuhashi and H. Hashimoto, pp. 441–448, University of Tokyo Press, Tokyo / University Park Press, Baltimore and London.
76 Kobayashi, F., Yamaguchi, M., Eda, J., Higashi, F., and Mitsuhashi, S. 1971. *J. Antibiot.*, **24**, 719–721.
77 Kobayashi, F., Yamaguchi, M., and Mitsuhashi, S. 1971. *Japan. J. Microbiol.*, **15**, 381–382.
78 Kobayashi, F., Yamaguchi, M., and Mitsuhashi, S. 1971. *Japan. J. Microbiol.*, **15**, 265–272.
79 Kobayashi, F., Yamaguchi, M., Eda, J., Hiramatsu, M., and Mitsuhashi, S. 1972. *Gunma Rep. Med. Sci.*, **5**, 291–301.
80 Kobayashi, F., Yamaguchi, M., Sato, J., and Mitsuhashi, S. 1972. *Japan. J. Microbiol.*, **16**, 15–19.

81 Kobayashi, F., Yamaguchi, M., and Mitsuhashi, S. 1972. *Antimicrob. Agents Chemother.*, **1**, 17–21.

82 Kobayashi, F., Koshi, T., Eda, J., Yoshimura, Y., and Mitsuhashi, S. 1973. *Antimicrob. Agents Chemother.*, **4**, 1–5.

83 Komura, I., Izaki, K., and Takahashi, H. 1970. *Agr. Biol. Chem.*, **34**, 480–482.

84 Komura, I. and Izaki, K. 1971. *J. Biochem.*, **70**, 885–893.

85 Komura, I., Funaba, T., and Izaki, K. 1971. *J. Biochem.*, **70**, 895–901.

86 Kondo, S., Okanishi, M., Utahara, R., Maeda, K., and Umezawa, H. 1968. *J. Antibiot.*, **21**, 22–29.

87 Kondo, S., Yamamoto, H., Naganawa, H., Umezawa, H., and Mitsuhashi, S. 1972. *J. Antibiot.*, **25**, 483–484.

88 Kono, M., Ogawa, K., and Mitsuhashi, S. 1968. *J. Bacteriol.*, **95**, 886–892.

89 Kono, M. and O'hara, K. 1976. *J. Antibiot.*, **29**, 176–180.

90 Kontomichalou, P., Papachristou, E. G., and Levis, G. M. 1974. *Antimicrob. Agents Chemother.*, **6**, 60–72.

91 Lai, C. and Weisblum, B. 1971. *Proc. Natl. Acad. Sci. U.S.*, **68**, 856–860.

92 Lai, C., Weisblum, B., Fahnestock, S. R., and Nomura, M. 1973. *J. Mol. Biol.*, **74**, 67–72.

93 Landy, M., Larkum, N. W., Oswald, E. J., and Streghtoff, F. 1943. *Science*, **97**, 265.

94 Laskin, A. I. and Chan, W. M. 1964. *Biochem. Biophys. Res. Commun.*, **14**, 137–142.

95 Le Goffic, F., Martel, A., and Witchitz, J. 1974. *Antimicrob. Agents Chemother.*, **6**, 680–684.

96 Le Goffic, F. 1975. *In* Drug-inactivating Enzymes and Antibiotic Resistance (2nd Int. Symp. on Antibiotic Resistance, Smolenice, 1974), ed. by S. Mitsuhashi, L. Rosival, and V. Krčméry, pp. 165–169, Avicenum, Czechoslovak Medical Press, Prague.

97 Levy, S. B. and McMurry, L. 1974. *Biochem. Biophys. Res. Commun.*, **56**, 1060–1068.

98 Maeda, K., Kondo, S., Okanishi, M., Utahara, R., and Umezawa, H. 1968. *J. Antibiot.*, **21**, 458–459.

99 Marengo, P. B., Chenowth, M. E., Overturf, G. D., and Wilkins, J. 1974. *Antimicrob. Agents Chemother.*, **6**, 821–824.

100 Matsumoto, H., Sawai, T., Tazaki, T., Yamagishi, S., and Mitsuhashi, S. 1972. *Japan. J. Microbiol.*, **16**, 169–176.

101 Matsushita, T., Suzuki, J., Sawai, T., Yamagishi, S., and Mitsuhashi, S. 1972. *Japan. J. Bacteriol.*, **27**, 231 (in Japanese).

102 Matthew, M., Harris, A. M., Marshall, M. J., and Ross, G. W. 1975. *J. Gen. Microbiol.*, **88**, 169–178.
103 Matthew, M. and Hedges, R. W. 1976. *J. Bacteriol.*, **125**, 713–718.
104 Miller, A. L. and Walker, J. B. 1969. *J. Bacteriol.*, **99**, 401–405.
105 Mise, K. and Suzuki, Y. 1968. *J. Bacteriol.*, **95**, 2124–2130.
106 Mitsuhashi, S., Kobayashi, F., and Yamaguchi, M. 1971. *J. Antibiot.*, **24**, 400–401.
107 Mitsuhashi, S., Kobayashi, F., Yamaguchi, M., O'hara, K., and Kono, M. 1972. *In* Adv. in Antimicrobiol and Antineoplasmic Chemother. (Proc. 7th Int. Congr. Chemother., Prague, 1971), ed. by P. Malek, pp. 561–564, Avicenum, Czechoslovak Medical Press, Prague.
108 Mitsuhashi, S., Inoue, M., Kawabe, H., Oshima, H., and Okubo, T. 1973. *In* Contributions to Microbiology and Immunology, Vol. 1, Staphylococci and Staphylococal Infections, ed. by J. Jeljaszewicz, pp. 144–165, Karger, Basel.
109 Mitsuhashi, S., Kawabe, H., Fuse, A., and Iyobe, S. 1975. *In* Microbial Drug Resistance, ed. by S. Mitsuhashi and H. Hashimoto, pp. 515–523, University of Tokyo Press, Tokyo / University Park Press, Baltimore and London.
110 Mitsuhashi, S. and Krčméry, V. 1975. *Zentralbl. Bakteriol.*, *I*, **242**, 528–546.
111 Mitsuhashi, S. 1975. *In* Drug-inactivating Enzymes and Antibiotic Resistance (2nd Int. Symp. on Antibiotic Resistance, Smolenice, 1974), ed. by S. Mitsuhashi, L. Rosival, and V. Krčméry, pp. 115–119, Avicenum, Czechoslovak Medical Press, Prague.
112 Mitsuhashi, S. and Kawabe, H. 1975. *In* Drug-inactivating Enzymes and Antibiotic Resistance (2nd Int. Symp. on Antibiotic Resistance, Smolenice, 1974), ed. by S. Mitsuhashi, L. Rosival, and V. Krčméry, pp. 157–163, Avicenum, Czechoslovak Medical Press, Prague.
113 Miyamura, S. 1961. *Japan. J. Bacteriol.*, **16**, 115–119 (in Japanese).
114 Miyamura, S. and Oketani, S. 1962. *Japan. J. Bacteriol.*, **17**, 294 (in Japanese).
115 Morel, C., Freymuth, F., and Villemon-Lemosquet, M. 1973. *Ann. Biol. Clin.*, **31**, 353–357.
116 Naganawa, H., Kondo, S., Maeda, K., and Umezawa, H. 1971. *J. Antibiot.*, **24**, 823–829.
117 Naganawa, H., Yagisawa, M., Kondo, S., Takeuchi, T., and Umezawa, H. 1971. *J. Antibiot.*, **24**, 913–914.
118 Nagai, Y. and Mitsuhashi, S. 1972. *J. Bacteriol.*, **109**, 1–7.
119 Nagate, T. and Mitsuhashi, S. 1976. *Antimicrob. Agents Chemother.*, in press.

120 O'hara, K., Kono, M., and Mitsuhashi, S. 1974. *J. Antibiot.*, **27**, 349–351.

121 O'hara, K., Kono, M., and Mitsuhashi, S. 1974. *Antimicrob. Agents Chemother.*, **5**, 558–561.

122 Okamoto, S. and Mizuno, D. 1964. *J. Gen. Microbiol.*, **35**, 125–133.

123 Okamoto, S. and Suzuki, Y. 1965. *Nature*, **208**, 1301–1303.

124 Okamoto, S., Suzuki, Y., Mise, K., and Nakaya, R. 1967. *J. Bacteriol.*, **94**, 1616–1622.

125 Okanishi, M., Kondo, S., Suzuki, Y., Okamoto, S., and Umezawa, H. 1967. *J. Antibiot.*, **20**, 132–135.

126 Okanishi, M., Kondo, S., Utahara, R., and Umezawa, H. 1968. *J. Antibiot.*, **21**, 13–21.

127 Ooka, T., Hashimoto, H., and Mitsuhashi, S. 1970. *Japan. J. Microbiol.*, **14**, 123–128.

128 Ozanne, B., Benveniste, R., Tipper, D., and Davies, J. 1969. *J. Bacteriol.*, **100**, 1144–1146.

129 Pato, M. L. and Brown, G. L. 1963. *Arch. Biochem. Biophys.*, **103**, 443–448.

130 Price, K. E., Chisholm, D. R., Misiek, M., Leitner, F., and Tsai, Y. H. 1972. *J. Antibiot.*, **25**, 709–731.

131 Richmond, M. H. and Sykes, R. L. 1973. *Adv. Microb. Physiol.*, **9**, 31–38.

132 Richmond, M. H. 1975. *Methods Enzymol.*, **XLIII**, 672–677.

133 Robertson, J. M. and Reeve, E. C. R. 1972. *Genet. Res.*, **20**, 239–252.

134 Saito, T., Hashimoto, H., and Mitsuhashi, S. 1969. *Japan. J. Microbiol.*, **13**, 119–121.

135 Saito, T., Shimizu, M., and Mitsuhashi, S. 1971. *Ann. N.Y. Acad. Sci.*, **182**, 267–278.

136 Sawada, Y., Yaginuma, S., Tai, M., Iyobe, S., and Mitsuhashi, S. 1975. *Antimicrob. Agents Chemother.*, **9**, 55–60.

137 Sawai, T., Mitsuhashi, S., and Yamagishi, S. 1968. *Japan. J. Microbiol.*, **12**, 423–434.

138 Sawai, T., Morioka, K., Ogawa, M., and Yamagishi, S. 1976. *Antimicrob. Agents Chemother.*, **10**, 191–195.

139 Sawai, T., Takahashi, K., Yamagishi, S., and Mitsuhashi, S. 1970. *J. Bacteriol.*, **104**, 620–629.

140 Sawai, T., Yamagishi, S., and Mitsuhashi, S. 1973. *J. Bacteriol.*, **115**, 1045–1054.

141 Schottel, J., Mandal, A., Clark, D., and Silver, S. 1974. *Nature*, **251**, 335–337.

142 Shaw, W. V. 1967. *Antimicrob. Agents Chemother.*, *1966*, 221–226.

143 Shaw, W. V. 1967. *J. Biol. Chem.*, **242**, 687–693.
144 Shaw, W. V. 1970. *In* Progress in Antimicrobial and Anticancer Chemother., Vol. II, ed. by H. Umezawa, pp. 552–555, University of Tokyo Press, Tokyo.
145 Shaw, W. V. 1973. Proc. Symp. Bacterial Plasmids (Soc. General Microbiol.), pp. 8–11.
146 Shaw, W. V. and Brodsky, R. F. 1968. *J. Bacteriol.*, **95**, 28–36.
147 Shemiyakin, M. M. 1961. Khimia Antibiotikov, Vol. I, Academy of Science, U.S.S.R., Moscow.
148 Sköld, O. 1976. *Antimicrob. Agents Chemother.*, **9**, 49–54.
149 Sköld, O. and Widh, A. 1974. *J. Biol. Chem.*, **249**, 4324–4325.
150 Smith, D. H. 1967. *Science*, **156**, 1114–1116.
151 Smith, D. H., Janjigian, J. A., Prescott, N., and Anderson, P. W. 1970. *Infect. Immunol.*, **1**, 120–127.
152 Smith, J. T., Bremner, D. A., and Datta, N. 1974. *Antimicrob. Agents Chemother.*, **6**, 418–421.
153 Summers, A. O. and Silver, S. 1972. *J. Bacteriol.*, **112**, 1228–1236.
154 Summers, A. O. and Lewis, E. 1973. *J. Bacteriol.*, **113**, 1070–1072.
155 Summers, A. O. and Sugarman, L. I. 1974. *J. Bacteriol.*, **119**, 242–249.
156 Suzuki, Y. and Okamoto, S. 1967. *J. Biol. Chem.*, **242**, 4722–4730.
157 Suzuki, Y., Okamoto, S., and Kono, M. 1966. *J. Bacteriol.*, **92**, 798–799.
158 Suzuki, I., Takahashi, N., Shirato, S., Kawabe, H., and Mitsuhashi, S. 1974. *In* Microbial Drug Resistance, ed. by S. Mitsuhashi and H. Hashimoto, pp. 463–473, University of Tokyo Press, Tokyo / University Park Press, Baltimore and London.
159 Sykes, R. B. and Richmond, M. H. 1970. *Nature*, **226**, 952–954.
160 Tai, K., Sawada, Y., Iyobe, S., and Mitsuhashi, S. 1975. *Japan. J. Bacteriol.*, **30**, 101 (in Japanese).
161 Takagi, Y., Miyake, T., Tuchiya, T., Umezawa, S., and Umezawa, H. 1973. *J. Antibiot.*, **26**, 403–406.
162 Takasawa, S., Utahara, R., Okanishi, M., Maeda, K., and Umezawa, H. 1968. *J. Antibiot.*, **21**, 477–484.
163 Tanaka, T., Nagai, Y., Sawai, T., Hashimoto, H., and Mitsuhashi, S. 1966. *Japan. J. Bacteriol.*, **21**, 591 (in Japanese).
164 Tanaka, N. 1970. *J. Antibiot.*, **23**, 469–471.
165 Tezuka, T. and Tonomura, K. 1976. *J. Biochem.*, **80**, 79–87.
166 Tonomura, K. and Kanzaki, F. 1969. *Biochim. Biophys. Acta*, **184**, 227–229.
167 Tonomura, K., Maeda, K., Futai, F., Nakagami, T., and Yamada, M. 1968. *Nature*, **217**, 644–646.

168 Tseng, J.-T., Bryan, L. E., and Van Den Elsen, H. M. 1972. *Antimicrob. Agents Chemother.*, **2**, 136–141.

169 Umezawa, H., Okanishi, M., Kondo, S., Hamana, K., Utahara, R., Maeda, K., and Mitsuhashi, S. 1967. *Science*, **157**, 1559–1561.

170 Umezawa, H., Okanishi, M., Utahara, R., Maeda, K., and Kondo, S. 1967. *J. Antibiot.*, **20**, 136–141.

171 Umezawa, H., Takasawa, S., Okanishi, M., and Utahara, R. 1968. *J. Antibiot.*, **21**, 81–82.

172 Umezawa, H., Doi, O., Ogura, M., Kondo, S., and Tanaka, N. 1968. *J. Antibiot.*, **21**, 154–155.

173 Umezawa, S., Tuchiya, T., Muto, R., Nishimura, Y., and Umezawa, H. 1971. *J. Antibiot.*, **24**, 274–275.

174 Umezawa, H., Umezawa, S., Tsuchiya, T., and Okazaki, Y. 1971. *J. Antibiot.*, **24**, 485–487.

175 Umezawa, S., Tuchiya, T., Jikihara, T., and Umezawa, H. 1971. *J. Antibiot.*, **24**, 711–712.

176 Umezawa, H., Nishimura, Y., Tsuchiya, T., and Umezawa, S. 1972. *J. Antibiot.*, **25**, 743–745.

177 Umezawa, H., Yamamoto, H., Yagisawa, M., Kondo, S., Takeuchi, T., and Chabbert, Y. A. 1973. *J. Antibiot.*, **26**, 407–411.

178 Umezawa, H., Yagisawa, M., Matsuhashi, Y., Naganawa, H., Yamamoto, H., Kondo, S., Takeuchi, T., and Chabbert, Y. A. 1973. *J. Antibiot.*, **26**, 612–614.

179 Umezawa, H., Matsuhashi, Y., Yagisawa, M., Yamamoto, H., Kondo, S., and Takeuchi, T. 1974. *J. Antibiot.*, **27**, 358–360.

180 Umezawa, S., Nishimura, Y., Hata, Y., Tsuchiya, T., Yagisawa, M., and Umezawa, H. 1974. *J. Antibiot.*, **27**, 722–725.

181 Umesawa, H. 1975. *In* Drug Action and Drug Resistance in Bacteria, Vol. II, Aminoglycoside Antibiotics, ed. by S. Mitsuhashi, pp. 3–43, University of Tokyo Press, Tokyo / University Park Press, Baltimore and London.

182 Umezawa, Y., Yagisawa, M., Sawa, T., Takeuchi, T., Umezawa, H., Matsumoto, H., and Tazaki, T. 1975. *J. Antibiot.*, **28**, 845–853.

183 Walker, J. B. and Skorvaga, M. 1973. *J. Biol. Chem.*, **248**, 2435–2440.

184 White, P. J. and Woods, D. D. 1965. *J. Gen. Microbiol.*, **40**, 243–253.

185 Wise, E. M., Jr. and Abou-Donia, M. M. 1975. *Proc. Natl. Acad. Sci. U.S.*, **72**, 2621–2625.

186 Witchitz, J. L. 1972. *J. Antibiot.*, **25**, 622–624.

187 Yagisawa, M., Naganawa, H., Kondo, S., Hamada, M., Takeuchi, T., and Umezawa, H. 1971. *J. Antibiot.*, **24**, 911–912.

188 Yagisawa, M., Naganawa, H., Kondo, S., Takeuchi, T., and Umezawa, H. 1972. *J. Antibiot.*, **25**, 495–496.

189 Yagisawa, M., Yamamoto, H., Naganawa, H., Kondo, S., Takeuchi, T., and Umezawa, H. 1972. *J. Antibiot.*, **25**, 748–750.

190 Yagi, Y. and Clewell, D. B. 1976. *J. Mol. Biol.*, **102**, 583–600.

191 Yaginuma, S., Sawai, T., Yamagishi, S., and Mitsuhashi, S. 1973. *Japan. J. Microbiol.*, **17**, 141–147.

192 Yaginuma, S., Sawai, T., Yamagishi, S., and Mitsuhashi, S. 1974. *Japan. J. Microbiol.*, **18**, 113–118.

193 Yaginuma, S., Terakado, N., and Mitsuhashi, S. 1975. *Antimicrob. Agents Chemother.*, **8**, 238–242.

194 Yamada, T., Tipper, D., and Davies, J. 1968. *Nature*, **219**, 288–291.

195 Yamagishi, S., O'hara, K., Sawai, T., and Mitsuhashi, S. 1969. *J. Biochem.*, **66**, 11–20.

196 Yamagishi, S., Sawai, T., and Kobayashi, T. 1975. *In* Microbial Drug Resistance, ed. by S. Mitsuhashi and H. Hashimoto, pp. 101–113, University of Tokyo Press, Tokyo / University Park Press, Baltimore and London.

197 Yamagishi, S., Nakajima, Y., Inoue, M., and Oka, Y. 1971. *Japan. J. Microbiol.*, **15**, 39–52.

198 Yamaguchi, M., Kobayashi, F., and Mitsuhashi, S. 1972. *Antimicrob. Agents Chemother.*, **1**, 139–142.

199 Yamaguchi, M., Koshi, T., Kobayashi, F., and Mitsuhashi, S. 1972. *Antimicrob. Agents Chemother.*, **2**, 142–146.

200 Yamaguchi, M., Mitsuhashi, S., Kobayashi, F., and Zenda, H. 1974. *J. Antibiot.*, **27**, 507–515.

201 Yamamoto, H., Kondo, S., Maeda, K., and Umezawa, H. 1972. *J. Antibiot.*, **25**, 485–486.

202 Yamamoto, H., Yagisawa, M., Naganawa, H., Kondo, S., Takeuchi, T., and Umezawa, H. 1972. *J. Antibiot.*, **25**, 746–747.

203 Yang, H. L., Zubay, G., and Levy, S. B. 1976. *Proc. Natl. Acad. Sci. U.S.*, **73**, 1509–1512.

204 Yokota, T. and Akiba, T. 1961. *Med. Biol. (Tokyo)*, **58**, 172–175 (in Japanese).

205 Yokota, T. and Akiba, T. 1962. *Med. Biol. (Tokyo)*, **63**, 160–164 (in Japanese).

206 Young, T. W. and Hubball, S. J. 1976. *Biochem. Biophys. Res. Commun.*, **70**, 117–124.

207 Zaidenzaig, Y. and Shaw, W. V. 1976. *FEBS Letters*, **62**, 266–271.

CLASSIFICATION OF R PLASMIDS

10 R FACTORS IN ENTEROBACTERIACEAE

Naomi DATTA
Royal Postgraduate Medical School, Hammersmith Hospital, London, U.K.

The R factors of the enterobacteria have proved to be very diverse. A classification of these plasmids into groups, based on their compatibility properties, is described in this chapter. That closely related plasmids are *incompatible*, *i.e.*, that they cannot co-exist in their bacterial host, has been known for many years (*17*). The subsequent history of plasmid, including R factor classification was reviewed by Datta (*7*). This chapter summarizes present knowledge of compatibility, describes the criteria used to define groups and discusses the applicability of incompatibility grouping in the study of plasmid evolution and ecology.

1. *Expression of Incompatibility*

The simplest expression of incompatibility is when the introduction of a second plasmid into a plasmid-bearing host leads to the elimination of the resident plasmid. This is *prima facie* evidence that the two plasmids are incompatible. Compatibility between the two is indicated by retention by the host of both incoming and resident plasmids. Compatibility testing must, of course, be carried out in standardized conditions, and qualifications of the simple statement above are necessary.

For reproducible results, plasmids must be classified by testing in one chosen host. There are known examples of compatibility relationships differing in different hosts (*32, 51, 52*). The classification described here is based on experiments using *Escherichia coli* K12, into which R factors and other plasmids from naturally occurring strains of many genera are transferable by conjugation. But many resistance plasmids, including all those identified in *Staphylococcus* and *Streptococcus* and some of those detected in *Pseudomonas, Proteus,* and *Serratia,* are not transmissible to *E. coli* K12, and so are not included in this classification scheme. Plasmids of a group designated V, identified so far only in strains of *Proteus mirabilis,* were transferable to *E. coli* K12, but were so unstable in that host that compatibility studies were impossible. On transfer to *E. coli* K12, they did not eliminate plasmids of any known group; this group was defined by compatibility studies in *P. mirabilis* (*28*). Incompatibility between pairs of plasmids is demonstrable in other genera and has been used in them as a method of plasmid classification (see, for examples Refs. *3, 48*).

2. Method for Incompatibility-grouping of Conjugative Plasmids in E. coli K12

The unknown R factor under test is transferred from its wild host to an auxotrophic strain of *E. coli* K12. The recipient must usually have chromosomally determined resistance to nalidixic acid or rifampicin, to allow its isolation from the mating mixture. Once the initial transfer is made, the new R+ strain is used as the donor in matings with a set of K12 cultures, whose nutritional requirements are distinct from those of the donor, and each of which carries a plasmid of known compatibility group. It is convenient to use *lac−* recipients with a *lac+* donor or *lac+* recipients with a *lac−* donor. The mating mixtures are plated on medium to select transconjugants, *i.e.,* plates containing the nutritional requirements of the recipient and an antibiotic whose resistance is specified by the incoming, but not the resident, R factor. The concentration of antibiotic (or other selective substance) used for selection should be the lowest possible to give complete inhibition of the R− recipient, thus allowing detection of plasmids conferring low levels of resistance. Because the activity of antibacterial drugs varies considerably in different media, the concentrations to be used should be determined in preliminary tests.

Colonies which appear on the selection plates require purifying by replating to obtain separate colonies. For this step, a medium that differentiates *lac+* from *lac−* colonies, such as MacConkey or EMB agar, may be used, incorporating the antibiotic that selects for the incoming R factor (but not the resident). This medium allows the growth of donor cells as well as R+ transconjugants, and is therefore suitable for purification of the latter. Where it is impossible to distinguish donor and transconjugant by their *lac* property, or where the drug of selection is a sulphonamide (SA), and therefore inactive in MacConkey or EMB agar, the transconjugants should be purified by restreaking to obtain well-separated colonies on plates of the same composition as the selection plates.

For each mating, a minimum of 10 transconjugant clones should be purified and tested for the presence of resistance genes of the incoming and resident plasmids. A convenient method of testing is to streak colonies from the purification plates across double ditch plates, the two ditches incorporating, respectively, drugs to indicate the presence of the two plasmids. Each R+ parent and an R− K12 are streaked in parallel as controls.

Three possible results are seen:

a)   In every transconjugant clone, the donor marker is present, the resident marker is lost. Transconjugants should be tested to show whether every marker of the incoming plasmid is present, and every distinguishable marker of the former resident is eliminated. The test for compatibility should then be repeated in the opposite direction, to see whether the plasmid that has been eliminated in the first test can, in its turn, eliminate the other. If it does so, in all clones tested, the two plasmids are assigned to the same group.

b)   Both plasmid markers are present in all transconjugant clones. When this is the result, at least one clone should be tested to show whether it carries all the distinguishable markers of both plasmids, besides the two indicator markers. The stable, and separate, co-existence of both plasmids is proof of compatibility. To test for this, a pure transconjugant clone is grown through many generations in liquid medium (growth to saturation from a small inoculum is convenient), plated, and colonies tested for the continued presence of markers of both plasmids. Instability of either plasmid indicates incompatibility (provided, of course, that the plasmid is stably maintained in the same conditions, when alone in the host). To test for the separate existence of the two plasmids, the transconjugant is used as a donor, separate selection plates being used to test for transfer of each plasmid. At least 10 transconjugants from each selective medium are purified and tested as described above. The separate transfer of *either* plasmid indicates the separateness, and therefore compatibility, of the two.

c) The resident plasmid is lost from some, but not all, of the transconjugant clones. This result on its own can be interpreted as indicating neither incompatibility nor compatibility of the two plasmids. The purified clones which possess resistance genes of both plasmids, should be tested, as described above, for the stability and separate transferability of each. If the two plasmids are stably inherited, and separate, they are compatible, despite the initially observed elimination of the resident (see below "Dislodgement"). If they are unstable, or have recombined, their incompatibility is indicated.

3. Definition of Compatibility Groups

To define a group, one must have at least two incompatible plasmids distinguishable by markers that can be used for selection in genetic crosses. Resistance genes are particularly easy to work with. In many cases, natural bacterial isolates have supplied a pair of prototypes to define the group. An example is provided by the F-like R factors, R_1 and R_{136} (Table I). These two plasmids are incompatible and are therefore assigned to a single incompatibility group, FII. In other cases, various genetic manipulations for the removal or addition of genes are required to make two plasmids distinguishable. The simplest of these is to find, by replica-plating the R+ strain, spontaneous loss of one resistance gene from a plasmid conferring multiple resistance. Such loss is usually irreversible, presumably resulting from deletion. An example is in the definition of group H (Table I) all of whose available members conferred resistance either to tetracycline (TC) alone or to TC, streptomycin (SM), chloramphenicol (CM), and SAs (TC. SM. CM. SA). Sometimes more complex manipulations are required, as in the definition of group J, all of whose known naturally

TABLE I. Plasmid Incompatibility Groups Represented by at Least Two Plasmids

Group	Plasmid	Genetic characters	Comments	Reference
C	R$_{40a}$	amp kan sul	Naturally occurring	10
	R$_{57b-1}$	cml sul	Spontaneous loss of markers of R$_{57b}$	10
FI	F-*lac*	lac$^+$	Recombination between replicons	40
	R$_{386}$	tet	Naturally occurring	15
FII	R$_1$	amp str cml kan sul	Naturally occurring	44
	R$_{136}$	tet	Naturally occurring	44
H	R$_{27}$	tet	Naturally occurring	21
	R$_{726-1}$	sul cml sul	Spontaneous loss of tet-res by R$_{726}$	14
I$_\alpha$	R$_{64}$	str tet	Naturally occurring	31
	R$_{144}$	tet kan Col Ib	Naturally occurring	31
I$_\gamma$	R$_{621a}$	tet	Naturally occurring	31
	ColIb-1M1420	Col Ib	Naturally occurring	39^a
J	R$_{391}$	kan	Naturally occurring	5
	R$_{391-3b-1}$	str tmp	Transposition of str tmp res: loss of kan res	—^{b}
L	R$_{472}$	amp	Naturally occurring	37
	R$_{831}$	str kan	Naturally occurring	37
M	R$_{446b}$	str tet	Naturally occurring	32
	R$_{930}$	amp	Naturally occurring	37
N	N3	str tet sul	Naturally occurring	8
	R$_{447b}$	amp kan	Naturally occurring	32
O	R$_7$	amp str tet sul	Naturally occurring	34
	R$_{724}$	str tet cml sul	Naturally occurring	14
P	RP4	amp tet kan	Naturally occurring	13
	R$_{702}$	str tet kan sul	Naturally occurring	35
S	R$_{478}$	tet cml kan	Naturally occurring	37
	R$_{477-1}$	str tet sul	Spontaneous loss of cml kan res by R$_{477}$	37
T	Rts1	kan	Naturally occurring	5
	R$_{401}$	amp str	Naturally occurring	5
W	S-a	str cml kan sul	Naturally occurring	29
	R$_{388}$	sul tmp	Naturally occurring	11

^{a} S. Howarth-Thompson, R. W. Hedges, and N. Datta, unpublished observations.
^{b} R. W. Hedges, unpublished.

occurring members have the same resistance pattern; they carry a single resistance gene (Table I). An R factor, R_{391-3b}, with the resistance pattern (kanamycin (KM). trimethoprim (TP). SM) was constructed by the transposition of resistance genes from R_{483} to R_{391} (see section below "Transposons"). A spontaneous segregant of this plasmid, $R_{391-3b-1}$, lacked KM resistance, and was therefore distinguishable from R_{391}. It was found to be incompatible, not only with its parent plasmid, R_{391}, but also with other KM resistance plasmids from the same natural source, which we had tentatively assumed to be of the same group (5).

Plasmid incompatibility was first observed between distinguishable F' factors, constructed by genetic manipulation, in that case, recombination with an unrelated replicon, the *E. coli* K12 chromosome. F' factors were used to define group FI, to which the F factor of *E. coli* K12 belongs (Table I). Other means of reducing or extending the genetic make up of plasmids may be used to make them distinguishable from one another. Examples not used in Table I are deletion of genes in transduction by a phage too small to accommodate the whole plasmid, "transductional shortening" (54) or addition of transduced genes by marker rescue (1).

4. *Difficulties Encountered in Classifying Plasmids by Compatibility*

There are difficulties in this classification scheme. Some of them are trivial, but others illustrate the genetic potentialities and evolutionary relationships of plasmids.

1) *Lack of distinguishable markers*
It may be impossible to classify a plasmid by the methods described above because its genetic markers overlap too much with those of a standard set of plasmids of known groups. Variants of the new plasmid may be sought by the methods described in the section above, "the definition of compatibility groups."

2) *Quantitative differences in compatibility properties*
An F' plasmid in an Hfr culture does not replicate, and is diluted out as the culture grows (16), but incompatibility is not always so clear-cut an all-or-none phenomenon. Some incompatible plasmids can co-

exist through many host-cell generations, which implies that both can replicate in the same cell, although their instability indicates that there is some interference in the replication of each by the presence of the other. Examples of complete and of partial incompatibility are observed among the I-like plasmids. The prototype I_α plasmids, R_{144} and R_{64} are completely incompatible, so that it is not possible to isolate clones of bacteria in which both are present (*31*). R_{483}, an R factor determining resistance to TP and SM (*33*), seemed to be compatible with typical plasmids of group I_α, although it resembled them in determining I pili and in being incompatible with R factor JR_{66a}. R_{483} was therefore assigned to a new compatibility group, I_β, and we suggested that JR66a (group I_ω) was an ancestral form from which both I_α and I_β compatibility groups had diverged (*31*). Recent work, however, has shown that the inheritance of R_{483} in cultures carrying the I_α plasmids R_{144} or R_{64} is not as stable as in cultures carrying R_{483} alone; R_{483} cannot, therefore, be considered as an example of a quite separate group, but rather as an atypical member of group I_α (*72*). The conclusion that JR66a may represent an ancestral form from which the prototype I_α plasmids and plasmids exemplified by R_{483} have diverged still holds, but we now accept that the divergence is not complete. A new compatibility specificity may be emerging.

Plasmid systematics thus resemble the systematics of other biological kingdoms. There exist well-separated, clearly defined groups, listed in Table I, but we may also expect to find examples of plasmids intermediate in their compatibility properties, the result of genetic divergence or convergence.

3) Hierarchies

MacFarren and Clowes (*43*) found that when two incompatible plasmids were introduced into a bacterium, their loss during growth of the culture was not always symmetrical. The plasmid less likely to be eliminated was considered as superior in a hierarchy. Extreme examples, in which the "superior" plasmid was never eliminated from the unstable double have been described (*12, 47*). The significance of such unilateral incompatibility is uncertain, but undoubtedly this, like the phenomenon described in the previous section, indicates variation, within groups, of the genes responsible for compatibility. Possibilities for genetic analysis of compatibility properties are thus opened.

4) Transposons

Transposons are defined as specific genetic sequences adapted for easy transposition between replicons, even where little or no DNA homology is demonstrable. The first was observed in RP4, an R factor conferring resistance to (ampicillin (APC). TC. KM). If RP4 was introduced into a culture carrying R_{702} (Table I), resistance pattern (SM. TC. KM. SA), the latter was always eliminated (evidence being the loss of (SM. SA) resistance). In the opposite cross, R_{702} did not appear to eliminate RP4, since its introduction never led to the loss of the APC resistance of RP4. This was because the APC resistance, as part of transposon A, was integrated in the host chromosome, so that the cell retained it, even though the plasmid, RP4, was eliminated by R_{702}. Transposon A, which includes the β-lactamase gene(s) of RP4, is readily transposable to other plasmids, as well as to the *E. coli* chromosome (*35*), which may explain why this type of β-lactamase gene is so widespread on plasmids, chromosomes and phages (*34, 38*).

Another example, transposon C, carries the information for resistance to TP and SM. Spontaneous transposition of this segment of DNA from R_{483} to the *E. coli* chromosome and to various plasmids has been observed (*1a, 31*). The use of this transposon allowed the definition of compatibility group J (see "Definition of Incompatibility Groups" above). Thus a phenomenon which is sometimes a hindrance in classifying plasmids by compatibility may also be exploited for that purpose.

5) Highly efficient recombination

When a plasmid is introduced into a host which carries an incompatible plasmid, recombination between the two may take place, rather than elimination of the resident. This is a usual outcome when selection is imposed due to the presence of both plasmids (*45*), but it is also seen to a variable extent when selection is only for the incoming plasmid (*5*). What determines the frequency of such recombination is not known, but it seems likely that the greater the extent of DNA homology between the two plasmids, the greater the liklihood of recombination. Thus, in experiments with two R factors, each derived by deletions from the same parent, R_1, no elimination of the resident was observed; all transcipients carried recombinant plasmids (S. Dennison and S. Baumberg, personal communication). The failure to observe any elimination could cause confusion.

6) *Powerful surface exclusion*

Surface exclusion, or the ability of a resident plasmid to prevent the entry, by conjugation, of another plasmid is correlated with incompatibility (*4, 59*), but the correlation is not perfect (*29, 31*).

Strong surface exclusion may interfere with tests for compatibility by preventing the entry of a second plasmid, which, if it succeeded in gaining entry, would prove to be compatible with the resident. In such a case, transfer frequency is very low; transfer to spontaneous R^- segregants in the predominantly R^+ recipient population will occur with disproportionate frequency, giving the impression that the resident plasmid has been actively eliminated.

Plasmids of the groups designated A and C (*10*) and A-C (*27*) provide examples of this difficulty. Group A is not included in Table I because experiments to elucidate the compatibility properties of these plasmids are still incomplete (N. Datta, unpublished).

7) *Dislodgement*

Elimination of a resident plasmid by the introduction of a second one is sometimes observed, even though the two plasmids prove to be compatible. This has been termed "dislodgement" (*5*). It is only effective immediately upon entry of the second plasmid; once established, doubles are quite stable. We have postulated that dislodgement may be the effect of an enzyme, specified by the incoming plasmid, necessary for its establishment in the cell, and thereafter repressed (*5*). One instance of dislodgement seemed to imply that the hypothetical enzyme recognized a DNA sequence of the dislodgeable resident that was present also in the incoming plasmid. This was in the case of R_{62}, a plasmid of group I_α, with a segment of DNA that was N-like in its homology properties (see below). R_{62} was compatible with plasmids of group N, but the introduction of an N plasmid often led, either to the dislodgement of R_{62}, or to excision of those markers which were believed to be specified by its N-like segment (*24*).

8) *Multiple plasmids and nonconjugative plasmids*

Many naturally occurring strains of bacteria carry several plasmids which may be very efficiently transferred together in conjugation. The presence of one can interfere with study of the compatibility properties of the others, especially where one (or more) is nonconjugative. Sometimes the only evidence that more than one plasmid is present in a culture is the biophysical demonstration of more than one plasmid molecular species. R factors R_{M413} and R_{721} were each allocated to newly-designated groups, I_ε (*34*) and I_δ (*41*), respectively, on the evidence that each determined the synthesis of I pili and was compatible with plasmids of all other known groups, including the I-like ones. Investigation at the molecular level, however, revealed that cultures carrying each of these R factors contained two kinds of plasmid DNA (*18*). The resistance plasmids in these cultures may have determined I pili, some other kind of transfer system, or have been nonconjugative. Until these systems are reinvestigated, therefore, the designations I_ε and I_δ should not be used.

Nonconjugative plasmids can be manipulated in genetic experiments using conjugation (mobilization), transduction, or transformation. A start has been made in investigating their compatibility properties (*56*).

9) Plasmids with more than one compatibility function

A laboratory recombinant between an FI plasmid, Col V, and an FII plasmid R_{538}, was found to be eliminated by plasmids of either group, *i.e.*, to have the compatibility specificities of both groups (*6*). Plasmids of this kind may occur in nature. Possible examples, described by Smith *et al.* (*55*) were plasmids of group H, incompatible with one another and also with the F factor, when the latter was replicating autonomously (though not in an Hfr culture). These plasmids showed little or no DNA homology with F. It was not an example of "dislodgement" as described above, since it was manifested by the instability of doubles as well as by elimination of a resident plasmid. A plasmid clone that had lost TC resistance had lost also the property of being incompatible with F. Whether the basis of this incompatibility was different from that between homologous plasmids was not known, but the authors emphasised that the phenomenon might be misleading in the classification of plasmids by compatibility.

5. *Correlation of Incompatibility with DNA Homology*

If the classification of plasmids into groups on the basis of incompatibility truly reflects their phylogenesis, a correlation between their incompatibility group and their physical and biological properties would be expected. Such correlation has indeed been shown in studies on DNA polynucleotide reassociation: plasmids within an incompatibility group almost always show extensive DNA homology, whereas plasmids of different groups rarely show significant homology (*18, 22, 23*).

An interesting exception has been reported among plasmids of group H, one example of which, TP116, although clearly incompatible with the other members, was quite different in DNA reassociation experiments. The DNA of other members of the group reassociated to at least 95% (*22, 55*).

Extensive DNA homology between plasmids of the same group is exemplified in the plasmids of compatibility group W, R factors, S-a, R_{7K} and R_{388}. They all determine different resistance patterns, and were detected in different bacterial genera, isolated in different parts of the world (*7*). The DNA of each hybridises with that of the others to at least 75% of its total length. Electron microscopy of heteroduplex molecules of these plasmids, and of their recombinants and deletion mutants, have permitted identification of the DNA loci encoding the various resistance genes (*20*) (Fig. 1).

An exception to the generalization that there is little, if any, DNA homology between plasmids of different incompatibility groups is found among the F-like plasmids, *i.e.*, those that determine F pili. Plasmids of groups FI and FII, although they are compatible, show extensive DNA homology. Almost all is explicable as residing in the genes of the *tra* region, determining the synthesis and control of the F pili (see Chapters 3, 5). Thus, FI and FII plasmids determine pili which must have a common evolutionary origin but this does not necessarily imply that their replication and compatibility determinants are derived from a common ancestor. The I-like plasmids of distinct incompatibility groups also share extensive polynucleotide sequences, which may be explained by the close similarity of their *tra* genes (*18*).

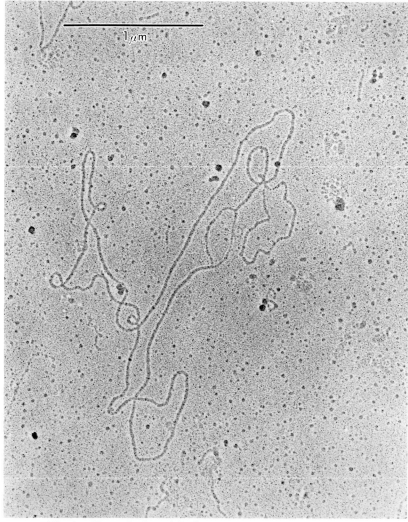

Fig. 1. Heteroduplex of R factors S-a and R_{288} of group W (see Table I). The two molecules reassociate throughout their lengths, except for a single deletion loop and a single substitution loop. Electron micrograph by courtesy of Professor S. Falkow.

6. Correlation of Pilus Type with Incompatibility Group

There is no known exception to the rule that all members of the same incompatibility group determine similar transfer mechanisms. Thus, all members of groups FI and FII (as well as the single plasmids assigned to groups FIII, FIV, and FV) determine F pili (*7*, *30*), plasmids of groups I_α and I_r determine I pili (*31*), plasmids of group P determine receptors for phage PRR1 (*50*) and plasmids of group N determine receptors for phage Ike (*42*). All known plasmids of group S are temperature-sensitive in respect of production of their transfer apparatus (*53*). For most of the plasmid groups listed in Table I, pili (or other conjugative organelles) have not been identified.

7. Correlation of Antibiotic Resistance Genes with Incompatibility Group

R factors of different groups frequently determine resistance to the same antibiotics or combinations of antibiotics. For example, the earliest R factors to be identified carried resistance to (SM. TC. CM. SA) (*46*); they belonged to group FII. The same resistance pattern is determined by R factors of other groups, *e.g.*, H and O (*14*). The pattern (APC. SM. TC. CM. SA) resistance is also common and found in many compatibility groups (*32*). Does this imply separate evolution in the different plasmid groups, with phenotypic convergence in response to the selective pressures imposed by the use of antibiotics by man? Or are the same genes distributed among plasmids of different groups? Studies on the mechanisms of plasmid-determined resistance give some answers to these questions. There is some degree of correlation of the carriage of particular genes (other than the pilus genes) with particular compatibility groups. For example, plasmid-determined SM resistance is usually associated with the synthesis of either SM phosphotransferase (SPT) or SM spectinomycin (SP) adenylate synthetase (SAS) (*2*). In general, R factors of groups F and N specify SAS, while I group plasmids specify SPT, but a few exceptions have been reported (*26*). R factor β-lactamase genes are not correlated with incompatibility group; genetic information for apparently identical enzymes is found in nearly all known groups (*34*), and the same seems to be true of neomycin (NM) phosphotransferase 1, the enzyme most commonly responsible for plasmid-determined resistance to NM and KM (J. Davies and R. W. Hedges, personal communication).

When R factors were first studied it was noted that CM resistance was specified only by fi^+, not fi^-, R factors (*60*). This was true of the

N group plasmids first studied in Japan and the I group ones in Europe. More recently, not only has CM resistance appeared, specified by many, diverse *fi⁻* R factors such as members of groups W (*29*), C (*10*), O and H (*14*), but this marker is also found in individual N group plasmids (*5*) and plasmids of group I_α (*57*). CM transacetylase of class 1 (*19*) is specified by plasmids of at least three different incompatibility groups. Thus there is sharing of resistance mechanisms between members of different groups, indicating considerable reassortment of resistance genes among naturally occurring plasmids.

8. Correlation of Incompatibility Group with Host Range

The distribution of plasmids among bacterial genera is correlated with compatibility. The first R factors to be discovered, and which belonged to group FII, were transmissible to all genera of the Enterobacteriaceae, but not beyond that tribe (*25*). Certain plasmid groups have an even wider range; group P is a notable example (*13, 36, 49*). Others have a narrower range, such as those mentioned in the introduction, as nontransferable to *E. coli* K12. Among the plasmids of enterobacteria, members of group I_α are not capable of transfer to the *Proteus-Providence* group (*9*); they are found most frequently in *Salmonella* but have also been reported in *Shigella, Escherichia,* and *Klebsiella*.

9. Mechanism of Incompatibility

The incompatibility of two plasmids may be explained by their having the same replicative mechanism, subject to the same control. Each plasmid exists in its host in a characteristic number of DNA molecules per host chromosome. The constancy of the number implies rigorous control of replication. Two plasmids in the same cell, with the same, or related, genes for the control of replication, would each be subject to control imposed by the other, and could not both continue to replicate normally. If the plasmid classification described here does indeed rest on this basis, then it reflects what is perhaps the most fundamental feature of the biology of plasmids.

For usefulness in epidemiological studies, compatibility properties should remain constant. It has been shown that certain resistance genes are readily transposable between unrelated plasmids. It does not seem likely that the same is true of the genes controlling replication and incompatibility; if it were, we should not expect DNA homology to be so extensive within groups as has been demonstrated, nor so little between groups.

That incompatibility is an expression of the specificity of replication control has never been conclusively proved. Plasmid mutants whose altered replication control was shown by their presence in the cell in increased numbers, were recently reported to be altered in their compatibility properties (*58*), which is good evidence for this view.

10. Role of Plasmid Classification in the Study of Ecology and in Epidemiology

Plasmids which are unrelated in compatibility properties and DNA sequences may determine the same resistance patterns; conversely plasmids closely related by these criteria may carry genes determining quite different bacterial characters. No understanding of the world-wide spread and distribution of plasmids would be possible, therefore, if their study were limited to a recognition of the phenotypes produced by them in their bacterial hosts. Classification by incompatibility would be incomplete without analysis and comparison of plasmid DNA, but DNA studies are too laborious and expensive to be used in all appropriate cases. Compatibility testing has allowed us to recognize the distribution of various plasmid groups geographically and among bacterial genera. Some groups (examples are FII, I_α, N) have been identified in bacterial strains isolated in all five continents. One, group L, has been found in only one bacterial species (*Serratia marcescens*) in a single ecological niche (*37*).

In epidemiology, classification of plasmids allows them to be traced. There are two ways in which R factors are spread: from one bacterium to another in the microenvironment, and carried within a particular bacterial host, from one environment (which may be a patient, a hospital, a farm, a river) to another. The tracing of these pathways requires identification of plasmids and of their host bacteria.

REFERENCES

1 Arai, T. 1974. Proc. Int. Symp. on Bacterial Resistance, Tokyo.

1a Barth, P. T., Datta, N., Hedges, R. W., and Grinter, N. J. 1976. *J. Bacteriol.*, **125**, 800–810.

2 Benveniste, R., Yamada, T., and Davies, J. 1970. *Infect. Immun.*, **1**, 109–116.

3 Bryan, L. E., Semaka, S. D., van den Elzen, H. M., Kinnear, J. E., and Whitehouse, R. L. S. 1973. *Antimicrob. Agents Chemother.*, **3**, 625–637.

4 Chabbert, Y. A., Scavizzi, M. R., Witchitz, J. L., Gerbaud, G. R., and Bouanchaud, D. H. 1972. *J. Bacteriol.*, **112**, 666–675.

5 Coetzee, J. N., Datta, N., and Hedges, R. W. 1972. *J. Gen. Microbiol.*, **73**, 543–552.

6 Cooper, P. 1971. *Genet. Res. Camb.*, **17**, 151–159.

7 Datta, N. 1974. *In* Microbiology—1974, ed. by D. Schlessinger, pp. 9–15, American Society for Microbiology, Washington, D.C.

7a Datta, N. T., and Barth, P. T. 1976. *J. Bacteriol.*, **125**, 796–799.

8 Datta, N. and Hedges, R. W. 1971. *Nature*, **234**, 222–223.

9 Datta, N. and Hedges, R. W. 1972. *J. Gen. Microbiol.*, **70**, 453–460.

10 Datta, N. and Hedges, R. W. 1972. *Ann. Inst. Pasteur*, **123**, 879–883.

11 Datta, N. and Hedges, R. W. 1972. *J. Gen. Microbiol.*, **72**, 349–356.

12 Datta, N., Hedges, R. W., Becker, D., and Davies, J. 1974. *J. Gen. Microbiol.*, **83**, 191–196.

13 Datta, N., Hedges, R. W., Shaw, E. J., Sykes, R. B., and Richmond, M. H. 1971. *J. Bacteriol.*, **108**, 1244–1249.

14 Datta, N. and Olarte, J. 1974. *Antimicrob. Agents Chemother.*, **5**, 310–317.

15 Dennison, S. 1972. *J. Bacteriol.*, **109**, 416–422.

16 Dubnau, E. and Maas, W. K. 1968. *J. Bacteriol.*, **95**, 531–539.

17 Echols, H. 1963. *J. Bacteriol.*, **85**, 262–268.

18 Falkow, S., Guerry, P., Hedges, R. W., and Datta, N. 1974. *J. Gen. Microbiol.*, **85**, 65–76.

19 Foster, T. J. and Shaw, W. V. 1973. *Antimicrob. Agents Chemother.*, **3**, 99–104.

20 Gori, J., Heffron, F., Hedges, R. W., and Falkow, S. Unpublished.

21 Grindley, N. D. F., Grindley, J. N., and Anderson, E. S. 1972. *Mol. Gen. Genet.*, **119**, 287–297.

22 Grindley, N. D. F., Humphreys, G. O., and Anderson, E. S. 1973. *J. Bacteriol.*, **115**, 387–398.

23 Guerry, P. and Falkow, S. 1971. *J. Bacteriol.*, **107**, 372–374.

24 Guerry, P., Falkow, S., and Datta, N. 1974. *J. Bacteriol.*, **119**, 144–151.

25 Harada, K., Suzuki, M., Kameda, M., and Mitsuhashi, S. 1960. *Japan. J. Exp. Med.*, **30**, 289–299.

26 Hedges, R. W. 1972. *J. Gen. Microbiol.*, **72**, 407–409.

27 Hedges, R. W. 1974. *J. Gen. Microbiol.*, **81**, 171–181.
28 Hedges, R. W. 1975. *J. Gen. Microbiol.*, **87**, 301–311.
29 Hedges, R. W. and Datta, N. 1971. *Nature*, **234**, 220–221.
30 Hedges, R. W. and Datta, N. 1972. *J. Gen. Microbiol.*, **71**, 403–405.
31 Hedges, R. W. and Datta, N. 1973. *J. Gen. Microbiol.*, **77**, 19–25.
32 Hedges, R. W., Datta, N., Coetzee, J. N., and Dennison, S. 1973. *J. Gen. Microbiol.*, **77**, 249–259.
33 Hedges, R. W., Datta, N., and Fleming, M. P. 1972. *J. Gen. Microbiol.*, **73**, 573–575.
34 Hedges, R. W., Datta, N., Kontomichalou, P., and Smith, J. T. 1974. *J. Bacteriol.*, **117**, 56–62.
35 Hedges, R. W. and Jacob, A. E. 1974. *Mol. Gen. Genet.*, **132**, 31–40.
36 Hedges, R. W., Jacob, A. E., and Smith, J. T. 1974. *J. Gen. Microbiol.*, **84**, 199–204.
37 Hedges, R. W., Rodriguez-Lemoine, V., and Datta, N. 1975. *J. Gen. Microbiol.*, **86**, 88–92.
38 Heffron, F., Sublett, R., Hedges, R. W., Jacob, A. E., and Falkow, S. 1975. *J. Bacteriol.*, **122**, 250–256.
39 Howarth-Thompson, S., Heffernan, H. M., and Buchan, M. D. 1974. *J. Gen. Microbiol.*, **81**, 279–282.
40 Jacob, F. and Adelberg, E. A. 1959. *Compt. Rend. Acad. Sci.*, **249**, 189–193.
41 Jobanputra, R. S. and Datta, N. 1974. *J. Med. Microbiol.*, **7**, 169–177.
42 Khatoon, H., Iyer, R. V., and Iyer, V. N. 1972. *Virology*, **48**, 145–155.
43 MacFarren, A. C. and Clowes, R. C. 1967. *J. Bacteriol.*, **94**, 365–377.
44 Meynell, E. and Datta, N. 1966. *Genet. Res. Camb.*, **7**, 134–140.
45 Meynell, E. and Datta, N. 1969. *In* Bacterial Episomes and Plasmids, ed. by G. E. W. Wolstenholme and M. O'Connor, pp. 120–133, Ciba Symposium, Churchill, London.
46 Mitsuhashi, S., Harada, K., and Hashimoto, H. 1960. *Japan. J. Exp. Med.*, **30**, 179–184.
47 Nordström, K., Ingram, L. C., and Lundbäck, A. 1972. *J. Bacteriol.*, **110**, 562–569.
48 Novick, R. P. and Richmond, M. H. 1965. *J. Bacteriol.*, **90**, 467–480.
49 Olsen, R. H. and Shipley, P. 1973. *J. Bacteriol.*, **113**, 772–780.
50 Olsen, R. H. and Thomas, D. D. 1973. *J. Virol.*, **12**, 1560–1567.
51 Palchoudhury, S. R. and Iyer, V. N. 1971. *J. Mol. Biol.*, **57**, 319–333.
52 Reeve, E. C. R. and Braithwaite, J. A. 1970. *Nature*, **228**, 162–164.
53 Rodriguez-Lemoine, V., Jacob, A. E., Hedges, R. W., and Datta, N. 1975. *J. Gen. Microbiol.*, **86**, 111–114.
54 Shipley, P. L. and Olsen, R. H. 1975. *J. Bacteriol.*, **123**, 20–27.

55 Smith, H. R., Grindley, N. D. F., Humphreys, G. O., and Anderson, E. S. 1973. *J. Bacteriol.*, **115**, 623–628.
56 Smith, H. R., Humphreys, G. O., and Anderson, E. S. 1974. *Mol. Gen. Genet.*, **129**, 229–242.
57 Terakado, N., Azechi, H., Koyama, N., Sato, G., and Mitsuhashi, S. 1974. Proc. Int. Symp. on Bacterial Resistance, Tokyo.
58 Uhlin, B. E. and Nordström, K. 1975. *J. Bacteriol.*, **124**, 641–649.
59 Watanabe, T. 1969. *In* Bacterial Episomes and Plasmids, ed. by G. E. W. Wolstenholme and M. O'Connor, pp. 81–97, Ciba Symposium, Churchill, London.
60 Watanabe, T., Nishida, H., Ogata, C., Arai, T., and Sato, S. 1964. *J. Bacteriol.*, **88**, 716–726.

11 R FACTORS IN *PSEUDOMONAS AERUGINOSA*

Shizuko Iyobe and Susumu Mitsuhashi
Department of Microbiology, School of Medicine, Gunma University, Maebashi, Japan

We isolated more than one hundred R plasmids from *Pseudomonas aeruginosa* strains of clinical origin using an intraspecies conjugation system in *P. aeruginosa*, and found that they were all nontransferable to *Escherichia coli* strains (*4, 11*); nontransferability to *E. coli* strains is, therefore, characteristic in *Pseudomonas* R plasmids. But few R plasmids were isolated from *P. aeruginosa*, which are conjugative to *E. coli* strains, and classified by incompatibility in the *E. coli* system (see Chapter 10). Bryan *et al.* (*1*) proposed an incompatibility classification of *Pseudomonas* plasmids in the *P. aeruginosa* system and classified R plasmids into four incompatibility groups, *i.e.*, P-1, P-2, P-3, and P-4. In addition to these R plasmids classified by Bryan *et al.* (*13*), we classified our R plasmids, an R plasmid R_{su38} (*6*) and a fertility factor FP2 (*3*) by incompatibility testing. Two isogenic strains of *P. aeruginosa* were used as host strains of R plasmids and the method of compatibility or incompatibility testing was almost the same as that described by Datta (see Chapter 10).

The incompatibility groups and members are listed in Table I, in which the transfer frequency of R plasmids between isogenic strains

TABLE I. Incompatibility Group of R Plasmids in *P. aeruginosa*

Group	Plasmid	Transfer frequency[a]	Transferability to *E. coli*[b]
P-1	RP4	10^{-1}	+
	R_{931} R_{130}	10^{-1}	−
	R_{su38}	10^{-1}	−
P-2	R_{ms159} R_{ms164} R_{ms178} R_{ms169} R_{ms170} R_{ms171} R_{ms172} R_{ms173} R_{ms174} R_{ms162} R_{ms146} R_{ms196} R_{ms197} R_{ms198} R_{ms199}	10^{-1}	−
	R_{ms161}	10^{-3}	−
P-3	R_{151}	10^{-1}	(−)[d]
P-4	R_{5265}	nt[c]	(+)[e]
P-5	R_{ms163}	10^{-2}	−
	R_{ms176}	10^{-1}	−
P-6	FP2	10^{-2}	−
P-7	R_{ms148}	10^{-1}	−
P-8	R_{ms149}	10^{-6}	−

The two letters "ms" are the abbreviation for the listing R plasmids isolated by our laboratory.

[a] Donor, *P. aeruginosa* ML4600; recipient, *P. aeruginosa* ML4262.
[b] Donor, *P. aeruginosa* ML4600; recipient, *E.coli* K12 χ1037 (*hsr*) or *E. coli* C.
[c] Not tested.
[d] Bryan *et al.* (1974) (*2*).
[e] Bryan *et al.* (1973) (*1*).

of *P. aeruginosa* and transferability of R plasmids to *E. coli* strains are described (*5*).

R plasmids belonging to the P-1 group are conjugally transmissible to *E. coli* and classified into the P group in the *E. coli* system (see Chapter 10). They confer susceptibility to bacteriophages such as PRR1, PRD1, PR3, and PR4 on their host bacteria (*9, 10, 14*). Sixteen among eighteen R plasmids isolated in Japan belong to the P-2 group and the prevalence of P-2 group R plasmids in *P. aeruginosa* has also been reported by Bryan *et al.* (*1, 2*). Conjugative transfer of these

R plasmids to *E. coli* strains has not been observed. These facts suggested that the P-2 R plasmids are representative as conjugative R plasmids in *P. aeruginosa*, and that the origin of R plasmids in *P. aeruginosa* is different from that of plasmids identified in other species of the family Enterobacteriaceae. P-2 plasmids inhibit the transfer of coexisting P-5 plasmids. The transfer of P-5 plasmids was strongly inhibited by some P-2 plasmids, but the transfer of P-2 plasmids was weakly inhibited. In the case of other P-2 plasmids, only the transfer of P-5 plasmids was inhibited by P-2 plasmids, but the transfer of P-2 plasmids was not inhibited by P-5 plasmids. Therefore, P-2 plasmids can be further divided into two groups; the transfer of one group of plasmids was inhibited by P-5 plasmids but that of another group was not.

The molecular weights of P-2 plasmids R_{931} and R_{130} were determined to be 25 and 23 Mdal., respectively, by Bryan *et al.* (*1*). These R plasmids seem to be characteristically small in size compared with R plasmids isolated from other species of strains (see Chapter 3).

The *Pseudomonas* R plasmids transferable to *E. coli* strains were isolated at a high frequency in Greece from strains highly resistant to gentamicin (GM) and carbenicillin (CPC), and classified into group C in the *E. coli* system (*7*). Bryan *et al.* (*2*) isolated an R plasmid R_{151} from *P. aeruginosa* which is incompatible with a C group R plasmid and classified into P-3 group in the *P. aeruginosa* system. The group P-3 in *P. aeruginosa* system, therefore, corresponds to group C in *E. coli* system, although R_{151} is not transferable to *E. coli* by conjugation.

R_{5265} was compatible with R plasmids belonging to P-1, P-2, or P-3 group, and classified into the P-4 group (*13*).

Two plasmids belonging to the P-5 group were detected from *P. aeruginosa* strains isolated in the same clinical ward in Japan. They are nonconjugative to *E. coli* but the resistance genes on R_{ms163} were found to be transferred to *E. coli* after integration into the RP4 plasmid (*12*).

The plasmid FP2 was isolated as a fertility factor in *P. aeruginosa* (*3*), and was found to carry resistance to mercuric chloride (*8*). The origin and direction of chromosome transfer by FP2 have already been reported (*3*).

Both P-7 and P-8 plasmids were isolated from the same strain in Germany (*11*). R_{ms149} is different from other R plasmids because of its low transfer frequency (Table I). But the transfer of R_{ms149} is facilitated by other R plasmids in *P. aeruginosa* and mobilized to *E. coli* by RP4, and R_{ms149} can replicate in *E. coli* by itself (5).

We could not perform complete incompatibility grouping for both R_{ms148} and R_{ms149} because the compatibility between the P-4 plasmid R_{5265} and either R_{ms148} or R_{ms149} could not be tested both because of the nontransferability of both R_{ms149} and R_{5265} to the same host cells, and because of masking of streptomycin resistance specified by R_{ms148} by R_{5265}. Therefore, there is a possibility that either R_{ms148} or R_{ms149} might belong to the same incompatibility group as R_{5265}.

REFERENCES

1 Bryan, L. E., Semeka, S. D., Van Den Elzen, M. H., Kinnear, J. E., and Whitehouse, R. E. S. 1973. *Antimicrob. Agents Chemother.*, **3**, 625–637.

2 Bryan, L. E., Shahrabadi, M. S., and Van Den Elzen, H. M. 1974. *Antimicrob. Agents Chemother.*, **6**, 191–199.

3 Holloway, B. W. 1969. *Bacteriol. Rev.*, **33**, 419–443.

4 Iyobe, S., Hasuda, K., Fuse, A., and Mitsuhashi, S. 1974. *Antimicrob. Agents Chemother.*, **5**, 547–552.

5 Iyobe, S., Sagai, H., Hasuda, K., and Mitsuhashi, S. 1976. 3rd Int. Symp. on Antibiotic Resistance, Castle of Smolenice, Czechoslovakia.

6 Kawakami, Y., Mikoshiba, F., Nagasaki, S., Matsumoto, H., and Tazaki, T. 1972. *J. Antibiot.*, **25**, 607–609.

7 Kontomichalou, P. and Papachristou, E. 1975. *In* Microbial Drug Resistance, ed. by S. Mitsuhashi and H. Hashimoto, pp. 329–348, University of Tokyo Press, Tokyo / University Park Press, Baltimore and London.

8 Loutit, J. S. 1970. *Genet. Res.*, **16**, 179–184.

9 Olsen, R. H., Siak, J., and Gray, R. H. 1974. *J. Virol.*, **14**, 689–699.

10 Olsen, R. H. and Thomas, D. D. 1973. *J. Virol.*, **12**, 1560–1567.

11 Sagai, H., Krčméry, V., Hasuda, K., Iyobe, S., Knothe, H., and Mitsuhashi, S. 1975. *Japan. J. Microbiol.*, **19**, 427–432.

12 Sagai, H., Iyobe, S., and Mitsuhashi, S. 1976. *J. Bacteriol.*, submitted for publication.

13 Shahrabadi, M. S., Bryan, L. E., and Van Den Elzen, H. M. 1975. *Can. J. Microbiol.*, **21**, 592–605.

14 Stanish, V. A. 1974. *J. Gen. Microbiol.*, **84**, 332–342.

ORIGIN OF R FACTORS

12 ORIGIN OF R FACTORS

Susumu MITSUHASHI
Department of Microbiology, School of Medicine, Gunma University, Maebashi, Japan

Most of the resistant strains of *Shigella* isolated prior to 1956 were resistant to only streptomycin (SM) or to tetracycline (TC), and no cases of the bacillary dysentery caused by multiple-resistant strains were reported from 1951 to 1956 in more than 10,000 isolates. The first isolation of a multiple-resistant *Shigella* in Japan was reported in 1952 (*94*) and the next isolation of a quadruple-resistant *Shigella* strain was reported in 1956 (*50*) (see Chapter 1).

The data collected by epidemiological surveys in Japan suggest that multiple drug-resistance did not appear in gradual stages but rather came at one time in an almost explosive manner. These facts strongly suggest that single or double resistance plasmids with resistance to TC, chloramphenicol (CM), SM, and sulfanylamide (SA) appeared at first and spread slowly. This can also be shown by the fact that most single or double resistance plasmids are nonconjugative. R plasmids encoding triple or quadruple resistance, *i.e.*, resistance to (TC. SM. SA), (CM. SM. SA), and (TC. CM. SM. SA), are conjugative and can spread rapidly by infectious transmission and by selective force as a result of the extremely widespread use of such drugs (*64, 65*).

The precise time of the first appearance of R factors cannot be pinpointed, but the first isolation of an R factor did not take place during the period of extensive SA use (beginning in 1945) and the beginning of the use of antibiotics, such as SM, TC, and CM (beginning in 1950). Although the first report of R factor isolation was made in 1959 in Japan, the existence of R factors can be traced more realistically to the period from 1951 to 1958 when multiple-resistant strains were isolated because of the high frequency of resistance R mostly to four drugs: TC, CM, SM, and SA. It should be noted, that R factors were also shown in *Shigella* strains isolated in Taiwan and Israel at that time (*81*). These facts strongly suggest that the world-wide distribution of R factors was not due to its spread by travellers moving from one country to another but rather its simultaneous independent appearance in many places in the world as a result of the increasing widespread use of antibiotics such as SM, TC, and CM.

Two possibilities concerning the origin of R factors have been advanced, *i.e.*, they are of either animal (*69*) or human origin. In Japan, however, human *Salmonella* infections were rare in comparison with *Shigella* infections and those of animal origin consequently, it might be surmised that the R factors occurring in Japan are mostly of human origin. As described in Chapter 2, however, the R factors have been demonstrated from livestock in Japan with high frequency since the adoption of the extensive use of antibiotics in animal foods. These facts could also indicate that the R factors appeared independently in human beings and in livestock as a direct result of the widespread use of antibiotics all over the world.

TABLE I. Isolation Frequency of R Plasmids from Resistant Strains to TC, CM,

Resistance pattern[a]	*Shigella*		*E. coli*	
	Resist. strains	R[+b] strains	Resist. strains	R[+] strains
Quadruple	75.7	75.5	64.2	60.5
Triple	4.7	86.7	5.7	59.1
Double	2.8	35.1	14.9	21.7
Single	16.8	9.6	15.2	4.5

Results based on surveys of 16,488 strains, including the *Shigella*, *E. coli*, *K. pneu-*
[a] Resistance patterns to resistance to TC, CM, SM, and SA.
[b] Demonstration frequency of R plasmids from the strains with the indicated re-

It is a known fact that the R factors have a wide range of hosts but are the most stable in *E. coli* and *Shigella* strains, followed by the *Proteus, Salmonella, Klebsiella, Serratia,* and *Vibrio (19, 54, 69)*. In *Salmonella* strains, for instance, the R factors can be lost spontaneously or eliminated at a high frequency by treatment with acridine dyes. Furthermore, they show a high frequency of segregation; R factors carrying multiple resistance are segregated into R(TC), R(SM. SA), R(TC. SM. SA), and R(CM. SM. SA) *(67, 100)*. These facts are in good agreement with the epidemiological features of the resistance patterns of R factors; the isolation frequency of R(TC. CM. SM. SA) factor being the highest in *E. coli* and *Shigella*, but lower in *Salmonella* and *Proteus*.

1. Easily Joinable Units Encoding Drug Resistance

Epidemiological data indicated that resistance patterns with reference to resistance to TC, CM, SM, and SA are characteristic in each bacterial species (Table I) but the demonstration frequencies of R(TC. CM. SM. SA) factors are the highest and followed by R plasmid encoding triple, double, and single resistance in that order. This fact can be interpreted by the following directions: (1) the R plasmids encoding multiple resistance are stable in their genetic structure, (2) the frequency of conjugal transferability of R plasmids with multiple resistance is rather high, and (3) wide spread by conjugation and by selection pressure due to multiple drugs. It should be noted further that the R plasmids possessing kanamycin (KM) or ampicillin (APC)

SM, and SA

K. pneumoniae		Salmonella		Proteus	
Resist. strains	R+ strains	Resist. strains	R+ strains	Resist. strains	R+ strains
66.4	56.4	2.8	88.6	21.9	54.1
8.2	65.4	15.9	73.6	24.3	39.0
5.8	25.0	12.6	39.9	24.0	16.3
20.6	6.6	68.6	2.2	29.9	14.3

moniae, Salmonella, and *Proteus* groups.

sistance pattern.

TABLE II. Resistance Patterns of R Factors Carrying KM or APC Resistance

R factor carrying	Resistance patterns	Number of R factors isolated
APC resistance	(TC. CM. SM. SA. KM. APC)	20
	(TC. CM. SM. SA. APC)	255
	Quadruple resistance	24
	Triple resistance	24
	Double resistance	6
	APC resistance	5
KM resistance	(TC. CM. SM. SA. KM. APC)	20
	(TC. CM. SM. SA. KM)	6
	Quadruple resistance	12
	Triple resistance	34
	Double resistance	9
	KM resistance	1

resistance appeared as plasmids encoding multiple resistance and R plasmids possessing double or single resistance are rather few in number (Table II and Fig. 1).

It was found further that the demonstration frequencies of R

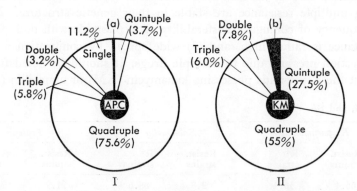

Fig. 1. Resistance patterns of APC- or KM-resistant strains of *Shigella*. Results based on surveys of 7,800 *Shigella* strains isolated in Japan. I. APC-resistant strains. Quintuple (TC. CM. SM. SA. KM); other resistance patterns, various combinations of the five drugs; (a) single APC-resistant strains. II. KM-resistant strains. Quintuple (TC. CM. SM. SA. APC); other resistance patterns, various combinations of the five drugs; (b) single KM-resistant strains.

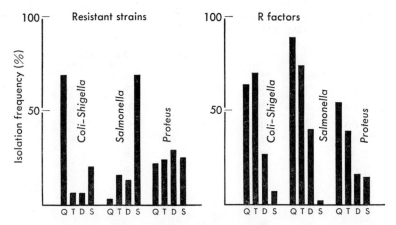

Fig. 2. Demonstration frequencies of R plasmids from drug-resistant strains. Q, quadruple (TC. CM. SM. SA) resistance; T, triple resistance; D, double resistance; S, single resistance.

plasmids are rather high from quadruple- and triple-resistant strains comparing with those from double- and single-resistant strains (Fig. 2). And the R plasmids from quadruple- and triple-resistant strains carried mostly quadruple and triple resistance. It should be noted further that most of the R plasmids encoding triple resistance are R(CM. SM. SA) and R(TC. SM. SA), and that there are only a few plasmids encoding other combinations with triple resistance.

Among the double-resistant strains, the (SM. SA)- and (TC. SA)-resistant strains are isolated most frequently and there are very few strains with other combinations of double resistance (Table III). The frequency of R plasmids demonstrated from double-resistant strains is low compared with those from triple- and quadruple-resistant strains except for those from (TC. SA)-resistant strains. Most R plasmids encoding double resistance are R(SM. SA) and the isolation frequency of R(TC. SA) is rather low from bacteria of human origin except for the few cases of R(TC. SA) plasmids from fish pathogens. Most of the plasmids demonstrated from (TC. SA)-resistant strains are R(TC), R(SA), r(TC), and r(SA). This indicates that there are some units encoding drug resistance that are easily joinable with each other, such as (SM) and (SA). The frequency of R plasmids encoding single resistance from single-resistant strains is rather low except for *Salmo-*

TABLE III. Isolation Frequency of R Plasmids from Single-(or Double-)resistant Strains to TC, CM, SM, and SA

Resistance pattern[a]	Shigella		E. coli		Salmonella		Proteus	
	Resist. strains	R+ strains	Resist. strains	R+ strains	Resist. strains	R+ strains	Resist. strains	R+ strains
SM. SA	74.2[b]	18.0[c]	71.2	22.0	93.0	12.4	75.0	24.0
TC. SA	21.1	88.9	21.0	76.6	40.9	75.3	15.0	0
TC. SM	0.9	(2/3)[d]	7.8	0.2	4.0	6.0	6.2	0
CM. SA	2.5	(5/7)	0	0	0	0	0	0
TC. CM	1.8	(4/5)	0	0	0	0	1.5	0
CM. SM	0.3	(1/1)	0	0	0	0	2.0	0
SA	97.8	5.6[c]	82.6	1.8	97.4	0.9	90.1	31.3
TC	2.1	34.6	1.4	11.1	2.0	68.2	6.2	0
SM	0.1	0	2.9	0	0.7	0	1.5	(1/11)
CM	0	0	0	0	0	0	3.2	0

Results based on surveys of strains, including the *Shigella, E. coli, Salmonella,* and *Proteus* groups.

[a] With reference to resistance to TC, CM, SM, and SA.

[b] Isolation frequency of the strains with the indicated resistance pattern among double-(or single-)resistant strains.

[c] Demonstration frequency of R plasmids from the strains with the indicated double resistance.

[d] Numerator, number of R+ strains; denominator, number of tested strains.

nella strains with single TC-resistance and for *Shigella, E. coli,* and *Salmonella* strains with (TC. SA) resistance. These data indicate that quadruple- and triple-resistant strains are mainly due to the presence of R plasmids encoding quadruple and triple resistance, *i.e.*, (TC. CM. SM. SA), (TC. SM. SA), and (CM. SM. SA). By contrast, the single-resistant strains are mostly due to presence of nonconjugative(r) plasmids, namely, r(TC), r(SA), and r(SM), and a few to the presence of R(TC), R(SM), or R(SA). Epidemiological and genetic studies of chromosomal genes encoding single resistance must still answer the questions of easily translocable resistance determinants and the origin of resistance plasmids. Other characteristics of the strains with single CM-resistance are that they are very few in number and the frequency of R(CM) and r(CM) plasmid demonstration is rather low. Based on these results we can postulate the evolutional process of the appearance of R plasmids with multiple resistance: first, the appearance of

R(SA), r(SA), R(SM), r(SM), R(TC), and r(TC) plasmids; second, the appearance of R(SM. SA) and r(SM. SA) plasmids; and finally, the appearance of R(TC. SM. SA), R(CM. SM. SA), and R(TC. CM. SM. SA) plasmids. Biochemical studies have disclosed that there are two types of mechanisms of plasmid-mediated SM resistance (see Chapter 9), *i.e.*, phosphorylation and adenylylation. Mechanisms of SM resistance mediated by R(SM. SA) and r(SM. SA) plasmids are mainly due to phosphorylation of the drug, even though the plasmids encode single SM-resistance or both SM and spectinomycin (SP) resistance (Fig. 3B). By contrast, SM is inactivated mainly by adenylylation by the SM-resistance determinants on R(CM. SM. SA), R(TC. SM. SA), and R(TC. CM. SM. SA) plasmids (Fig. 3A) (*48, 77*).

Recent studies have also disclosed that there are two types of mechanisms of SA resistance, *i.e.*, decrease in permeability of SA through the cell membrane and the formation of SA-resistant dihydropteroate synthetase (see Chapter 9). The mechanism of SA resistance mediated by r(SA), R(SA), r(SM. SA), and R(SM. SA) plasmids is mainly due to the formation of SA-resistant dihydropteroate synthetase (Fig. 3B). But the mechanism of SA resistance mediated by R plasmids encoding triple and quadruple resistance is explained as a decrease in the permeability of the drug through the cell membrane

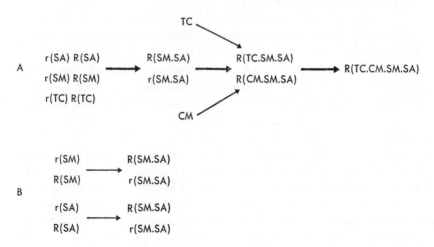

Fig. 3. The possible process of the formation of plasmids with multiple resistance. R, conjugative; r, nonconjugative.

(Fig. 3A) (*79*). These results indicate that there are at least two evolutional routes of the formation of R plasmids encoding multiple resistance: one with a group consisting of plasmids encoding SA, SM, and (SM. SA)-resistance, and the other with a group consisting of R(TC. CM. SM. SA), R(TC. SM. SA), and R(CM. SM. SA) plasmids. The results are summarized in Fig. 3.

2.   *Transposable Resistance Determinants on Plasmids*

It is generally accepted that R factors consist of two major segments: one responsible for the expression of drug-resistance, and the other capable of conferring ability, such as replication, self-regulation, and sexual transfer. In the transduction of R(TC. CM. SM. SA) factors with bacteriophage P1, the R factors were transduced as a whole, and most were conjugally transferable and able to confer four-drug resistance (*51*, *82*). By transduction of the R(TC. CM. SM. SA) factor in group E *Salmonella* with phage ε or P22, which is much smaller than phage P1, the resistance determinants of R factor were all segregated, and segregation was found between TC and other remaining resistance markers (CM. SM. SA) (*20*, *98*). The resistance determinants in transductants, *i.e.*, *tet* and (*cml str sul*) were found to be integrated into the chromosome (*20*).

An unstable mutant R factor conferring only CM resistance was obtained by spontaneous segregation. After storage in broth, a stable CM-resistant mutant was obtained and the *cml* gene governing CM resistance was integrated into the *E. coli* chromosome, closely linked with the *met* B locus (*35*). We further obtained mutants of the *E. coli* K12 strain, in which the *cml* gene of an unstable R(CM) factor was integrated into the chromosome, one (*cml₂*) being located between *str*-r and *his*, and the other (*cml₃*) between *mal* B and *thr* (*36*).

During an investigation on the transduction of an R factor with phage P1, a phage lysate was obtained which could transduce CM resistance at an extremely high frequency. The transduction of the CM-resistant character with this lysate was consistently accompanied by lysogenization with phage P1. Moreover, a single infection with the phage permitted plaque formation with the formation of CM-resistant lysogenic cells at the center of the plaque. Both the transducing and plaque activities of the lysate were lost by neutralization with anti-

P1 phage serum. These observations led us to the conclusion that a derivative of phage P1 that had retained its fundamental genetic properties had been isolated but had become specifically associated, presumably by recombination, with the CM-resistance gene (*cml*) of an R factor, called P1 *CM* (or P1-*cml*) (*52*).

Nonconjugative(r) plasmids that encode TC, CM, or macrolide antibiotics (Mac) resistance were transduced with bacteriophage S1 in staphylococci. We obtained a derivative of S1 phages that transduce TC^r, CM^r, or Mac^r and infect productively. Furthermore, the resistance genes (*tet cml mac*) of plasmids were found to be a part of the genome of bacteriophage S1. These recombinants between S1 particle and the resistance determinants on nonconjugative(r) plasmids are called S1*ptet*, S1*pcml* and S1*pmac* (*32–34, 78*). The same type of converting bacteriophage with APC and KM resistance in *Proteus* (*9*), CM or TC resistance in *E. coli* (*63*), and APC resistance in *E. coli* (*91*) was reported.

During a transductional analysis of an R(TC. CM. SM. SA) factor with the bacteriophages P1 and ε_{15}, phage lysates were obtained which were capable of transducing TC, CM, or (CM. SM. SA) resistance at high frequency. The transducing agents were defective (*d*) elements, like P1*d*1 (*56*), called εdTC, εd(CM. SM. SA), and P1*d*CM, which lacked certain bacteriophage functions. After lysogenization with normal phage and ultraviolet induction, strains carrying the defective transducing elements produced lysates which had a high frequency of transduction (HFT). These resistance determinants which interact with other replication systems are generally only R-factor segments, since they are defective in certain functions such as replication and transfer (*43, 53*). These facts led us to the conclusion that the resistance determinants of plasmids have a rather wide range of homology with other plasmids, such as F, F′, T, and Col, and bacteriophages, such as P1, ε, and P22. The resistance determinants regain their lost properties or assume a new pace and mode of replication once they become part of a host chromosome or of plasmids. The fact that the drug resistance determinants on plasmids are easily translocable has been recently explained by the presence of the insertion sequence (IS) (see Chapter 4).

According to the studies on the biochemical mechanisms of R-factor resistance, APC resistance of R factor can be accounted for by the formation of β-lactamase that causes the splitting of β-lactam ring of APC (*10*). It is well known that β-lactamase is widely distributed among both gram-positive and gram-negative strains of bacteria which are resistant to penicillins (PCs). It was found, moreover, that the penicillinases (PC β-lactamases, PCase) produced by R factor-resistant strains are divided into four subgroups in their substrate specificity (see Chapter 9). The most common R factor PCase was found to be similar to that produced by *Klebsiella* in its substrate specificity (*11*), and enzymological and immunological properties (*15, 90*). This fact is sufficient to postulate the origin of APC-resistance determinant of the R factors. It was reported that the strains of *E. coli* carrying an R factor capable of conferring CM resistance inactivates the antibacterial activity of CM by acetylation in the presence of acetyl CoA (*94*). CM acetyltransferase is detected in CM-resistant strains of both *Staphylococcus aureus* and gram-negative enteric bacteria (*73, 86, 95*). These facts strongly suggest that the resistance determinants of the R factors are widely distributed among the resistant strains of clinical origin and may be derived from them, resulting in the formation of the R factor by integration into some plasmids.

3. Transfer Factors

We (*42*) proposed three theories on the initial appearance of R factors: (a) R factors were present in microbial populations prior to the use of antibacterial agents. They have become manifest by selection as a result of the extensive use of antibacterial agents. (b) Conjugative plasmids, which did not carry drug-resistance determinants, were initially present in microbial populations. R factors were formed by recombination between the conjugative plasmids and the drug-resistance determinants in microorganisms and became manifest after the introduction of antibacterial agents. (c) Extrachromosomal genetic elements, which did not carry drug-resistance genes and were conjugally nontransferable, acquired first, drug resistance by the following three possibilities: (a) spontaneous mutation, (b) transduction, and (c) recombination. Consequently, the nontransferable (r) plasmids carrying a drug-resistant determinant acquired the ability of conjugal transference by recombination with other plasmids that were originally transferable.

According to a report on the CsCl density gradient analysis of R factors, they consist of two genetic elements, the transfer factor responsible for autonomy of plasmid and the drug-resistance determinants capable of conferring drug resistance (*17*, *89*).

As stated in Chapter 3, we obtained an R factor segment by transduction of R(TC. CM. SM. SA) factor with bacteriophage ε (*20*). This R factor segment was found to be capable of conferring TC resistance on its host bacteria, not eliminated by acridine dyes and not transferable by conjugation, suggesting that the determinant for TC resistance was integrated into the host chromosome (*22*). This R factor segment was referred to as the resistance determinant carrying TC resistance, *i.e.*, *tet*. The *tet* determinant acquired conjugal transferability by infection of *Salmonella tet* with the F factor. *E. coli tet* to which only *tet* was separately transferred by conjugation could not transfer its *tet* determinant. However, *E. coli tet* F⁺ conjugants, to which both F and *tet* were transmitted simultaneously by conjugation, were also capable of transferring F, *tet*, and F-*tet*. The recombinant F-*tet* was formed as a result of interaction between F and *tet* determinant (*21*). By cross analysis of *E. coli* Hfr *tet* with *E. coli* K12 F⁻ or by reciprocal crossing, it was found that the *tet* determinant was located on the *E. coli* K12 chromosome between *lac* and *pro*, near *lac* (*22*). Two possibilities were advanced regarding the acquisition of transferability of the *tet* determinant that was integrated into the host chromosome, (a) transfer of *tet* accompanying the host chromosome by sex factors, (b) formation of the recombinant F-*tet* factor by interaction between the F factor and the *tet* determinant in the host bacterium. Similarly, the otherwise nontransmissible *tet* determinant in *E. coli* K12 *tet* acquired transmissibility by conjugation by infection with either F-*lac* or the wild-type R factor, resulting in the formation of the recombinants F-*lac tet* (*24*) and R-*tet* factors, respectively (*23*). Similar findings were also reported by the formation of F-*cml* and P1-*cml* which are capable of transferring CM resistance (*52*, *53*). These facts are in keeping with other evidence that the R factor consists of resistance determinants plus the genetic determinants responsible for autonomous activities such as replication, self-regulation, and transfer.

Since the known sex factor F can apparently combine with the nontransferable R factor derivative, *tet*, to form a functional, infectious F-*tet* factor, we made a survey of the distribution of genetic elements (termed transfer factor, T factor) among clinical isolates which were capable of conferring conjugal ability on noninfectious drug-resistance determinants. Two noninfectious drug-resistance determinants in *E. coli* K12 were employed. As described above, *tet* is integrated into the *E. coli* chromosome, and the *tra⁻* R_{530} factor, capable of conferring TC resistance, differs from the *tet* in that it can be eliminated by acriflavin. From this fact we infer extrachromosomal existence in the *E. coli* host strain. Numerous enteric strains were tested for the presence of T factors by mixed cultivation experiments employing *E. coli* carrying the *tra⁻* R_{530} factor. After overnight incubation of *E. coli* $R_{530}{}^+$ with an appropriate organism to be tested, the mixed culture and strain *E. coli* 58–161 F⁻ NAʳ, which is a final recipient of TC resistance and resistant to nalidixic acid (NA), were inoculated into nutrient broth and incubated at 37°C. After 16 hr of incubation, the mixed culture was plated onto BTB-lactose agar containing both NA and TC. After incubation for 48 hr, the colonies that had acquired TC resistance, were picked, purified, and used for further analysis, including conjugal transferability. The T factors, which are capable of transferring the nontransferable *tet* determinant on R_{530} factor, were detected at high frequency from many clinical isolates belonging to the Enterobacteriaceae, including *E. coli, Shigella, Salmonella, Proteus, Klebsiella,* and *Aerobacter (44, 66, 74)*.

When *E. coli* K12 carrying *tet* was mixed with *E. coli* K12 $T_{95}{}^+$ carrying one of the T factors, the otherwise nontransferable *tet* determinant acquired transmissibility by conjugation, resulting in the formation of a new conjugative plasmid, T-*tet*. By mixed cultivation of *E. coli* K12 carrying nontransmissible *tra⁻* R(KM) factor with *E. coli* K12 T⁺, the T-*kan* factor was formed. By interaction between *kan* determinant of *tra⁻* R(KM) factor and T-*tet* factor, we obtained the recombinant T-*tet kan* plasmid. These are new plasmids which are capable of conferring drug resistance, transferable by conjugation, and, consequently, newly formed conjugative resistance factors, *i.e.*, R(TC) and R(TC. KM) *(24, 44–46)*.

Using a stock culture of *Aerobacter cloacae* which was isolated from a clinical specimen before the introduction of penicillin G (PC-G) to Japan, and which exhibited lowered resistance (12.5 µg/ml) to APC and produced only a low titer of PCase (1.7 units/mg dry weight bacteria), we obtained a resistant mutant *A. cloacae* APCʳ by overnight incubation on an APC-plate; this mutant being resistant to 200 μg/ml of APC and capable of producing PCase (16 units/mg of dry weight bacteria). When *A. cloacae* APCʳ was infected with T-*tet* factor by mixed cultivation with *E. coli* K12 T-*tet*⁺, the T-*tet amp* factor was formed by recombination of the *amp* determinant with T-*tet* factor (*80*). The T-*tet amp* factor was found to be transduced jointly as single unit with phage P1, transferable by conjugation, and capable of conferring resistance to both TC and APC on its host. The APC resistance conferred by the T-*tet amp* factor is due to increase in the production of PCase (13.5 units/mg of dry weight bacteria). By interaction between the T-*tet amp* factor and the T factor, the T-*amp* factor, capable of conferring only APC resistance and transferable by conjugation, was formed. These facts imply that the origin of the R factor carrying APC resistance came about by the acquisition of the resistance determinant of some mutants by conjugative plasmids. Similarly, we have obtained several recombinants, *i.e.*, T-*tet cml*, T-*tet cml str sul*, T-*tet str sul*, and T-*cml str sul* (*44–46, 74*). These recombinants are new conjugative plasmids that are capable of conferring multiple resistance and transferring their resistance by conjugation.

Consequently, it was concluded that there are three possibilities that should be considered regarding the acquisition of nontransferable resistance determinant in cooperation with conjugative plasmids: (a) transfer of resistance determinant integrated into the host chromosome along with the transfer of host chromosome by sex factors, *i.e.*, by F-mating, R-mating (*93*), T-mating (*44–46*) and by *Δ*-mating (*5*), (b) formation of the recombinant factors by interaction between resistance determinants and conjugative plasmids, such as F (*21, 99*), F'(*24*), R(*75*), and T (*44–46, 66, 74, 75*), and (c) transfer of nonconjugative resistance(r) plasmid by complementation with conjugative plasmids, *i.e.*, F(*21*), R(*23*), T(*44*), Col (*27*), and *Δ* factor (*1*).

This fact, *i.e.*, complementation, first reported by Ozeki *et al.* (*87*), showed that the readily transmissible factors Col I and Col B in some ways resemble the F factor of *E. coli*, and the presence of Col I or Col B in *Salmonella typhimurium* LT2 enables it to transmit the otherwise nontransmissible Col E2 and Col K. In this case, however, both factors were transferred to a cell after a long period of incubation but only one of the two factors was transferred separately after a short period of mixed cultivation (*87*), suggesting their separate existence in a cell.

It is quite interesting to note that the transfer frequency of the T-*kan* or T-*tet kan* factor is 10^2- to 10^3-fold higher than that of T-*tet* (probably T_{95}) factor and *E. coli* K12 carrying T-*kan* or T-*tet kan* factor becomes sensitive to male phages, although *E. coli* K12 T_{95}^+ or T-*tet*$^+$ is resistant to male phage (*24*). According to the reports by Meynell and Datta (*62*), these facts can be explained by assuming the production of repressor substances in the mating system: (a) R, T_{95} and T-*tet* factors are in a self-repressed state for pili formation in contrast to the derepressed state of F factor for pili formation, and (b) T-*kan* and T-*tet kan* factors become derepressed for pili formation following the recombination between the *kan* determinant and the T_{95} or T-*tet* factor, resulting in the increase in transfer frequency and becoming sensitive to male phages. *E. coli* K12 harboring both T-*kan* (or T-*tet kan*) and *ifm*$^+$ (the determinants responsible for the inhibition of F-mating) R factors becomes resistant to male phages and the transfer frequency of T-*kan* (or T-*tet kan*) factor is decreased. This fact can be explained by the following procedure (*40*): (a) T_{95} and T-*tet* factors are *ifm*$^+$ and in self-repressed state for pili formation, (b) the mating (or conjugal transfer) loci consist of a regulator (*i, 13; ifm*), and (*tra*) or (*rmt*) (R-mating) genes, and (c) the T-*kan* (or T-*tet kan*) factor has lost the regulator gene following recombination between the *kan* determinant and the T_{95} (or T-*tet*) factor, resulting in the formation of new conjugative plasmid in a derepressed state for pili formation. But the function of the T-*kan* (or T-*tet kan*) factor that contributes to pili formation could be inhibited by a repressor produced in the cytoplasm by the presence of the *ifm*$^+$ R factor in *E. coli* K12 T-*kan*$^+$ (or T-*tet kan*$^+$) *ifm*$^+$R$^+$ (*24*).

Accordingly, the high frequency of isolation and world-wide spread of the R factors carrying multiple resistance, especially the quadruple-resistant R factors, can be explained in the following way: (a) increase in the transfer frequency of plasmids by the recombination with resistance determinant and by increasing the resistance pattern, (b) selective force by the wide use of multiple drugs, including TC, CM, SM, and SA, favoring the survival of the R factors carrying multiple drug-resistance, and (c) increase in the stability of R factors in the host strains.

The transfer factor ($\mathit{\Delta}$) is an agent that changes the phage type of *S. typhimurium*. It crosses into *S. typhimurium* in which the resistance determinant is transferred but lost, and produces drug-resistant lines not showing the characteristic change of phage type and unable to transfer their resistance. Such resistance determinants may be integrated into the chromosome, but it seems more probable, because of the case in which they are mobilized by $\mathit{\Delta}$, that they are located in the cytoplasm. When *Salmonella* strains carried the *tet* determinant, it became attached to $\mathit{\Delta}$, resulting in the formation of $\mathit{\Delta}$-*tet*. The transfer of *tet* into *Salmonella* with an *amp* determinant introduces $\mathit{\Delta}$, to which the *amp* determinant becomes attached. This attachment is independent of that of *tet* but most copies of $\mathit{\Delta}$ will carry *tet* because of their close association. Consequently, most particles harboring *amp* will already possess *tet* and the resulting progeny will be of the *tet amp* type. When these cells are mated with a sensitive recipient, they will transfer *amp*, (*amp tet*) and *tet*, but the *amp* class will be detected easily only early in the crossing (*1*). A determinant for resistance to neomycin and KM was isolated from a strain of phage type 29 of *S. typhimurium* (*3*) in which the *kan* determinant was associated with an *ifm*+ transfer factor, referred to as X. The X-*kan* factor belongs to a class of dissociable resistance factors first observed in *S. typhimurium* (*1*). In this class the resistance determinant and the transfer factor are basically independent plasmids occupying different cellular attachment sites (*4*). They have a reversible association with each other, and it is only when they are in the associated state that the determinant can be transferred to a new host. Because of the dissociability of the complex, the whole transmissible resistance determinant, or the resistance determinant alone, or the transfer factor alone may enter the recipient during transfer. This factor in the *S. typhimurium* type 29 strain consists of a determinant for resistance to APC (*amp*) and the transfer factor.

The F+ *kan* strain was prepared by introducing the F-*kan* factor into prototrophic K12F−. The F-*kan* factor was also transferred into K12HfrH to produce the Hfr *kan*; in this crossing the invading F factor was lost but the *kan* determinant was retained in the recipient strain (*2*).

Anderson *et al.* (*5*) investigated the conjugal analysis of the transfer frequency of the *kan* determinant, and the *pro*, *trp*, and *his* markers in K12F$^+$ *kan* and K12Hfr *kan*. The results are summarized as follows: (a) the *kan* determinant was transferred by the K12 F$^+$ *kan* at a much higher frequency than were chromosomal markers, (b) most recombinants receiving *kan* or chromosomal markers also acquired the F factor, (c) the *kan* determinant was transferred from the K12 HfrH *kan* and the K12F$^+$ *kan* at the same frequency to K12 F$^-$, (d) in the Hfr *kan* F$^-$ crosses, the recipient colonies remained F$^-$ and could not transfer the *kan* determinant, and (e) the frequency of appearance of the unselected markers in the *kan* recombinants was in accordance with what is known of the K12 linkage map and of transfer from HfrH. These results suggested that the attachment of *kan* to F is independent of the integration of F into the chromosome and that the association between *kan* and F can be regarded as identical in both F$^+$ and Hfr strains, establishing the hypothesis that the *kan* determinant is covalently bonded to F and that such bonding occurs after the opening up of F before transfer to a new host (*5*).

During the life cycle of the *kan* determinant in K12 F$^+$, the association of both the *kan* determinant and the F factor was demonstrated but both the F factor and the *kan* determinant of K12 F$^+$ *kan* were eliminated with high frequency by acridine dyes. The acridine treatment yielded the following classes from the original F$^+$ *kan* strain: F$^-$ *kan*, F$^+$ *kan*-s, and F$^-$ *kan*-s. It was thus evident that F and *kan* determinants were independently removed by acridine dyes, which is further support for the hypothesis that they are ordinarily independent of each other in the host cell (*5*). Thus, it was postulated that the Δ (or X) factor and resistance determinant exist separately in a cell and association between both factors takes place either in a cell or during the course of conjugal transfer, implying that the association between the X or F factor and resistance determinant is easily dissociable.

We reported that the determinants governing resistance to PC, CM, SM, TC, SA, and Mac in staphylococci are located extrachromosomally, namely, on nonconjugative(r) plasmids. Each plasmid generally carries a single resistance determinant; there are relatively few plasmids carrying multiple resistance (*25, 68, 72, 76, 84, 88*). We were able to find, however, jointly transduced resistance to (TC. SM), (TC. SM. SA), (CM. TC), and (Mac. PC) in staphylococci at a high frequency. According to studies on transduction, transformation, and molecular analysis, we concluded that plasmids are easily associated and dissociated in a cell, and an associated plasmid is capable of joint transduction (*30, 31, 33, 47, 71, 76, 78*).

4. *Prophages*

A prophage is the genetic material of a bacteriophage and is generally attached to the bacterial chromosome. Lysogeny, therefore, is an example of the integration of a virus into its host; other situations in which a permanent association between a virus and its host cell exists are known as latent virus infections. Among chronic viral infections which have been reported in vertebrates, insects, and plants, some appear to be a permanent association between the virus and certain cells (*41*). According to detailed studies of prophages, the new problem of the possible existence of proviruses in vertebrates, insects, and plants has been raised and has become one of today's most important biological problems (*6, 38, 57*). The term "moderate viruses" has been proposed by Dulbecco (*12*) in analogy with the temperate bacteriophages to designate viruses which can exist in the host cells.

It is a well-known fact that most temperate phages in *E. coli* K12 are located on specific sites of the bacterial chromosome. However, there are other findings showing that mating experiments have not revealed any such specific sites for prophages (*7, 39*). There are two possible explanations for this: (a) the prophage P1 associates with any of several chromosomal sites and is readily detached from the chromosome, and (b) it exists extrachromosomally without any chromosome-associated phase. Ikeda and Tomizawa (*28, 29*) analyzed the P1 DNA of a lysogenic bacteria based upon the principle that the bacterial DNA of a lysogenic bacteria should behave differently depending on whether the prophage P1 is associated with the bacterial chromosome or not. They demonstrated that P1 DNA is not in physical association with the bacterial chromosome and exists extrachromosomally. Sucrose zone centrifugation and electron microscopic examination, demonstrated that the prophage P1 DNA is circular and that the conversion from a linear (*28*) to a circular molecule takes place during the process of lysogenization, resulting from recombination between single, terminally redundant DNA molecules that lose the redundant part of the molecule. The replicating prophage DNA is not associated with the host chromosome and rarely interacts with the bacterial chromosome indicating that the prophage P1 is physically independent of the host chromosome and replicates autonomously. There is an average of one prophage P1 per bacterial chromosome and the lysogenic cells rarely segregate from nonlysogenic cells. This can be explained by the fact that the replication of the prophage P1 does not occur randomly and must be strictly controlled, the number of prophages in a cell being determined by the number of specific cellular sites. In contrast, P1 genomes replicate to a great extent in the vegetative state. This fact suggests that vegetative replication is regulated by a phage function(s) and prophage replication by a cellular function(s). According to the results described above, it can be concluded that phage P1 lysogenizes without integration into the host chromosome; it is the type of lysogeny in which a prophage exists as a plasmid called the "extrachromosomal lysogeny" (*29*). The genetic material of a temperate bacteriophage gives an example of the genetic structure which is added to the genome of a cell and which exists inside the cell in two distinct forms, the autonomous state and the integrated state.

Matsubara (*58, 60*) isolated the *λdv* plasmid from the bacteriophage *λ*. The *λdv* plasmid, an autonomously replicating DNA fragment originating from the *λ* phage genome, represents a simple self-controlled replication system, *i.e.*, a replicon (*37, 42*). A replicon is the fundamental genetic unit for autonomous replication and self-regulation. Recent analyses have shown that plasmid *λdv* has three indispensable genes, *O*, *P*, and *tof*, all of which are the under control of a

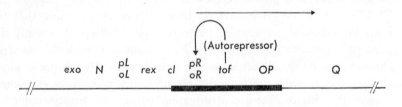

Fig. 4.   A portion of the *λ* phage genome (*60*). Arrows indicate the origin and direction of transcription. The bold line represents a segment of the genome which can be extracted to form the *λdv* plasmid. For symbols of the phage *λ*, see Campbell (*8*).

single promoter operator, *pRoR* (*58, 61*). The products of the *O* and *P* genes act cooperatively and positively in the replication of the λ genome (*97*). It has been inferred that the *tof* gene product is a new type of repressor which acts on the *pRoR-tof-OP* operon, interacting at the *pRoR* (*14, 18, 59, 96*). A portion of the λ phage genome is illustrated in Fig. 4.

Jacob and Wollman (*37*) proposed the term "episomic elements or episomes" to designate genetic elements carrying such genetic properties, such as temperate bacteriophages, the sex factor of bacteria, and colicinogenic factors. They summarized the properties of bacterial episomes as follows: (a) they are genetic elements which may or may not be present, (b) when absent from a bacterium, they can only be acquired from an external source, (c) when present in a bacterium, they may be either in an autonomous or in an integrated state, (d) their behavior in the autonomous state and the phenotypic expression of this state are specific attributes of a particular type of episome, (e) in the integrated state, they are located on the bacterial chromosome, but do not appear to form part of its linear structure, (f) they alternate between the integrated and the autonomous state, and the integrated state, in general, appears to be naturally exclusive, and episomic elements in the integrated state may undergo genetic recombination with the neighboring region of the bacterial chromosome.

The role of the cytoplasm in heredity has been studied by many investigators since the advent of genetics (see review, Ref. *16*). It is generally admitted that as cytoplasmic self-reproducing units extrachromosomal units, such as plastids, centrosomes, various organelles, and mitochondria, are capable of reproducing from pre-existing identical structures carrying the properties of the units. Lederberg (*55*) proposed the term plasmid to designate all extranuclear structures that are capable of reproducing in an autonomous fashion.

Jacob and Wollman (*41*) postulated that episomic elements are of viral origin and described the possible variations of episomes. The ability of a temperate bacteriophage to integrate is determined by the genes that control the specific attachment of the phage genome to the bacterial chromosome. As a result of a single mutation, the ability of lysogenization is lost and the mutant phage loses its episomic character; it behaves as an obligatory virus that can reproduce autonomously. On the other hand, a mutation or deletion of any one of the genes essential to the obligatory virus state causes the suppression or loss of a function essential for vegetative multiplication. Such a defective phage genome can only exist in the integrated state (*41*) or as a plasmid (*28*).

It was found that bacterial plasmids, *i.e.*, F, Col, R, T, (or X) factors, generally have common genetic properties such as conjugal transfer of host chromosome, replication, and sexual transferability. But the origin of sex factors is still obscure, and they are different from bacteriophages in several functions: (a) ability of transfer of the host chromosome, (b) ability of sexual transfer between two cells, and (c) ability of infectivity of the conjugative plasmid itself. The most important properties of the conjugative plasmids different from those of bacteriophages, therefore, are the ability to cause pili formation and the loss of both infectivity and virulence to their host.

It is known that some of the Col factors and the staphylococcal plasmids (*25, 68, 70, 83*) have no power of the independent transmissibility and they are different from the conjugative plasmids in the sense of sex factors. However, Hayes (*26*) stated that the F, Col, R factors, staphylococcal plasmids, *etc.*, belong to the same general category of elements, whatever their mode of expression and irrespective of their transmissibility. Most of the attributes by which they were originally distinguished can be gained or lost by mutation. He, therefore, suggested the designation "plasmid," instead of episomes, as an all-embracing substitute. The term plasmid was introduced by Lederberg in 1952 before the possibility of a chromosomally-inserted state was conceived, and was defined simply as an extrachromosomal element. Hayes (*26*) further stated that a distinction cannot be made between cytoplasmic elements on the basis of whether they can or cannot be inserted into the chromosome, but only on the basis of frequency of insertion. I agree with this opinion, because the definition was essentially an operational and descriptive one referring to a dispensable genetic element that, in a given cellular species, may be found in either a chromosomal or an extrachromosomal state (*101*).

It was my intention, however, to make a distinction between conjugative and nonconjugative plasmids, because the nonconjugative plasmids have no ability for independent transmissibility and cannot gain the transmissible character by mutation. In other words, the nonconjugative plasmid is simply an extrachromosomal element, that is conjugally nontransferable, *i.e.*, not the *tra⁻* mutant from the *tra⁺* ele-

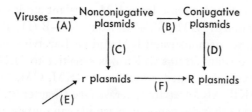

Fig. 5.   Possible relations of virus, and nonconjugative and conjugative plasmids. A, the loss of virus virulence in a mutation which loses
the virus virulence; B, a mutation which acquires conjugal transferability; C, acquisition of a resistance determinant by mutation on
its replicon or from some other genetic element; D, acquisition of
resistance determinant(s) by mutation on its replicon or from some
other genetic element; E, recombination between transducing phage
and its parent phage; F, recombination between nonconjugative(r)
plasmid and a sex factor(s).

ment. It seems to me that an operational distinction between prophages, nonconjugative plasmids, and conjugative plasmids, will be
meaningful in biology before the precise understanding of the phylogenetical situation of the extrachromosomal elements can be achieved.
The possible relations between these dispensable genetic elements are
shown in Fig. 5.

As described in Chapter 9 it should be noted that the mechanism
of the R factor-resistant strains is rather common in many resistant
strains regardless whether they are gram-positive or gram-negative
bacteria, *i.e.*, β-lactamase, CM acetyltransferase, aminoglycoside-phos-
photransferase, -acetyltransferase, and -adenylyltransferase. Except
for β-lactamase, such enzymes need coenzymes, such as acetyl CoA
and ATP. These facts implied that the resistant determinants of plasmids would be mutated genes derived from those distributed widely
among most genera of bacteria and which are physiologically functional in their metabolic process by using either acetyl CoA or ATP.
These mutated genes would become capable of splitting β-lactam ring,
and of acetylating, phosphorylating and adenylylating antibacterial
agents, including their normal metabolic substances. Isolation of several types of β-lactamase produced by R factors favored the view that
the genes would mutate to act on a substance that is newly introduced
by changing their substrate profile. We were able to demonstrate, in

fact, first KM(NM) acetyltransferase from KM-resistant strains which was sensitive to gentamicin (GM), 3′, 4′-dideoxy KM-B (DKB), and AK (amikacin). Next, we demonstrated KM and GM acetyltransferase from KM- and GM-resistant strains which was sensitive to DKB and AK. Thus, such bacteria developed resistance to (KM. GM. DKB)-, and to (KM. GM. DKB. AK)-acetyltransferase (see Chapter 9).

These facts indicate that the genes on plasmids can mutate and increase their substrate number, resulting in the formation of plasmids capable of inactivating multiple drugs. These mutations cannot be held accountable for changes caused by multi-steps of gene mutation, and can occur easily in strains which are isolated most frequently from clinical specimens. They also can survive even in a noxious condition of extensive use of antibacterial agents. In other cases, plasmids acquire new resistance determinants and confer extensive multiple resistance on their host, resulting in the formation of plasmids with multiple resistance.

The resistance genes of plasmids are derived from the genes of bacteria which can easily acquire resistance following mutation, or are naturally resistant strains, resulting in the increase in isolation frequency from clinical specimens by the selection of antibacterial agents.

The nonconjugative plasmids may be of bacteriophage origin. But it seems more likely that nonconjugative plasmids are different from conjugative plasmids in their biological properties, such as conjugal transfer and ability to transfer their host chromosome, *i.e.*, the genetic characters such as *tra+*, *mat+* and ability to form sex pili. It seems more plausible to me that the evolutional sequences are the following: bacteriophages→nonconjugative plasmids→conjugative plasmids. The acquisition of conjugal transferability, *i.e.*, sexual transfer and mating ability, by the nonconjugative plasmids is a very fascinating problem for both geneticists and microbiologists, and it still remains to be speculated upon and ultimately solved.

The facts showing that the transfer factors are widely distributed among most genera of the Enterobacteriaceae are quite interesting and bring to mind my emphasis of the problems of lysogeny, and the latency of virus infection in bacteria, plants, insects, and higher organisms. Parasitism is the most common biological features in higher organisms (*92*) and an organic union consisting of two units of an organism will be a fascinating new problem in biology (*49*). The presence of the nonconjugative and conjugative plasmids favor microorganisms with their ability to survive the changes in their circumstances, and the appearance of the R (or r) factors shows the rapid changes in gene evolution and the exchange of genes between the many strains of bacteria which exist as a normal flora.

REFERENCES

1 Anderson, E. S. and Lewis, M. J. 1965. *Nature*, **208**, 843–849.
2 Anderson, E. S. 1966. *Nature*, **212**, 795–799.
3 Anderson, E. S., Pitton, J. S., and Mayhew, J. N. 1968. *Nature*, **219**, 640–641.
4 Anderson, E. S., Kelemen, M. V., Jones, C. M., and Pitton, J. S. 1968. *Genet. Res. Camb.*, **11**, 119–124.
5 Anderson, E. S., Mayhew, J. N., and Gridley, N. D. F. 1969. *Nature*, **222**, 349–351.
6 Berg, D. 1974. *Virology*, **62**, 224–233.
7 Bioce, L. B. and Luria, S. E. 1963. *Virology*, **20**, 147–157.
8 Campbell, A. 1971. *In* The Bacteriophage Lambda, ed. by A. D. Hershey, pp. 609–620, Cold Spring Harbor Laboratory, New York.
9 Coetzee, J. N. 1975. *J. Gen. Microbiol.*, **87**, 173–176.
10 Datta, N. and Kontomichalou, P. 1965. *Nature*, **208**, 239–241.
11 Datta, N. and Richmond, M. H. 1965. *Biochem. J.*, **98**, 204–209.
12 Dulbecco, R. 1955. *Phys. Rev.*, **35**, 301–335.
13 Egawa, R. and Hirota, Y. 1962. *Japan. J. Genet.*, **37**, 66–69.
14 Echols, H., Green, L., Oppenheim, A. B., and Honigman, A. 1973. *J. Mol. Biol.*, **80**, 203–216.
15 Egawa, R., Sawai, T., and Mitsuhashi, S. 1967. *Japan. J. Microbiol.*, **11**, 173–178.
16 Ephrussi, B. 1953. *In* Nucleo-cytoplasmic Relations in Microorganisms, Oxford University Press (Clarendon), London and New York.
17 Falkow, S., Citarella, R. V., Wohlhieter, J. A., and Watanabe, T. 1966. *J. Mol. Biol.*, **17**, 102–116.
18 Hampachepova, M., Koutecka, E., and Neuwbauer, A. 1973. *Mol. Gen. Genet.*, **120**, 133–137.
19 Harada, K., Suzuki, M., Kameda, M., and Mitsuhashi, S. 1960. *Japan. J. Exp. Med.*, **30**, 289–299.
20 Harada, K., Kameda, M., Suzuki, M., and Mitsuhashi, S. 1963. *J. Bacteriol.*, **86**, 1332–1338.

21 Harada, K., Kameda, M., Suzuki, M., and Mitsuhashi, S. 1964. *J. Bacteriol.*, **88**, 1257–1265.

22 Harada, K., Kameda, M., Suzuki, M., Shigehara, S., and Mitsuhashi, S. 1967. *J. Bacteriol.*, **93**, 1236–1241.

23 Harada, K., Kameda, M., Suzuki, M., and Mitsuhashi, S. 1967. *Japan. J. Microbiol.*, **1**, 143–151.

24 Harada, K., Kameda, M., Suzuki, M., Shigehara, S., Nakajima, T., and Mitsuhashi, S. 1970. *Japan. J. Microbiol.*, **14**, 423–426.

25 Hashimoto, H., Kono, M., and Mitsuhashi, S. 1964. *J. Bacteriol.*, **88**, 261–262.

26 Hayes, W. 1969. *In* Bacterial Episomes and Plasmids, ed. by H. Hayes, pp. 4–11, Ciba Foundation, J. and A. Churchill, Ltd., London.

27 Iijima, T. 1961. Abstr. 33rd Meet., Genet. Soc. Japan, p. 7.

28 Ikeda, H. and Tomizawa, J. 1965. *J. Mol. Biol.*, **14**, 85–109.

29 Ikeda, H. and Tomizawa, J. 1968. *Cold Spring Harbor Symp. Quant. Biol.*, **33**, 791–798.

30 Inoue, M., Hashimoto, H., Yamagishi, S., and Mitsuhashi, S. 1970. *Japan. J. Microbiol.*, **14**, 261–268.

31 Inoue, M., Oshima, H., Okubo, T., and Mitsuhashi, S. 1972. *J. Bacteriol.*, **112**, 1169–1176.

32 Inoue, M. and Mitsuhashi, S. 1975. *Virology*, **68**, 544–546.

33 Inoue, M., Okubo, T., Oshima, H., and Mitsuhashi, S. 1975. *In* Microbial Drug Resistance, ed. by S. Mitsuhashi and H. Hashimoto, pp. 153–164, University of Tokyo Press, Tokyo / University Park Press, Baltimore and London.

34 Inoue, M. and Mitsuhashi, S. 1976. *Virology*, **72**, 322–329.

35 Iyobe, S., Hashimoto, H., and Mitsuhashi, S. 1969. *Japan. J. Microbiol.*, **13**, 225–232.

36 Iyobe, S., Hashimoto, H., and Mitsuhashi, S. 1970. *Japan. J. Microbiol.*, **14**, 463–471.

37 Jacob, F. and Wollman, E. L. 1958. *Compt. Rend. Acad. Sci.*, **247**, 154–156.

38 Jacob, F. 1964. *In* Les Bactéries Lysogénes et la Notion de Provirus, Pasteur Institute, Masson and Co., Paris.

39 Jacob, F. and Wollman, E. L. 1959. *In* Recent Progress in Microbiology (7th Int. Congr. Microbiol., Stockholm, 1958), pp. 15–30.

40 Jacob, F. and Monod, J. 1961. *J. Mol. Biol.*, **3**, 318–356.

41 Jacob, F. and Wollman, E. L. 1961. *In* Sexuality and the Genetics of Bacteria, ed. by F. Jacob, Academic Press, New York and London.

42 Jacob, F., Brenner, S., and Cuzin, F. 1963. *In* On the Regulation of

DNA Replication in Bacteria, ed. by F. Jacob, pp. 329–348, Cold Spring Harbor Laboratory, New York.

43 Kameda, M., Harada, K., Suzuki, M., and Mitsuhashi, S. 1965. *J. Bacteriol.*, **90**, 1174–1181.

44 Kameda, M., Harada, K., Suzuki, M., and Mitsuhashi, S. 1969. *Japan. J. Microbiol.*, **13**, 255–262.

45 Kameda, M., Suzuki, M., Nakajima, T., Harada, K., and Mitsuhashi, S. 1970. *Japan. J. Microbiol.*, **14**, 339–349.

46 Kameda, M., Harada, K., Suzuki, M., Nakajima, T., and Mitsuhashi, S. 1972. *Japan. J. Microbiol.*, **16**, 205–213.

47 Kasuga, T., Hashimoto, H., and Mitsuhashi, S. 1968. *J. Bacteriol.*, **95**, 1764–1766.

48 Kawabe, H., Tanaka, T., Inoue, K., and Mitsuhashi, S. 1976. *Antimicrob. Agents Chemother.*, in press.

49 Kawakita, Y. 1963. *In* Infection, Iwanami Press, Tokyo.

50 Kitamoto, O., Takigami, T., Kasai, N., Fukaya, I., and Kawashima, A. 1956. *Japan. J. Infect. Dis.*, **30**, 403–405 (in Japanese).

51 Kondo, E., Harada, K., and Mitsuhashi, S. 1962. *Japan. J. Exp. Med.*, **32**, 139–147.

52 Kondo, E. and Mitsuhashi, S. 1964. *J. Bacteriol.*, **88**, 1266–1276.

53 Kondo, E. and Mitsuhashi, S. 1966. *J. Bacteriol.*, **91**, 1787–1794.

54 Kuwabara, S., Akiba, T., Koyama, K., and Arai, T. 1963. *Japan. J. Microbiol.*, **7**, 61–68.

55 Lederberg, J. 1952. *Physiol. Rev.*, **32**, 403–430.

56 Luria, S. E., Adams, J. N., and Ting, R. C. 1960. *Virology*, **12**, 348–390.

57 Lwoff, A. 1953. *Bacteriol. Rev.*, **17**, 269–337.

58 Matsubara, K. and Kaiser, A. D. 1968. The Bacteriophage Lambda, ed. by L. Frisch, pp. 769–775, Cold Spring Harbor Laboratory, New York.

59 Matsubara, K. 1972. *Virology*, **50**, 713–726.

60 Matsubara, K. 1974. *Virology*, **13**, 596–602.

61 Matsubara, K. 1976. *J. Mol. Biol.*, **102**, 427–439.

62 Meynell, E. and Datta, N. 1965. *Nature*, **207**, 884–885.

63 Mise, K. and Arber, W. 1975. *In* Microbial Drug Resistance, ed. by S. Mitsuhashi and H. Hashimoto, pp. 165–167, University of Tokyo Press, Tokyo / University Park Press, Baltimore and London.

64 Mitsuhashi, S. 1963. *Protein, Nucleic Acid, Enzyme*, **8**, 216–228 (in Japanese).

65 Mitsuhashi, S. 1965. *Gunma J. Med. Sci.*, **14**, 169–209.

66 Mitsuhashi, S. 1969. *J. Infect. Dis.*, **119**, 89–100.

67 Mitsuhashi, S., Harada, K., and Kameda, M. 1961. *Japan. J. Microbiol.*, **31**, 119–123.

68 Mitsuhashi, S., Morimura, M., Kono, M., and Oshima, H. 1963. *J. Bacteriol.*, **86**, 162–164.

69 Mitsuhashi, S. and Takahashi, H. 1964. *Gunma J. Med. Sci.*, **13**, 129–134.

70 Mitsuhashi, S., Hashimoto, H., Kono, M., and Morimura, M. 1965. *J. Bacteriol.*, **89**, 988–992.

71 Mitsuhashi, S., Oshima, H., Kawaharada, U., and Hashimoto, H. 1965. *J. Bacteriol.*, **89**, 967–976.

72 Mitsuhashi, S., Hashimoto, H., Kono, M., and Morimura, M. 1965. *J. Bacteriol.*, **89**, 988–992.

73 Mitsuhashi, S., Kono, M., and Harada, K. 1967. 5th Int. Congr. Chemother., Vienna, Austria, C2/9, pp. 499–509.

74 Mitsuhashi, S., Kameda, M., Harada, K., and Suzuki, M. 1969. *J. Bacteriol.*, **97**, 1520–1521.

75 Mitsuhashi, S. 1971. *Ann. N.Y. Acad. Sci.*, **182**, 141–152.

76 Mitsuhashi, S., Inoue, M., Kawabe, H., Oshima, H., and Okubo, T. 1973. *In* Staphylococci and Staphylococcal Infections, ed. by J. Jeljaszewicz, pp. 144–165, Karger, Basel.

77 Mitsuhashi, S., Hashimoto, H., Tanaka, T., Iyobe, S., and Kawabe, H. 1974. *In* Progress in Chemotherapy (Proc. 8th Int. Congr. Chemother. Athens), ed. by G. K. Daikos, pp. 35–47.

78 Mitsuhashi, S., Inoue, M., Oshima, H., and Okubo, T. 1976. *In* Staphylococci and Staphylococcal Infections, ed. by J. Jeljaszewicz, pp. 253–274, Gustav Fisher Verlag, Stuttgart and New York.

79 Nagate, T., Inoue, K., Tanaka, T., and Mitsuhashi, S. 1976. *Antimicrob. Agents Chemother.*, in press.

80 Nakajima, T., Suzuki, M., Kameda, M., Harada, K., and Mitsuhashi, S. 1973. *Japan. J. Microbiol.*, **17**, 251–256.

81 Nakaya, R. 1960. *Recent Adv. Med. Biol.*, **1**, 109–139 (in Japanese).

82 Nakaya, R. 1961. *Japan Clinic*, **19**, 1151–1159 (in Japanese).

83 Novick, R. P. 1963. *J. Gen. Microbiol.*, **33**, 121–136.

84 Novick, R. P. 1967. *Fed. Proc.*, **26**, 29–38.

85 Okamoto, S. and Suzuki, Y. 1965. *Nature*, **208**, 1301–1303.

86 Okamoto, S., Suzuki, Y., Mise, K., and Nakaya, R. 1967. *J. Bacteriol.*, **94**, 1616–1622.

87 Ozeki, H., Stocker, B. A. D., and Smith, S. M. 1962. *J. Gen. Microbiol.*, **28**, 671–687.

88 Richmond, M. H. and John, M. 1964. *Nature*, **202**, 1360–1361.

89 Rownd, R., Nakaya, R., and Nakamura, A. 1966. *J. Mol. Biol.*, **17**, 376–393.

90 Sawai, T., Mitsuhashi, S., and Yamagishi, S. 1968. *Japan. J. Microbiol.*, **12**, 423–434.

91 Smith, H. W. 1972. *Nature*, **238**, 205–206.
92 Smith, T. 1934. *In* Parasitism and Disease, Princeton University Press, Princeton.
93 Sugino, Y. and Hirota, Y. 1962. *J. Bacteriol.*, **84**, 902–910.
94 Suzuki, S., Nakazawa, S., and Ushioda, T. 1956. *Chemotherapy*, **4**, 336–338 (in Japanese).
95 Suzuki, Y., Okamoto, S., and Kono, M. 1966. *J. Bacteriol.*, **92**, 798–799.
96 Takeda, Y., Matsubara, K., and Ogata, K. 1975. *Virology*, **65**, 374–385.
97 Tomizawa, J. 1971. *In* The Bacteriophage Lambda, ed. by A. D. Hershey, pp. 769–775, Cold Spring Harbor Laboratory, New York.
98 Watanabe, T. and Fukasawa, T. 1961. *J. Bacteriol.*, **82**, 202–209.
99 Watanabe, T. and Ogata, C. 1966. *J. Bacteriol.*, **91**, 43–50.
100 Watanabe, T. and Lyang, K. 1962. *J. Bacteriol.*, **84**, 422–430.
101 Wollman, E. L. 1969. *In* Bacterial Episomes and Plasmids, ed. by H. Hayes, Ciba Foundation, J. and A. Churchill, Ltd., London.

NAME INDEX

SUBJECT INDEX

A

Acetyl CoA 4, 299
Acetyltransferase 299
Acriflavin 19
Adenylylation 284
Adenylyltransferase 299
Aerobacter 16
Aeromonas liquefacience 40, 42
Aeromonas salmocida 40, 42
Aminoglycoside 299
Angilla japonica 39
Antibiotic-resistant 14
Antibiotics 43
APC 36
  resistance 37, 282
Arizona 17
Artificial elimination of R (or r)
  plasmids 50
Atabrine 153
ATP 299
att$_\lambda$ 94
Autonomous replication (*rep*) 157

B

Bacillary dysentery 9
Bacterial chromosome 18
Bacteriophages 8, 76
Bordetella bronchiseptica 20
5-Bromouracil 153

C

Calves 38
Cell-to-cell contact 19
Centrosome 297
  mobilization 60
CM acetyltransferase 177, 178,
  299
Cointegration 79
Col Ib-P9 182
Col B-*tet* 77
Coli-Shigella 34
Colicin plasmids 181
Con$^-$ 113, 126
Conjugal transfer 136
Conjugal transferability 73, 135
Conjugative 25, 89, 298
  plasmids 298
Covalently closed circular (CCC)
  174, 180
Cultured fish 39, 41
Cytoplasmic existence 50

D

Delta
  Δ 124, 166
  Δ-mating 291
  Δ-*tet* 293
  dna 187
  *dna*A 187

*tra*H   92, 93
*tra*J   93
*tra*K   92, 93
*tra*L   92
*tra*I   93, 124
*tra*O   96
*tra*S   93, 112
Transition   172
Transposable   286
Transposons   82, 83
Trionyx sinensis japonicus   39
Triple resistance   26, 283

Trypanosome brucei   3
Tuberculosis inpatients   16
Turning off   171
Turning on   171

V

Vibrio   20, 40, 42
  comma   20

X

X-*kan*   293